6/9 5

IBS
A Complete Guide to Relief from Irritable Bowel Syndrome

Christine P. Dancey is Senior Lecturer in Psychology at the University of East London and writes regularly for scientific journals. **Susan Backhouse** suffered from IBS for many years and is co-founder of the IBS Network, a self-help group for sufferers. She was also for five years the editor of the Network's journal, *Gut Reaction*.

Contents

A Note on the Contributors

SUSAN BACKHOUSE co-founded the self-help organization, the IBS Network, and was the editor of its journal, *Gut Reaction*, for nearly six years. She has written articles about irritable bowel syndrome and, together with Christine Dancey, wrote the self-help manual *Overcoming IBS* (1993) and edited and contributed to the follow-up book, *Treating IBS* (1995).

CHRISTINE P. DANCEY is Senior Lecturer in Psychology at the University of East London. Her research is concerned with the psychological effects of living with chronic disorders such as IBS, and she has published work (some in collaboration with Susan Backhouse) in scientific journals. She is co-founder of the IBS Network and sub-editor of *Gut Reaction*.

RACHEL FOX graduated from the University of East London with a BSc (Hons) in psychology in July 1994. At present, she is working as a research assistant on various projects relating to IBS.

NICK READ is Professor of Gastrointestinal Physiology and Nutrition at the University of Sheffield. He has been seeing patients with Irritable Bowel Syndrome in a specialist capacity for over 20 years and has published three books and over 300 papers on the condition. His career, developing through medicine, physiology, nutrition and latterly psychotherapy, provides a broad base for the development of more holistic concepts of understanding and treating IBS.

CLAIRE RUTTER graduated from the University of East London

with BSc (Hons) in psychology in July 1994. In September of that year, she started work as a research assistant, investigating the psychological effects of living with IBS in childhood.

MARGO STEEDEN graduated from the University of East London with BSc (Hons) in psychology in July 1996. She has worked with Christine Dancey on the problems faced by women suffering from endometriosis who had initially been misdiagnosed as having IBS.

ALAN STEWART qualified as a doctor in 1976. For the last 14 years he has specialized in nutritional medicine and is actively involved in teaching other doctors on the subject. He has published widely on nutrition.

MARYON STEWART studied preventative dentistry and nutrition and worked as a counsellor with nutritional doctors for four years. She founded the Women's Nutritional Advisory Service in 1987. She has written several books on nutrition, including, together with Dr Alan Stewart, *Beat IBS through Diet* (1994).

ELIZABETH E. TAYLOR has been using hypnotherapy and psychotherapy for over ten years and has specialized in treating people with gut disorders for much of that time. She worked alongside Dr Peter Whorwell of Manchester's Withington Hospital for three years. She is the founder of the Register of Approved Gastrointestinal Psychotherapists and Hypnotherapists.

BRENDA TONER is currently head of the Women's Mental Health Research Programme at the Clarke Institute of Psychiatry and Associate Professor at the University of Toronto. Her research interests include the psychosocial assessment and treatment of irritable bowel syndrome, and gender issues in functional gastrointestinal disorders. At present, she is completing a randomized treatment outcome study on cognitive–behavioural group therapy for IBS. The treatment manual used in this study has been incorporated into a book by Drs Toner, Segal, Emmott and Myran, entitled *Functional Gastrointestinal Disorders: A Cognitive–Behavioural Perspective* (1994).

Foreword

Dr James Le Fanu

Virtually everyone buying this book will have in common a similar experience. They will, at some time in the past, have been discomforted by a combination of unpleasant abdominal symptoms – colicky pains, flatulence, distension and diarrhoea alternating with constipation. They will have lost count of their numerous, often unsatisfactory, medical consultations where doctors have prodded their tummies and nodded knowingly on detecting a tender (and to them painful) site. They will almost certainly have been referred for a specialist opinion and undergone a series of uncomfortable and embarrassing tests where tubes have been stuck up their bottoms and they have been tilted around on the X-ray table while having a barium enema. And at the end of all this they will have been told: 'we can find nothing wrong', 'we have excluded organic disease' (i.e. you don't have cancer), 'you have a disturbance of bowel motility', 'you have irritable bowel syndrome.' And what then? IBS is a catch-all diagnosis, perhaps best described as a dustbin diagnosis into which all those whose symptoms are not readily explained by some physical change in the lining of the bowel are tossed. There is no specific treatment though virtually everything – psychotherapy, hypnosis, dietary manipulation – may help some sufferers. In such circumstances doctors tend to be therapeutically rather nihilistic, usually recommending a high fibre diet, anti-spasmodics for the pain, and appropriate drugs for the constipation and diarrhoea. They then leave patients to get on with their lives as best they can.

That at least was the discouraging situation that most IBS sufferers found themselves in up until 1993 when Christine Dancey and Susan Backhouse published their book *Overcoming IBS*. In retrospect the original idea that inspired them was now so obvious, so sensible, it is astonishing that nobody had thought of it before – the experts on IBS are not doctors or gut specialists, but the patients themselves. The questionnaire sent out to a network of fellow sufferers that forms the basis of the book generated a whole series of fascinating and important insights into the illness.

The first and most alarming message is just how devastating IBS can be – not only in the physical distress it causes, but also because of the effect it has on people's social and working lives. For those afflicted with IBS the realization that they are not alone in their misfortune, and in the failure of their doctors to provide much in the way of help or support, is itself very encouraging.

Secondly the variation in symptoms of IBS is very striking. For some, pain is the most disabling symptom, for others excess wind, and for others again the disturbance in bowel habits. Thus, by definition there can be no blanket or standard treatment such as the oft recommended high fibre diet but rather one that is tailored to the individual.

Thirdly, the self-discovery – usually through trial and error – by those with IBS of what has proved helpful widens considerably the range of therapeutic options available. Some have been helped, often dramatically, by changing their diet and excluding certain foods, others by hypnotherapy and others again by types of complementary medicine such as acupuncture. Just as significantly it is important to realize (and not to be discouraged by) the fact that in some cases certain treatments either do not work or indeed may make matters worse.

The final story about IBS is still to be written. Personally, I suspect the main underlying explanation remains to be discovered and may well have something to do with the gut peptides, the complex series of neurotransmitters in the gut wall which control its functions. Then the psychological problems so often associated with IBS, such as anxiety and depression, will be seen to be an effect rather than a cause of the disturbance of bowel function.

In the meantime, though, we have this book whose true importance can best be appreciated by trying to imagine what life was like for those with IBS before it was published. People can turn to it for the help, support and advice that sadly the medical profession has, it seems, been unable to provide.

James Le Fanu, G. P.

From Christine: I would like to dedicate this book to Jo Johnstone and Maureen O'Hara, for all their support and practical help over many, many years. Thanks also for all the envelope-stuffing and reading of my IBS articles over the past seven years.

From Sue: To my son Ken, for all I've learned being with him.

Acknowledgements

We are grateful to the Neal's Yard Bakery Co-operative for permission to reproduce the following recipes from *The Neal's Yard Bakery Wholefood Cookbook* by Rachel Haigh: hummus, gluten-free muesli, guacamole, Caribbean stew, swede and orange pie, strawberry mousse and dairy-free mayonnaise. We are also grateful to Rider Books for permission to reproduce the recipe for aubergine pie from *Greek Vegetarian Cookery* by Jack Santa Maria; to the Henry Doubleday Research Association for permission to reproduce recipes from *Good Food, Gluten Free* by Hilda Cherry Hills; to Berrydales for permission to use the recipe for chocolate cake from their newsletter; to the Ashgrove Press for permission to use the recipes for tofu burgers, brown rice digestive biscuits, potato shortbread and mock cream from *The Foodwatch Alternative Cookbook* by Honor J. Campbell; and to J. M. Dent & Sons for permission to use the recipes for millet and peanut cookies and carob fudge from *The Cranks Recipe Book* by David Canter, Kay Canter and Daphne Swann.

Preface

In 1990, there were no organizations, no self-help or support groups, nothing catering for the needs of IBS sufferers. Early in 1991, we decided to set up such an organization, which became known as the IBS Network. Our main aim was to help alleviate the isolation of people diagnosed as having IBS by providing a means of contact with fellow-sufferers. This was achieved by way of the quarterly journal *Gut Reaction*, and later through our previous two books. The IBS Network, run from our homes in Sheffield and London in the early days, is now a registered charity, with two offices, trustees, workers and volunteers. We even have our own IBS web pages! *Gut Reaction*, once a black-and-white four-page newsletter, is now a professionally published 16-page colour journal, with a circulation of 4,000 (1996) and growing all the time.

When we wrote our first two books, both of us had experienced bowel symptoms, one of us for over 20 years. Once we had contacted others with IBS, we quickly realized that what people wanted most of all was to be able to read about the experiences of others with the same disorder. They needed to know that other people were suffering the same ordeals, and were coping with them. The very few books on IBS describe the symptoms and speculate on its causes, yet none of them describe what it is like from the sufferer's point of view. Consequently, although people can read about the tests they have undergone and what may have caused their IBS, they cannot read about how painful the tests were, the feelings the tests gave rise to, and how, when each test was shown to be negative, they felt as if they were a fraud; IBS has never had the validity of a 'real' disease. They have not been able to read about the embarrassment that the loud noises in the digestive system can bring, the lack of control felt when rushing to the toilet numerous times a day, and so on. Sufferers had no way of knowing how common their feelings were.

Apparently IBS was first described in 1820 by a gastro-enterologist called Powell. Since then it has been called by various names, including spastic colon, spasmodic stricture of the colon, membranous enteritis and vegetative neurosis. IBS is a diagnosis of exclusion: once other, more serious diseases have been discounted (cancer of the bowel, Crohn's disease, colitis, coeliac diseases), and there are no signs of parasites or enzyme deficiency, IBS is diagnosed. It has no known causes, and no cure which is lastingly effective. Sufferers experience continuous or recurrent symptoms of abdominal pain, altered bowel habits, flatulence, early satiety, and bloating or a feeling of abdominal distension. Altered bowel habits may give rise to diarrhoea, constipation, or an alternation of both. Often there is straining or urgency, and a feeling of incomplete evacuation of the bowel.

IBS is responsible for a significant loss of work time, a large number of visits to doctors and frequent hospital admissions; it accounts for 30 to 50 per cent of consultations to gastroenterologists. However, despite the prevalence of this disorder, there is incomplete agreement on its definition and its status as a valid diagnostic entity and is not taken seriously by many doctors – something that can be very distressing if your life is being ruined by it.

For this book, we have written two new chapters, one about women and IBS, the other on adolescent sufferers of the condition. In the Western world, twice as many women than men are diagnosed as having IBS. Knowing this fact sometimes leads people to the conclusion that IBS may be a result of differing hormone levels. While hormones can have an effect on the gut, this explanation doesn't account for the finding that prevalence rates depend on the country in question – we know that more men than women are diagnosed as having IBS in India, for instance. So while the symptoms of some women may be worse at different times in the menstrual cycle, the different prevalence rates are probably due to what is called 'consulting behaviour' – that is, more women than men attend the doctor for most complaints in the UK, probably because it is more acceptable for women to go to the GP with their problems than it is for men. This is not the whole explanation, though, because even with people who suffer from symptoms of irritable bowel but who do *not* go to their doctor, more women than men seem to be affected. Again, this is probably because it is more acceptable for women to admit to these symptoms than it is for men.

Whatever the reason for the different prevalence rates between men and women, it is clear that many more women have a diagnosis of IBS. Because of this, IBS is often seen as a 'woman's complaint' and, like other women's problems, it may be trivialised by others. Researchers have found that women suffering from what are labelled 'women's problems' are often treated with less seriousness than those with other ailments. The belief that IBS is a woman's complaint affects men, too, of course, for if they believe it is a woman's complaint, it will be that much harder for them to cope. And while women may talk to other women about their IBS, sharing their problems and worries, men are less likely to do so. It's not something they will want to discuss in the pub!

While women are readily diagnosed with IBS on the basis of symptoms alone, a greater proportion of men are thoroughly investigated before a diagnosis of IBS is made. While some men with serious diseases such as Crohn's disease or colitis may initially be given a diagnosis of IBS, there is more scope for women to be misdiagnosed because of confusion with gynaecological diseases such as endometriosis and pelvic inflammatory disease (PID). Discussion of these issues is in Chapter 11.

While the symptoms of both men and women may be affected by such things as stress, diet and major life events (bereavement, moving house, marriage, divorce, etc.), women have the added problems of operations such as hysterectomies and laparoscopies, and normal events such as pregnancy and childbirth. Operations have been shown to have a link with abdominal symptoms, and pregnancy also affects and is affected by IBS.

When we started researching into younger people with IBS, we were told by one medical practitioner, 'We know that children don't suffer from IBS.' Our work with IBS Network members, however, showed that nearly half said that they had suffered some symptoms of irritable bowel between the ages of 11 and 17. Some of these sufferers say their childhood was being marred by suffering from this disorder. At the University of East London, researchers have investigated young people (11–17) who had been diagnosed as suffering from IBS.

As far as we know, there is no other written information (for the lay reader) on IBS in children – and yet it is clear that many parents would like information about this. One thing that stood out in the interviews with IBS Network members was that parents of children with IBS wanted to meet others in the same situation, and the teenagers themselves would have found it helpful to have someone of a similar age (and sex) with whom to share their problems.

You will notice that some of the views expressed by the contributors in this book differ widely. This is because, although we now know a good deal about IBS itself, the way it is treated depends partly on views about what causes it. And however much any particular expert is convinced that his or her view is the correct one, at present there is no consensus. Information is power, so gather as much of it about IBS as you can, and try to decide which is the best way for you to tackle your IBS. We hope this book will enable you to do exactly that.

Chapter 1

What Is IBS?

Christine P. Dancey and Susan Backhouse

'*My problems start with a pain, like a dull ache, in the lower abdomen, followed by the most incredible bloating ever seen in a non-pregnant woman, constipation, pain and a feeling of general malaise. This is eventually relieved by strong doses of Colpermin and laxatives.*'

Irritable bowel syndrome (IBS) is a collection of symptoms (syndrome) including, especially, unexplained abdominal pain, varying in intensity from mild to extremely severe, and altered bowel habits, which can include diarrhoea, constipation or an alternation of both, together with other symptoms discussed later in this chapter. The disorder can be fairly persistent, but is often characterized by times when the symptoms become very bad and remissions where the symptoms are much more manageable. IBS is termed a 'functional' disorder – which means that there is no actual disease which can account for the symptoms experienced.

IBS is probably a catch-all label for a variety of conditions with a variety of causes linked by a bowel disorder which doctors cannot identify or understand, nor treat effectively. In the past for instance, symptoms caused by lactose intolerance have come under the heading of IBS. Some researchers believe there are more IBS 'sub-groups' to be discovered and they are trying to develop tests to identify them. There is unlikely to be a miracle cure round the corner which will help all IBS sufferers.

IBS is one of several disorders grouped under the term

'invisible chronic illness' (ICI) by Drs Donoghue and Siegel in their book aptly titled *Sick and Tired of Feeling Sick and Tired*. Other invisible chronic illnesses include lupus erythematosus (lupus), Lyme disease, migraine and thyroid disease. IBS shares certain characteristics with these other ICIs – pain, fatigue, bladder urgency, constipation, diarrhoea and sleep disorders, among others.

How does IBS start?

Henry describes how his IBS started:

'I'm 30 now, and have had IBS to varying degrees for about seven years. I was never aware of having any bowel problems when a child. On a few occasions at school when I was 17 or 18 I remember feeling the need to go to the toilet during the day, but in general there was no urgency and I was able to last out until I got home. I had one period of a few months when I suffered severe flatulence which made me feel as if I needed a bowel movement but wasn't actually able to do anything. I also became aware of occasionally needing to go to the toilet twice in the morning, or in the late afternoon or early evening, particularly if I was on holiday or had gone out for the day. A few years later, when I was in a job which I enjoyed, I found I only just had time to open the post before I needed to go to the toilet. It rapidly got worse, and I soon reached a situation where I was having to go three times in quick succession in the morning, and often suddenly at other times of the day as well, which quite worried me, as I thought it might be something serious. For a month or so the IBS was probably as bad as it ever has been since. I have never really had any clear idea of why IBS developed at this time.'

However, different people experience the start of their IBS in different ways – there is no common pattern of onset. Here some other sufferers describe how their IBS started.

'It all began a year ago while I had what I thought was indigestion. I took some antacids. On getting up the next day I still had the indigestion, but started having bowel problems. This went on for two weeks; I felt unwell and couldn't eat. My bowel motions began becoming looser and looser till everything started going right through me. The GP suggested I go on a liquid diet for three or four days, but I lost a stone and felt weaker. I was also suffering from nausea. I had all the tests, and my GP said it was my nervous disposition that was making me ill. I tried everything to get better, but it became worse. I had pain, loss of appetite and eventually depression.'

Some people link their IBS to a period of stress:

'I have always suffered from a "nervous stomach" at times of stress but it went back to normal once the stressful situation had passed. But a little while ago I was off work for four months with various medical problems, and it was all too much for me to cope with. During this time my nervous stomach was completely out of control. The diarrhoea was so bad I couldn't leave the house, I felt very nauseous and had a lot of stomach pain. I also had this most peculiar sensation in my stomach as if there was something alive in there and it was chewing at my insides. I have had all the tests and have been prescribed all sorts of medications, but nothing helps.'

Others can become totally puzzled by their IBS, which seems to have come on suddenly, without any warning:

'Mine came on very suddenly. In the night I woke up with severe pains in my stomach and upper abdomen and started being violently sick, with excessive diarrhoea. My GP took me into hospital where they took my gallbladder away, but after the operation I was still suffering very bad pains and still vomiting and having diarrhoea. I lost my job because I was unwell. After eight times in and out of hospital I was told that all I had was IBS. It made me feel that no one believed I was ill because it was made out that it was nothing important.'

'About four years ago when I was 55 diarrhoea started suddenly, and when it didn't clear up I went to the doctor. He gave me tablets but that didn't work. I lost two and a half stone, and was very worried. I pass wind a lot, which is embarrassing and out of control at times.'

'My IBS started just after the war. I tend to have spells of trouble on and off which last from a few days to several months. I never know what really triggers off an attack which comes when I am not stressed or anxious. I do not get bad diarrhoea, mainly looseness or constipation, but I do have a great deal of pain, particularly with the looseness. Also, wind is very troublesome and seems to be the cause of much of the pain. The pain often wakes me at night.'

Some sufferers found that their IBS started after an abdominal operation:

'I have suffered for six years. After a hysterectomy in 1985 I had problems with constipation and severe spasms. It took 12 months of going to the hospital before they told me it was IBS.'

About a quarter of those people suffered with IBS after having gastroenteritis or food poisoning:

'Just over three years ago I suffered food poisoning. This went, but some time after I started to have griping pains and my bowel pattern became irregular – alternate constipation with small pellet motions and then larger motions, sometimes a bit loose, but not really diarrhoea. My stomach rumbled and I started to have bloating and pain, mainly on the left-hand side of the abdomen, with muscle spasm and a feeling of being over-full after a large meal.'

It can be seen that there is no clear pattern in the way IBS starts. In some people the symptoms creep up gradually; in others, they come suddenly after gastroenteritis or a stressful event.

What are the symptoms of IBS?

You can see from the above accounts that IBS is made up of many different symptoms. People classified as having IBS may have some or many of the following problems.

Abdominal pain and spasm
Pain can be experienced throughout the abdomen and in different sites at different times. IBS sufferers usually find the pain is in the lower abdomen, although some also experience it in the upper abdomen. Some people find the pain is worst in the early hours of the morning.

Diarrhoea, constipation or an alternation of both
In IBS, diarrhoea is caused by food moving too quickly through the system. However, some studies have shown that, although transit times tend to be a little faster in those with diarrhoea, the major feature of the diarrhoea is an increased frequency of small amounts of stool. In fact, stool weight per day in IBS patients may be exactly the same as people without IBS – it's just that sufferers with diarrhoea pass motions far more frequently.

'Constipation' means infrequent or difficult bowel movements. Food moves too slowly through the system, so there is too much water absorption and faeces become dry and hard.

People with long-term IBS frequently tell us they no longer know whether their bowel habits are normal or not. Thus, sufferers often worry because they feel they have too many or too few bowel movements. There is in fact a wide variation in the bowel habits of people without IBS – some people go once every three days, some three times a day, and there are many whose bowel habits vary from week to week. It is hard to say what is normal. Bowel habits also depend on what part of the world you live in – by Western criteria, all Ugandan villagers have diarrhoea because they produce more than 400 g of unformed stool every day (the rate in the West is 300 g per day). **Researchers have tried to** define constipation and diarrhoea precisely – for instance, some researchers may define constipation as not more than three hard stools per week, with straining, and diarrhoea as more than 21 unformed stools per week – but such precise definitions cannot work. Someone who has watery motions and has to get to a toilet urgently may be certain they have diarrhoea, even if their bowel patterns do not strictly conform to the 'over 21' criterion.

People who have alternating diarrhoea and constipation perhaps find this harder to cope with – they never know from one minute to the next how their bowels are going to work, and those taking medication may find this difficult. Any laxative for constipation may bring on an episode of diarrhoea, and an anti-diarrhoeal drug may cause constipation. This is a difficult problem.

Bloated stomach, rumbling noises and wind

Most sufferers have to put up with the digestive system making loud rumbling noises at random times of the day. Although it is said that other people rarely notice these noises, the people we talked to were very bothered by them. Again, while the average person passes wind 17 times a day without noticing it, IBS sufferers are generally aware that they are passing wind and are worried that other people know too. The embarrassment adds to their other discomforts. Some IBS sufferers also have to wear loose clothes if they suffer from a bloated stomach:

'I cannot fit into any of my clothes, and tend to find that I cannot finish a meal because I feel bloated and full.'

'I am becoming desperate. This condition is so embarrassing. I constantly need to go to the loo and I suffer from terrible bouts of wind. In my job I deal with people all the time so you can imagine how difficult it is. I have to refuse to go out because of it.'

'After having my second child I noticed that I felt bloated and wanted to pass wind, as well as having gurgles and cramps. They came on suddenly after a meal and often I would have to rush to the loo, where I would have very runny motions. As you can appreciate it is very embarrassing, especially if you're in somebody else's house. I would be terrified they would hear me passing wind and I'd be scared to get off the loo in case I had to go back five minutes later.'

'I broke wind one day at work, and someone laughed. I felt so humiliated I felt like walking out.'

Urgency and incontinence

Once the sufferer has the urge to go to the toilet, he or she has to get there pretty quickly! Sixteen per cent of IBS sufferers have experienced bowel incontinence at some time or another. Most sufferers are very aware of toilets – their life revolves around them, and it is difficult for them to arrange any journey without knowing exactly where the toilets will be situated.

A feeling of incomplete emptying of the bowels

Quite often, sufferers will find that they leave the toilet feeling that they have not done all that they could have. Many people find that, within a few minutes, they have to rush to the toilet again. This may happen three or four times in succession, or even more. Needless to say, this is very disruptive to normal everyday life!

A sharp pain felt low down inside the rectum

Pain attacks can be mild or severe enough to make you almost faint. Luckily, most people find this pain passes off in less than five minutes, and in some it is over in a few seconds. It also sometimes happens to people without IBS. The cause of this *proctalgia fugax*, as it is called, is unknown. Although IBS sufferers are more likely than non-sufferers to get this feeling, it is not one of the more common symptoms.

Nausea, belching and vomiting

Again, these are not common symptoms, although some sufferers experience nausea to a degree which leaves them feeling weak and unable to eat.

How many people have IBS?

Estimates vary as to the number of people who have IBS. Some researchers say it affects 15 per cent of the population in developed countries. Others say that it could be as high as 35 per cent. In any case, IBS accounts for almost half of all consultations to gastroenterologists, making IBS a very expensive complaint – and most gastroenterologists do not feel able to treat patients effectively.

Researchers found symptoms of bowel disorders in over 300 apparently healthy subjects, although few people had bothered to consult a doctor – those seen by physicians are just the tip of the iceberg. People usually go to the GP and receive a diagnosis of IBS when their symptoms become more frequent, or more painful. There are twice as many women as men diagnosed as having IBS in Britain, although this may be because women in this country tend to go to the doctor more than men anyway. In India the situation is reversed – four times more men than women being diagnosed as having IBS.

In the past it has been difficult to diagnose someone as having IBS; different doctors used different criteria. However, many researchers and doctors now use the Manning Criteria. In 1978 Manning and his team defined IBS as abdominal pain associated with three or more of the following symptoms:

- Pain relieved by defecation.
- More frequent stools with pain onset.
- Looser stools with pain onset.
- Abdominal distension.
- Mucus in the stool.
- Feeling of incomplete evacuation after defecation.

A patient is likely to be diagnosed as having IBS if she or he has pain along with at least three of the above symptoms, and in the absence of any other disease. If you have abdominal pain without any bowel disturbance, and you are told you have IBS, you should question the diagnosis. IBS is a syndrome – that is, a collection of symptoms – and it should not be diagnosed on the basis of only one symptom. In our experience this sometimes happens. If you have constipation only, you are not considered to have IBS.

Symptoms that are not due to IBS

In women
It is sometimes the case that women are diagnosed as having IBS when their problem is really gynaecological. For instance, women have been told they have IBS when they actually have pelvic inflammatory disease (PID) or endometriosis.

PID is an inflammation of the pelvic organs which can be due to infection of the Fallopian tubes, ovaries, or both. PID can cause a sharp pain throughout the abdomen, although sometimes the pain may be dull. Someone with PID is likely to have other symptoms: pain or bleeding from the vagina during or after intercourse and an abnormal vaginal discharge.

Endometriosis is a condition in which parts of the womb lining (endometrial cells) migrate to other organs – for example, the bladder or the bowel. These cells act as though they are still in the womb, so they respond every month to the hormones produced during the menstrual cycle – they thicken, enlarge and bleed. This can cause great pain in the abdomen and sometimes in the back. Intercourse is often extremely painful; periods are heavy as well as painful, and they often become worse towards the end. Because adhesions may have stuck the bowel to the womb, a woman can have bowel symptoms as well. In research carried out by the Endometriosis Society in the US, nearly 3 per cent of women subsequently diagnosed as having endometriosis had been previously diagnosed as having IBS. Treating endometriosis frequently brought relief of their gastrointestinal symptoms.

In a survey carried out by Britain's National Endometriosis Society and published in 1996, 7 per cent of a large sample – 2,463 sufferers! – had been diagnosed as having IBS or Crohn's disease. Most of the research into the misdiagnosis of endometriosis as IBS states that it is symptom similarity that causes problems.

However, symptoms such as sharp pain during sexual penetration, bleeding in between periods and muddy discharge are not typical of IBS, and yet women experiencing these symptoms have been misdiagnosed.

Writing in a scientific journal in 1996, a nurse wrote that healthcare workers should show caution when any woman complains of weight-loss, nocturnal diarrhoea, bowel incontinence or blood in the stools. She believes that they should be referred for further testing straightaway, and that a careful history is needed to differentiate IBS from other disorders.

Both PID and endometriosis are treatable. If you have bleeding from the vagina in between periods, if your period pains become worse at the end of the period, if you have an unusual discharge, insist that you see a gynaecologist. While IBS symptoms are often worse during a menstrual period, IBS does not cause the symptoms mentioned above. Neither should sex be extremely painful! If it is, do not accept a diagnosis of IBS without seeing a gynaecologist. This is the story of one person wrongly diagnosed as having IBS:

'I had what was called IBS for three years. My main symptom was pain. I did have some bowel problems. I also had bleeding in between periods, and painful sex. My periods were so painful I sometimes fainted. The GP said my symptoms were due to stress. Over the years the pain was sometimes so excruciating I called doctors out or went to casualty. They always told me it was IBS. In the end, it was so bad I paid privately for a laparoscopy – they found I had one of the worst cases of endometriosis ever. Once I was cured of the endometriosis, all the "IBS" symptoms disappeared.'

In women and men

Other symptoms which should be checked before IBS is confirmed are rapid loss of weight and rectal bleeding. These are two symptoms which could be due to other, more serious diseases. Having said that, however, some people with IBS do lose quite a bit of weight, either because of constant diarrhoea or because of the worry associated with having an illness, especially before it is diagnosed as IBS. Bleeding from the rectum can be due to haemorrhoids or more serious causes, so it is important to go to your GP to have this checked out.

Will IBS lead to cancer?

IBS is not associated with any other disease; it cannot lead to cancer and there are no fatalities. This may be one reason why IBS is not taken seriously. However, IBS is a very common condition which causes misery to hundreds of thousands of people, costs the National Health Service vast sums of money and affects employers whose employees lose time from work. It is therefore important to take IBS as seriously as any other illness.

What sort of people have IBS?

According to research, the average age at which symptoms become apparent is about 29, although the range is about 1 to 63. However, the people we talked to ranged from 20 to 78 years old. Most were women who had suffered from IBS for anything between six months and 50 years! The majority of people, however, had suffered from IBS for less than ten years. The people we spoke to were of all ages, both sexes, and with all sorts of occupations.

What causes IBS?

IBS can be considered as a disease of function, rather than of structure – in other words, there is nothing physically wrong with any specific part of the digestive system, it is the way the system works that is wrong. IBS has been considered by many practitioners to be a motility disorder ('motility' meaning 'movement') – that is, the contents of the gut move either too quickly or too slowly through the system. However, the case for IBS being a motility disorder is not really established. In IBS, contractions of the muscles of the digestive tract may be quite normal and if they are not, the responses are often exaggerated rather than, strictly speaking, abnormal. IBS is therefore really a disease of exaggerated gut reaction, although this aspect of it may not afflict all patients.

People may be puzzled when they are told they have IBS, as it often comes on suddenly and they can see no good reason for it. The causes of IBS are still largely unknown, and there are no cures which are lastingly effective. While there are various theories as to what causes it, none of them is very satisfactory.

Here we give you a brief outline of the various theories which attempt to explain why people suffer from IBS. These theories are discussed in more detail in the chapters to follow. However, in order to understand the theories fully, it is important to have some knowledge of your digestive system

Physiology of the gut

The term 'gut' encompasses all of the digestive system, from the mouth to the anus. It thus includes the oesophagus ('gullet'), stomach, small intestine, colon and rectum. The gut has its own nervous system, called the enteric nervous system, the activity of which is modulated by the brain via the autonomic nerves and hormones.

The gut is basically a hollow tube which is made up of smooth muscle tissue that is not under voluntary control. Although some people believe it is only active when you eat, this is not true – the gut is almost always active. It does not, of course, work on its own – it is controlled by the nervous system. This is the system which relays information from the outside and from internal organs to the brain so that it can process this information and act accordingly. The nervous system can be divided into two: the central nervous system (brain and spinal cord) and the peripheral nervous system (which includes the enteric nervous system). Your digestive system is controlled by a complex interaction of these systems, with paths of nerves linking the brain and gut. Your hormonal system also works to keep the gut functioning normally, various circulating hormones exerting powerful effects on its muscle.

The oesophagus is about 20 cm (8 in) long, and leads from the

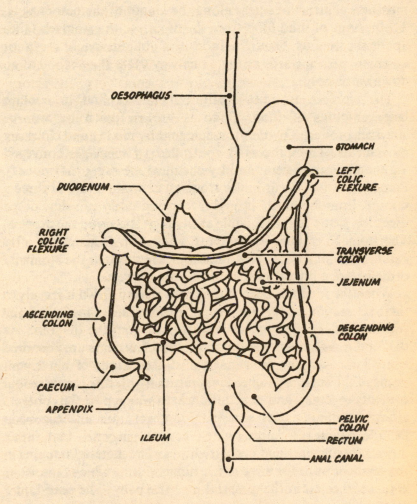

OESOPHAGUS

STOMACH

LEFT COLIC FLEXURE

DUODENUM

RIGHT COLIC FLEXURE

TRANSVERSE COLON

JEJENUM

ASCENDING COLON

DESCENDING COLON

CAECUM

APPENDIX

PELVIC COLON

ILEUM

RECTUM

ANAL CANAL

The digestive system, or gut

mouth to the stomach. It secretes mucus and transports food to the stomach. When you eat, food is moved down the oesophagus by an involuntary muscular process called peristalsis in which waves of muscular contractions pass along the length of the oesophagus. The passage of solid food from the mouth to the stomach takes about six seconds. Once the food is in your stomach, it cannot normally pass upwards again; a one-way valve allows food to go downwards only.

The stomach is quite small, but can expand to contain large amounts of food. Food is broken down by various enzymes produced by the stomach, and by mixing and churning movements. This process is controlled by messages conveyed via the nervous system, and by chemical messages (hormones). Peristaltic waves occur in the stomach at a rate of about three a minute. Emotions such as anger, fear or anxiety can slow down digestion in the stomach, while excitement speeds up the process. The stomach empties its contents within two to six hours after eating. Carbohydrates pass most quickly through the stomach, proteins are a little slower, and fats are slowest.

When the food has been sufficiently broken down it travels to the next section of the gut, the small intestine. This is 6 m (20 ft) long but is coiled up, as you can see from the diagram. As the food travels down the small intestine, nutrients are absorbed from it through the intestinal walls. Two kinds of movement occur in the small intestine: movements which mix the intestinal contents together, and peristaltic waves which pass the contents along. Intestinal juices secreted for absorption and digestion include pancreatic juices, which contain enzymes that break down proteins, fats and carbohydrates. The material remains in the small intestine for three to five hours, during which time water is reabsorbed from the material into the body. The semi-liquid material is called chyme.

The large intestine, or colon, is about 1.5 m (5 ft) long. Much of the pain associated with IBS is likely to derive from the colon. The nutrients have mostly been absorbed by the time food enters the colon. Waste material is prepared for elimination by the action of bacteria known as the gut flora. These bacteria ferment any remaining carbohydrates and release various gases which contribute to flatulence. The material remains in the large intestine for three to ten hours, and should at this time be solid or semi-solid, as the water from the waste material should have been reabsorbed by this time. Muscular contractions ensure the faeces are pushed along the large bowel to the rectum. Whether they are solid or semi-solid depends on the length of time they are exposed to this process of absorption.

As the rectum (20 cm/8 in long) fills up with waste material, it triggers the urge to expel the faeces. About 100 g (4 oz) of faeces are passed daily, mostly composed of water, inorganic matter, cellulose, fatty substances, mucus and bacteria – the latter comprising 80 per cent of faecal solids. The anal sphincter, which keeps the bowel shut, is under voluntary control, and if you relax it, the waste material will be allowed out. If the rectum is not emptied, it will relax and the desire to defecate will pass.

This is how the normal gut works. It may sound simple, but in fact, the process is very complicated. The nervous system of the brain and the gut, and hormones and other chemicals all have to work in harmony if everything is to go according to plan.

Causes of IBS: The theories

Physiological factors

The brain–gut link The gut has its own nervous system which gastroenterologists sometimes think of as the 'little brain'. This means that is incorrect to think of the gut as being controlled directly by your brain as the gut itself is capable of having some control, although what happens in your gut will be passed through to the 'big brain' in your head and vice versa. Digestive functions are controlled by an interaction between the big brain and the little brain. It could be that IBS is due to a failure in the way the brain–gut relationship functions.

Disorder of the smooth muscle tissue It has been suggested that some IBS patients may have hyper-reactive, or oversensitive, bowel muscle. This could be genetically determined (inherited), or it could be acquired (for instance, from an attack of gastro-enteritis). According to this theory, IBS could be a disorder of the smooth muscle tissue. Being born with such a disorder, or acquiring it later in life, would mean that you are likely to get IBS, which could be triggered by factors such as some types of food, stress, or hormone abnormalities. People without the underlying abnormality of the smooth muscle tissue would not get IBS even when the same triggers were present. People with IBS often have bladder problems such as the need to pass water very frequently. This would tie in with the above theory, as the bladder is also made up of smooth muscle tissue.

New techniques of measuring motility in the gut (the speed at which digested food is moved along) have shown that there are abnormalities in the electrical pattern in the gut in some people with IBS; these abnormalities can be triggered by stress or certain drugs, but they are also present without triggering factors. For instance, researchers recorded gut movements while people played computer games, drove in London traffic, and heard their own voices through headphones. These activities are acknowledged as being stressful. One or more abnormalities was seen in 19 out of 22 IBS patients, but only one in ten non-IBS people. This leads to the conclusion that IBS sufferers have hyper-reactive bowels which react more to any sort of stress than those of normal people.

Fatty meals have also been shown to provoke a different pattern of motor activity (movements) in the small intestines of IBS patients.

Other researchers measured motor activity in the small intestines of people going about their own business (i.e. not doing specific tasks set by the researchers). These studies found that there were differences in the motor activity in the gut between IBS sufferers and healthy people. It is poss-ible that the disturbed motility produces the symptoms of distension, discomfort and an inappropriate urge to go to the toilet.

Professor Read, Professor of Gastrointestinal Physiology and

Nutrition at the University of Sheffield Northern General Hospital, explains that some people have an oversensitive rectum, which makes them feel as if they need to go to the toilet when physically there really is no need. Some people may have the opposite problem; they may have an undersensitive rectum so that they do not realize when they need to go, leading to constipation. Professor Read also states that some people suffer from an oversensitive or undersensitive bowel, not just the rectum, and believes that most people with IBS can be placed in one of these categories.

Sometimes people blame themselves for having IBS – 'If only I could cope better with stress,' they say, or 'I realize I have to control it with my mind.' Often they feel guilty because they still have the symptoms even when they are leading a relatively stress-free life. They may feel that there is something wrong with them if they cannot control their symptoms. This is why it is important for you to know that there is evidence that the tendency to have IBS is biological. That is, you have a predisposition to IBS, and there is nothing you can do about that!

Genetic predisposition There is some debate about whether the predisposition to IBS is inherited. One study has shown that symptoms are more likely to develop when there is an abnormality in the autonomic nervous system, which makes the gut more susceptible to sudden changes in blood flow. Such increases in blood flow are associated with attacks of pain. A disorder of the autonomic nervous system also gives rise to migraines, and it has been found that families of IBS patients have a higher rate of migraine headaches. This gives support to the view that IBS might be due to a dysfunction of the autonomic nervous system, and that such dysfunction might be inherited. However, the study was conducted on people with recurrent abdominal pain, which may or may not have been IBS.

Trigger factors

A response to stress The most common assumption by laypeople – and some medics – is that IBS is a reaction to the stress of life events. Some think it is due to an inability to cope, either part of the sufferer's personality or a 'conversion' symptom – in other words, because you cannot cope with a bad marriage or major relationship, and find this difficult to deal with, you convert your problems into bodily symptoms, in this case IBS. Certainly, sufferers often *do* suffer psychologically – they may be anxious and depressed, and research has found that some sufferers remember being under a lot of stress before the IBS started. The problem with these retrospective accounts, however, is that many people can recall a stressful episode if asked to do so, even if they are not suffering from any symptoms, and people who are ill have a tendency to look back to find 'causes' which can explain their illness. Also, if IBS sufferers are told again and again that IBS is a result of stress (and most articles on IBS and books written on it for the layperson include stress as a major factor), the repetition can be very convincing! It is clear that stress can aggravate any illness, not just IBS, and it may worsen already existing symptoms; whether or not it actually causes or triggers symptoms of irritable bowel when the sufferer is in remission is less clear.

Some sufferers have given up work, thinking it is work-related stress which is causing their IBS; this helps some people, but others feel that it hasn't made any difference to them. Some sufferers say that their symptoms worsen when they are under pressure. However, many others have gone to great lengths to reduce the stress in their lives, only to find that their symptoms remain – or, paradoxically, that they suffer badly during relatively stress-free periods. This is what Maureen, who is in her seventies, found:

'My life is very curtailed by this condition which is a great pity as, after a very stressful life, I have now reached much calmer waters, and it seems very perverse that I coped with the stress and then develop this stressful condition when my life has become so much freer. I could live a much fuller and more outgoing life were it not for this condition.'

The colon normally moves food by moderate contractions or spasms. If a person with IBS becomes excited or anxious, the colon reacts with either too few or too many contractions, leading to either constipation or diarrhoea. The trigger factor theory accepts that there could be a predisposition to IBS, either hereditary or acquired, and that stress of any kind acts as a trigger. Consequently counselling or stress control could be of benefit. Stress is covered in more detail in Chapter 4.

Although many IBS sufferers report that stress triggers their IBS, and much research supports such an association, in 1996 Professor Whitehead, an expert in gastrointestinal disorders at the University of North Carolina, stated that carefully controlled studies have shown that the association between stress and IBS is weak, much weaker than you would expect, having listened to the frequency with which people talk about stress and IBS. He concluded that people tend to exaggerate the importance of stress in order to explain the inexplicable.

Dietary factors It used to be thought that IBS was due to too little fibre in the diet. Fibre decreases the transit time and also the reabsorption of water from the faeces in the colon. This increases the volume of the faeces, makes them pass more easily through the colon, and also results in increased frequency of defecation. However, since IBS people do not generally differ from non-IBS people in their intake of fibre, this is not now thought to be the cause of IBS. See Chapters 4 and 7 for more information on diet.

Many people feel that certain foods make their IBS worse. This is not the same as saying that these foods cause IBS. Although some researchers feel that food intolerance can cause IBS, this is not the consensus of medical opinion. However, certain foods could act as a trigger, setting off an attack of IBS in people already predisposed to it.

Hysterectomy One study attempted to find out whether hysterectomy patients have an increased risk of IBS. Symptoms were measured in over 200 women six weeks before, and then again six months after, their operation. One in five women had symptoms of IBS (mostly the constipation type) before their operation, and over half these women actually improved after their hysterectomy. However, one in five women had increased symptoms. One in ten women who had been symptom-free before their operation showed signs of IBS afterwards, most of these cases being constipation-predominant IBS.

The researchers found that many women who already have symptoms when they go for hysterectomy improve afterwards, but some women who have no IBS symptoms beforehand can be expected to have IBS problems later. It seems that hysterectomy can act as a trigger for IBS in some women, but it is not known why this is.

Another study found that women who had had a hysterectomy were more likely to have constipation than other women. This is thought to be because altered hormone concentration may affect bowel habit after hysterectomy, especially in women who have also had their ovaries removed. It is also possible that the operation on the pelvic area may have caused damage to the nerves in that region.

Gall bladder trouble Some of the people we spoke to said their IBS began after their gall bladders were removed. According to Professor N. W. Read this can give rise to IBS because the bile acid can leak into the duodenum, and if it is not absorbed, it can have a laxative effect. A 'faulty' gall bladder can provoke the same response.

Mercury poisoning Some people believe that IBS can be triggered by mercury poisoning. Roger Dyson, a homoeopath, has studied the work of homoeopath Pritam Singh and some of the writings of J. G. Levenson, President of the British Dental Society for Clinical Nutrition. Roger Dyson now believes that mercury (used for filling teeth) gives off a vapour which, when swallowed, combines with hydrochloric acid to form mercuric chloride; this destroys gut bacteria and allows an overgrowth of candida. The formation of this compound may leave the body deficient in hydrochloric acid so that digestion cannot proceed efficiently. Roger Dyson says that the effects of mercury poisoning can be slow, taking perhaps five years or more to show.

Why, then, doesn't everyone with mercury fillings have the symptoms of IBS? Dyson says that some people are more resilient than others, and not everyone is sensitive to the effects of mercury. According to Dyson, you do not need to rush to the dentist to have your fillings out – homoeopathic remedies may, he says, help this condition. In fact, having your fillings removed may cause even more mercury damage.

Hormones Oestrogen and progesterone affect the function of the colon and the movement of food through it. There are some women whose symptoms fluctuate with the menstrual cycle, which is governed by these hormones. However, this is not likely to be a major contributory factor in IBS – although twice as many women as men are diagnosed as having IBS in Britain, this is not the case in other countries. It is possible, though, that in some women these hormones can make IBS worse at certain times of the month.

Disturbance of gut flora The balance of different bacteria in the gut can be altered by taking antibiotics, or by a bout of gastroenteritis. Some researchers believe that IBS may be a result of the gut flora becoming disturbed – the 'good' bacteria are pushed out, allowing the 'bad' bacteria or yeasts (such as candida) to take over. You will find more about this in Chapter 4.

Is there a link with sexual abuse? Over the past six years or so, there have been several studies that suggest a link between childhood sexual abuse and later gastrointestinal complaints, including IBS. For instance, patients with IBS are more likely to report sexual abuse than patients with inflammatory bowel disease. However, it is not possible to compare the studies enquiring into the link between IBS and sexual abuse, mainly because they use different criteria for assessing abuse; also the prevalence rates refer to different types of abuse and different timespans. Comparison of prevalence figures, however, is much less important than the finding that all the studies suggest that there is a link between childhood sexual abuse and some gastrointestinal problems.

Psychological factors
Many studies find IBS patients to be more anxious and depressed than non-IBS patients. Some researchers have concluded that their IBS is thus due to anxiety and depression. (See Chapter 4 for more on this.) In other words, IBS occurs as a result of the psychological disorder. At the moment there is no way of knowing whether this is the case, or whether having a disorder like IBS causes the anxiety and depression.

Researchers at St Bartholomew's Hospital, London, in a study published in 1996, found that inpatients with emotional disorders were more likely to have IBS than other people. However, their IBS almost invariably *preceded* their emotional disorder, and their symptoms had become worse since their emotional problems had begun. The researchers concluded that emotional problems affect the severity of symptoms, but do not play a major part in causing them.

A particular type of personality? To find out whether IBS sufferers have a distinct personality, scientific studies have compared them with other groups of patients such as sufferers of Crohn's disease. Both groups were tested on psychological measures such as neuroticism, extroversion, hostility, fatigue, depression, anxiety and so on, and differences between the groups were compared. Studies sometimes contradicted each other, but IBS patients did tend to be more anxious than other people. However, no distinctive personality type has yet been pinpointed. Dr Paul Latimer, a professor of psychiatry in the US, says: 'Psychological studies have found patients to be compulsive, over-conscientious, dependent, sensitive, guilty and unassertive . . . Little evidence exists that IBS patients have a distinctive personality profile.' Other studies have come to the same conclusion.

All in the mind Living with a chronic disorder for which the medical profession and others have little sympathy can lead to psychological problems. For instance, ulcerative colitis, a disease with a definable pathology which causes diarrhoea, pain and general ill-health, may take some time to diagnose correctly, during which time sufferers may be told that their symptoms are a manifestation of stress, depression or anxiety. One patient, before a correct diagnosis of colitis was made, was told he had underlying worries. When the patient said that he was unaware of this, he was told that he was worrying about something although he did not know it (from *Colitis* by Michael Kelly, 1992). Studies have been conducted which have shown that colitis patients have psychological problems; however, these also show that the problems tend to subside after correct treatment, suggesting that the disturbance results from the disease rather than the other way round.

This may well be the case for many IBS sufferers. Ascribing psychological causes to illnesses is not a trivial matter for people who are suffering with obvious physical symptoms. Attributing a psychological cause to a disorder has both advantages and disadvantages. If someone believes that stress has caused their disorder or illness, then the solution for preventing a recurrence and becoming healthy lies within themselves. For patients with irritable bowel, attributing their disorder to stress means that they feel that they can, or should be able to, control it. The disadvantage is that, if symptoms remain despite all strategies for reducing stress (and this is most likely), depression and anxiety can result. Of course, if stress really *does* cause, or trigger, IBS, then such knowledge must not be withheld from sufferers; however, it is the case that at present *this really is not known*. While there is no doubt that emotional and psychological well-being contributes to physical health, it is common to hear people with IBS cite the stresses they have been through without any worsening of their symptoms.

Attributing a chronic disorder to 'stress' puts the onus firmly on the patient to change and recover, and is often an easy answer for professionals to give when at a loss to know how to explain irritable bowel. Medical practitioners have been found to attribute illnesses to stress when there is no *apparent* organic cause for a patient's distress. One study by two psychologists cited several examples of the reversal of cause and effect by health-care professionals when searching for causes of illnesses: multiple sclerosis sufferers are often told their symptoms are psychological or psychosomatic, and their strange behaviours labelled as neurotic or malingering, as are sufferers with chronic fatigue syndrome (CFS), primary dysmenorrhoea, diabetes and even cancer. The researchers noted these views particularly affect women, often assumed by medical practitioners to be more likely to be neurotic. Sufferers from endometriosis (a gynaecological disease) take an average of eight years to be correctly diagnosed. During the course of their illness they suffer severe abdominal pain, and their bowels may be affected – having a bowel movement can be painful, and they may suffer from diarrhoea. Three per cent of these women have previously been diagnosed as having irritable bowel, but their symptoms tend to disappear once the endometriosis is treated.

Health-care workers can be very dismissive of patients when they think patients have nothing organically wrong with them. Patients with IBS, often believing themselves to be the cause of their own disorder, and having only a few minutes to discuss their problems with the doctor, may leave the surgery feeling more miserable and 'stressed' than ever. The debate as to whether IBS is caused by stress, or whether having to live with it causes the stress, will no doubt continue for some time to come.

Can IBS be cured?

There is nothing that cures all the symptoms of IBS, but there are various treatments which can ease some of them. People do recover from IBS. You can help yourself by finding out as much as possible about IBS, including the theories of how IBS starts, and what treatments are available. Self-help groups are very useful because they can help sufferers feel less alone and more in control of themselves and their symptoms, and they are often a good source of tips on useful treatments. In the following chapters we will describe the medical investigations IBS sufferers undergo, the various treatments, and the physical and psychological consequences of having IBS. We will also look at how IBS sufferers cope with the condition, and the roles played by stress and lifestyle. The people quoted in this book all suffer, or have suffered, from IBS. It is to be hoped that their stories of how they coped will help you understand IBS and be able to deal with the disorder more effectively.

Chapter 2

The Physical and Psychological Consequences

Susan Backhouse and Christine P. Dancey

'I live from hour to hour and avoid making plans in advance. IBS has changed my life – I work, travel and so on around my symptoms.'

Living with IBS can mean a very restricted life. It may prevent you doing things other people take for granted – for instance shopping, car and bus journeys, long-distance travel, going for walks or visiting friends. It may prevent you from doing the sort of work you'd like to do, or even working at all.

If diarrhoea is a problem, you may find yourself having to plan around the availability of toilets in everything you do. If pain is one of your symptoms, you may be stopped from doing things because the agony keeps you at home in bed. If you are constipated, you may find you have to keep to a specific routine. If you suffer from wind, you may only want to see people in the open air, or not at all. Women with bloating sometimes have to put up with people asking them when their baby is due! Some of the symptoms of IBS can be a great embarrassment: wind, incontinence, having to rush to the toilet, being doubled up with pain – these alone can prevent sufferers from socializing. Isolation and depression can follow.

Many IBS sufferers will tell of the psychological effects of having to live with the condition. It may be hard to cope with for a number of reasons. IBS lacks validity and a sufferer may find that doctors and family are far from understanding and sympathetic. It seems to be the luck of the draw whether you get support and useful information from your GP or from gastroenterologists, although specialists with a particular interest in IBS, and their staff, can be more sympathetic. At the moment, the medical profession has little to offer in the way of effective treatment. 'There are no known clinical tests that will confirm or refute the diagnosis with certainty and there is no specific therapy for the condition,' say researchers on a study into IBS. Although medical professionals are advocating that IBS is diagnosed on a positive basis – i.e. on the basis of the presence of particular symptoms – it is still, in practice, a diagnosis of exclusion: in other words, it's what you've got if you haven't got anything else! You may go through a series of uncomfortable or painful tests only to be told there's nothing wrong with you, try a high fibre diet, take these anti-spasmodics or this bulking agent, and there's not much else that can be done to help you. You may be given tranquillizers or anti-depressants and told to reduce the stress in your life, but as Louise, a 32-year-old housewife, says, 'It's having to live with IBS that causes me the most stress.'

Family and friends may not understand and you may feel they see you as lazy or wanting attention, or being unable to cope with life. Because of the attitudes of others, and sometimes of the medical profession, it is not uncommon for IBS sufferers to blame themselves or feel guilty about their condition. However, a supportive GP, relative or friend can make all the difference.

The symptoms themselves are hard to cope with. Quite apart from the main symptoms of diarrhoea and/or constipation, abdominal pain, bloating and wind, there may be secondary ones. For instance, many people with IBS experience panic attacks – a racing heart, difficulty in breathing, sweating, a feeling of faintness and sickness. This can be a very frightening experience that can make you think twice about putting yourself in the same situation again. The panic attack may be caused by the fact that you were in a place where no toilet was nearby and you feared you were going to have an accident. Indeed, you may not have made it to the toilet in time – incontinence is more common than people realize. Thereafter, that location – whether it was in a supermarket, on the street, or even at home – can bring on feelings of panic because you fear it happening again. Consequently you avoid those situations, or suffer great anxiety when you are forced into them.

Sufferers may develop obsessions or other behaviour that seems strange to non-sufferers. You may feel safer or more comfortable in certain clothes, you may take to wearing incontinence pads or sanitary towels, you may not be able to leave the house without going to the toilet many times, you may not be able to eat in public, you may not feel able to stay at friends' homes, you may have to avoid morning appointments or events in the evening, you may develop routines in the morning or at bedtime that cannot be broken without causing you anxiety. These limitations will be understandable to other IBS sufferers, but you may not feel able to explain why you can't go out for a meal with a friend or for a drink with work colleagues, for example. Therefore, you may resort to elaborate behaviour patterns. You make bizarre excuses to avoid situations that make you anxious: you'd rather be thought to be unfriendly or unsociable than explain why you can't go out for a meal; you go out of your way to avoid someone you know in the street in case she stops to talk and you want to go to the toilet, or are in pain, or need to fart . . .

Needless to say, if people with IBS feel that they cannot be open about their symptoms they can become isolated and depressed and may feel ashamed of their behaviour, or inadequate about their inability to cope. But coping is just what you are doing – coping in the ways that are available to you (see Chapter 3 for more on coping).

When sufferers do not feel they cope well with their IBS, depression can be the result. Says Sheila:

'I cope very badly. I'm in tears most days as it's so bad when I get up and continues through the day and night. I get very frightened of going to work and sitting all day with so much congestion and pain, with nowhere to go to alleviate it.'

Some people have sought psychiatric treatment because of the stress and anxiety they suffer. Many do not feel optimistic that their IBS will improve, especially if they've had it some time and it hasn't got better, or has even got worse.

Other secondary symptoms include fatigue and lethargy, when you are unable to do anything but curl up with a hot-water bottle. This adds to the frustration, as you feel that your life is passing you by. There are so many things you want to do, but are prevented from doing. Pat, a 37-year-old secretary, feels like that:

'I feel that four years out of the five I've had IBS have been ruined, wasted. I don't have any leisure activities at all. I gave them all up. For four years I didn't go anywhere on holiday, or go to a restaurant; I didn't eat in the street in case I couldn't find a loo, I didn't visit anyone, and I stood at the back of the church where the loo was. In the cinema, I have to sit in the end seat, just in case.'

Many sufferers worry about the future. How will they cope with their IBS? What jobs will they be able to do? They worry about having panic attacks, about incontinence and pain, about not being in control of their own body.

Why is it so common to find that people with IBS feel somehow it is their fault, and why does guilt often accompany an attack?

'I get so depressed and fed up with myself because it's not fair on my son to find me in bed all the time when he gets home from school.'

'I always felt like a hypochondriac, so played down my symptoms at consultations.'

'The doctors were pleasant but made me feel inadequate because I couldn't cope with IBS.'

'I would probably have felt too guilty at being stupid enough to have IBS to join a self-help group. I always feel I should cope better.'

It is usually the attitudes of people who don't have IBS that trigger these feelings in us.

> 'I'm fed up with being told, however indirectly, that I'm some kind of stressed-up failure who likes to be the way I am because I either want to avoid life or am lazy!'

> 'I am fed up with having a reputation for being late or thought of as being lazy. It is impossible to explain to someone who is "normal" how you can have been up since before 7 am but still find it difficult to get out by 9 am.'

Embarrassment is common. Bowels and their problems are, at best, an unglamorous subject. Some people find having IBS more embarrassing than others. Claudia describes how she feels:

> 'I would die if anyone knew about it. To even my closest friends this is top secret and I spend my life inventing excuses for why I can't do things. The distressing thing is that I would love to join in and do things other people do, but my life depends on my stomach.'

Claudia, now 42, has had IBS since she was 16. She was only diagnosed three years ago, and during the previous 23 years, she presumed she was a 'nervous wreck'.

> 'When I was eventually referred to a specialist I was quite relieved that it was a recognized problem. Perhaps someone somewhere had had it before!'

She goes on to describe how it all began:

> 'We moved south when I was 16. I joined the sixth form down here and then the problems started. I had to leave school after three months of hell, much to my parents' disappointment. Like them, I too expected I would go on to university and get a good job, but now I couldn't even sit in a classroom for 30 minutes. Even sitting in the doctor's waiting room was a trial. No one

understood. I began to feel I was mental and made up all sorts of reasons about having to leave school to look after my sick mother. I was taken to see psychiatrists and diagnosed as having "nerve problems".

'When I was a teenager I think I was regarded as a freak as I always wanted the TV or radio on to drown my stomach. I am still the same now but, being a housewife, at least I am in charge of the situation at home. The problems start at other people's houses. People began to think I had a fear of "quiet" so I had to let them think that. It was less embarrassing. Saying you are claustrophobic gets you a seat on the end of the row in a theatre or restaurant so that you can dash to the loo. Having a migraine is useful for getting out of things you just can't face.

'I now have three children and they have been marvellous to hide behind. You can always leave anywhere to take a child to the loo (and go yourself) and you can always talk and make noises with a child in a quiet situation – for example, doctors' and dentists' waiting rooms.

'I find it impossible to attend talks at the children's schools. I dread parents' evenings. In fact, I don't eat for three days beforehand in case that will help. I dread things months ahead because I don't know how I can get out of them.

'I can't go to church because I can't sit through the sermon. They asked me to be a school governor but I had to leave the meeting to go to the loo so I made excuses to get out of that. People think I'm afraid of commitment – but it's not that.

'All in all, to everyone else, I am a likeable person, but because of all these problems they probably think I am a bag of nerves. I am not. All I need is a new stomach.'

Having IBS in this society can, as Claudia describes, seriously influence a person's behaviour. Dora, who has had it for 14 years, writes about the lasting effects on her:

'After all these years the actual bouts of IBS are rare and short-lived but unfortunately, what is almost worse, I have been left with a terrible phobia about being in any situation where I do not have easy access to a toilet. The panic caused by the threat of being in such a situation is indescribable and causes instant, terrible diarrhoea.'

Sex and relationships

In the study we carried out among IBS Network members, nearly half of our respondents (46 per cent) said IBS directly affected their sex lives. Sometimes IBS can make sex painful for both women and men. 'Painful sex with my husband was never really examined by doctors for IBS. I was told it was just one of those things,' says Tina, a 33-year-old who has had symptoms since she was 25.

Other times the symptoms a person is suffering can take away all desire. Sex may also be affected by embarrassment, as Judy, a 41-year-old housewife who has had IBS for ten years, says:

'I worry that I might pass wind during intercourse. I was brought up to believe that passing wind just wasn't the thing to do and I get very embarrassed about it. Men make fun of it between themselves, but if a woman does it, it's a different thing.'

Andrea, a 26-year-old administrator who has suffered the condition since she was 13, says:

'Regrettably, I've never had the chance to find out if IBS would make sex painful for me. Apart from embarrassment, it often makes you feel too ill to care about the opposite sex.'

'I've never had a relationship as I never go out. By the evening I am in too much pain and bloated,' says Megan, a 42-year-old ex-teacher who has had IBS since she was 21. Dorothy, an admin officer in her thirties who has had IBS ever since she can remember, finds sex painful:

'I have no partner at present. Most positions are painful. I only seem to be comfortable on my side with absolutely no pressure on my abdomen.'

And Rita, who has suffered from IBS for 22 years, says:

'Sex has for some time not been attempted for fear of being "caught out" at a highly personal moment in time, but after 24 years of marriage, love, hugs and kisses make up for an awful lot of missed sex life!'

IBS often causes a lot of friction and tension between the sufferer and those with whom they live closely. This is almost inevitable unless the loved ones are particularly understanding – or suffer themselves! In extreme cases, relationships are ruined and marriages break down. Gail remembers:

'I felt a failure in coping with IBS. When the children were small, and my husband's workload permitted a family outing, it always, so it seemed, "played up". He would say, "I knew this would happen," and I felt devastated. I did become depressed and anxious largely due to the IBS – not the other way round as my current GP imagined. I would go as far as to say I think it played a part in our consequent divorce.'

For Claudia, the worst occasion was:

'. . . when my husband's boss invited several people and their wives to his house for dinner and I just couldn't face the embarrassment of my stomach and refused to go. He went on his own and said I had to babysit for someone. I really felt I let him down and I'm sure his boss must have thought our marriage was on the rocks.'

IBS can also affect one's self-confidence, as Sarah, who is 53 and has had it since she was in her mid-thirties, writes:

'IBS has had a profound effect on my love life! I used to feel very sexually confident and outgoing. However, since developing IBS, I have had very few relationships and have become pretty reclusive. I have recently been contemplating the possibility of starting a new relationship with someone, but am very aware that embarrassment about wind etc. has left me feeling it's not worth going through all the anxiety, so I haven't done anything about pursuing the relationship.'

IBS has prevented Lorna from leaving her husband:

'My marriage is not terribly happy, and if I was "normal", I would probably have left my husband several years ago, but I don't have the courage to do so. He may have his faults, but he has always been absolutely super regarding my problems. He never minds how many times I need to visit the loo, and is very understanding. I feel it would be awful to have to start again with someone else, and try to explain. Imagine being with someone new, perhaps the first time you make love, then having to rush off to the loo! Also, if I left I would have nowhere to go. I would have to rent a flat or house, and I cannot afford it on what I earn. I could share with another girl if I were "normal", but I couldn't even think about sharing the way things are. So I continue in a dead marriage. We don't argue a lot, I can't say it is stressful, we just live in the same house but don't communicate a lot. We have nothing in common, he goes out, I spend a lot of time on my own. I feel there is more to life than this, but what can I do about it?'

Lack of self-confidence can be a problem for men as well as women. Steven, a 24-year-old admin assistant, explains how he feels:

'I don't dare have a girlfriend. I lack self-confidence in that I'm dependent often on being near a toilet. I feel different, abnormal and frustrated in not being able to do what I want.'

Henry echoes Steven's sentiments:

'It makes it difficult to develop relationships with the opposite sex – what girl would want to go out with a man who daren't go out of reach of the loo? How can I be open with them about it?'

Maisie, on the other hand, doesn't feel that her IBS has had any great effect on her relationships:

> 'I live alone and am not at present in a long-term relationship. I make a point of not telling new friends about my IBS. I want them to know me first as Maisie and not "the girl with the IBS". Nobody has run off yet when I've told them! I still have a lot of interest from men as I did before I got IBS and I'm glad to say I haven't lost interest in them!'

How work is affected

Maisie is 34 and has had IBS for the past three years. Her working life as a civil servant has been severely affected, because pain prevents her from sitting down for more than ten minutes at a time.

> 'For the first seven months, the pain was on and off. I underwent the usual medical tests which meant time off. My employers were very sympathetic. After seven months, the pain became and has remained continuous. Every minute of every day I'm either in bad or very bad pain and discomfort. There is no relief except for when I sleep.
>
> 'After seven months I decided to go on indefinite sick leave to concentrate all my energy into getting well. It was becoming impossible to do my job properly, as it entailed a lot of travelling and sitting in court and in interviews. Sitting had become, and still is, unbearably uncomfortable. I have reached the stage now where most of my day is spent either on the move or standing up. That's not to say that I'm in very much less discomfort when I'm on the move. It's just more easy to bear, pacing about.'

After the hospitals had told her they couldn't help any more, Maisie decided to try complementary medicine. She spent £1000 on trying to find a cure but nothing helped even in the slightest. Her symptoms gradually got worse. She continues:

'After seven months of being on sick leave, I had a chat with my boss and decided to accept a completely different job. I had got worse while I was on sick leave, but as I couldn't see an end to this problem I knew I just had to go back to survive. I don't just mean financially – but I couldn't afford to give in to it.

'The job I do now is very much less demanding. It enables me to walk around a fair bit, but at the end of the day, it is still a desk job and I'm just so uncomfortable sitting down that I can't concentrate.

'I'm unhappy and frustrated at work now. Every day I don't feel well enough to go in but I make myself. I haven't missed a day since I went back two years ago, but there are times when I've had to continue work lying on the floor in pain. When I get home, I give myself a pat on the back for getting through the day. Very occasionally I allow myself a good cry, take a deep breath and start again. There is never a morning when I don't wake up full of renewed hope that maybe today's the day.

'I'm three years behind as far as promotion is concerned and it is very frustrating seeing my contemporaries pass me by. Having said that, IBS has made me take stock of my life and sort out my priorities. I value my health, family and friends even more now.'

Maisie is tired of the daily struggle and is considering a complete change of career. She explains it this way:

'If a typist loses her arm, she doesn't go back to typing – she sits down and thinks what else she can do with what she has left. Maybe it is time for me to accept that I have got a disability which prevents me from doing a desk job. Also, so much of my energy goes into battling against IBS that I don't currently need such a demanding job. Doing routine work stretches me. I'm trying to do something which I'm not fit to do, and this is causing me stress and in turn must be affecting my IBS.'

Maisie's decision not to apply for promotion because she needs all her energy to cope with IBS has meant loss of pride and self-esteem.

Sheila, a finance clerk, has had IBS for five years. Her main symptom is severe bloating and wind. She describes what it's like at work:

'I'd love to change my job but don't know how I would cope as I spend so much time in the toilet. It's difficult now at work with people noticing. I spend most of my time lying on the floor trying to pass wind or bent double in pain. I have to hold or suppress the symptoms, which makes it worse, or keep going out to the toilet. I am worried about how I can hold a job down in this condition. It's becoming increasingly difficult for me to hide the symptoms.'

Rita is 44 and works as a local government officer. This year she has lost three months due to her IBS. She suffers from continuous diarrhoea and abdominal pain.

'Travelling to work is a major problem on bad days – I am in constant fear of any hold-up in transport in case I need to rush to the toilet. Sitting in on meetings or even travelling to them is also a problem. What if I need to leave in a hurry and cannot find the cloakroom? (I usually arrive extra early and try to do this first!)

'Part of my job is to meet and talk to the public, which I usually find rewarding, but not feeling 100 per cent for the best part of my working day causes stress; I feel as if I am on stage, and put on my best face and performance for my customers, the public. Career promotion has twice been put on one side as I was unable to fulfil the obligations of the posts offered, because of IBS. If you are working as a team, you cannot expect your colleagues to cover or carry you for long periods. This again I feel stressed and angry about – angry with myself for not being in control. My present head of section has always been very kind and thoughtful about my condition, but when he leaves later on this year, I fear his replacement will not be so easy. I have already had the unkind remarks about people pulling their weight, etc.!'

For those sufferers whose symptoms are worse in the morning, nine-to-five jobs can be very difficult. Edwina has always suffered with her bowels but did not worry too much about it until she started working in an office.

'I was working in a bingo hall where I didn't have to be in work until 1 pm and that gave me the time to go to the loo as many times as I needed. It was when I got into the claustrophobic office atmosphere that the symptoms really flared up. I was getting up at 6.30 am and still going to the loo at 9 am. It would start with windy crampy pains and spasms that would double me over. Then the stools would start. When I thought the bowel was empty, the whole process would begin again, sometimes up to eight or nine times in the morning, maybe more. Luckily, my work was on flexi-time but I was finding it hard to make it for 9.30 am. I would put my coat on to leave and have to rush back to the loo. It was the same at work. By 10 am, my stomach would be empty and the foul wind would start. I would then have to think of excuses to leave the office and rush to the loo. I had to start going home at lunchtime as I could not eat at work because, as soon as I did, the wind would begin again. My work did suffer. I was warned about my sick leave and was in constant debit with my flexi-time.

'The symptoms were often accompanied by hot flushes and panic attacks, especially in pubs, shops, buses and in the office. When I'm out, I need my space – claustrophobia brings my symptoms on.

'At Christmas I went to my doctor and asked for a sick note, as I felt so bad I think if I had continued working I would have had a nervous breakdown. I was physically and mentally exhausted with the whole thing. My employers, the Department of Social Security, were very good. They sent a welfare officer every month to see how I was and to offer advice. By the September I decided to resign as I could not see myself returning and I have been on

Invalidity Benefit ever since. I'm feeling better now I'm at home but if I have to go anywhere like the doctor's or for a night out, the severe symptoms begin again.'

For Adele, who has had IBS for nine years, the pressure of work aggravated her symptoms.

'I became a temporary veterinary nurse, a job I had not done for 12 years and a solo position as opposed to a team one as I had done previously. I found the vet I worked for very abrupt and unfriendly, with very high standards. Before operations were due to begin each morning I frequently had to go to the loo with diarrhoea.'

At present she is a part-time youth and community worker. She goes on to say:

'I have had diarrhoea before leaving home for difficult meetings which seems daft, but I am OK once I get there. It is a job which I enjoy and I am determined not to let my IBS stop me.'

Even working from home isn't without its problems, as Brenda, a 63-year-old writer, explains:

'I can't leave the house before 10 am. This interferes with professional appointments, conferences, etc. I have two to four wasted hours daily because of urgent visits to the lavatory, 6 to 10 am.'

Giving up work

Nearly 5 per cent of those taking part in our survey were unable to work at all because of their symptoms. Another survey carried out by Gail Rees of South Bank University, London, revealed that 8 per cent were not working due to IBS.

Amy has tried everything over the last 20 years in the hope of finding a cure. She had to give up her job as a teacher and is no longer able to work, but her enforced rest hasn't eased the symptoms. When she was working she was off continually and is now on Invalidity Benefit. She says:

> 'I am very slow and get tired easily. I am always battling against the pain. There is so much I want to do but the pain stops me.'

Being unable to work has meant lack of money and an insecurity that causes anxiety, and also prevents her from doing things she would like to.

Andrea also had to give up her job and now works from home in a family business:

> 'Despite a fairly positive attitude to "making the best of it", I have found my working life very curtailed, right from having to drop out of doing science A Levels because I was too ill to concentrate properly. I was an able student but have had to adapt to doing what my body is capable of rather than my mind.'

Graham is 56 and was a milkman for 24 years. He enjoyed the work, being outside in the fresh air, meeting people every day and, best of all, being able to plan the workload to suit himself. After an operation for haemorrhoids, he found that he had trouble with diarrhoea. He went to the doctor and, after having to undergo various investigations, was told that he 'probably' had IBS, as they couldn't find anything wrong! He was prescribed an anti-diarrhoeal drug.

> 'I was able to carry on with my outside job, although I had to be aware of the locations of all the toilets on my round. I found that I needed to go while working more and more often.'

He coped for quite a long time, but in October 1990 had very severe stomach pains that kept him off work for five weeks. It was found that he had a disease of the small intestine which cleared up with antibiotics. The following February he was off work for a further three weeks. Various tests were given, including ones for food allergies, but all were negative. By October his condition had worsened and he was forced to stop work.

> 'During one of my frequent visits, my GP told me, "You will have to accept that you may be unable to continue with your outside job, and should ask your employers if they are able to offer you an inside job." This wasn't possible and it was suggested that I apply for early retirement.'

At the time of writing Graham is on sick pay, but his employer is trying to hasten his retirement.

Mick is 55 and has suffered from constipation for many years. For 16 of them he took a laxative that his doctor assured him had no long-term ill-effects. When he started to get pains in his right abdomen his doctor decided perhaps he should not be taking the laxative after all. Eventually IBS was diagnosed. Mick remembers how, six years ago, the doctor advised him to give up work.

> 'My doctor suggested it would be advisable for me to give up work in view of my continued ill health, and as my job was stressful, this would help my condition. After six years of being home with no stress (except the illness), I have continued to gradually get worse and life has become a misery only consoled by a loving and considerate family without whose help I could not cope. I gave up a successful career with excellent prospects.'

What follows is an account of how ignorance and intolerance have forced Lorna to leave two jobs.

> 'I was getting very depressed and bored at home after my family left home and my marriage was going through a sticky patch. I had had IBS problems for many years though didn't at the time know what the problem was, medically speaking. I decided to get a job.
> 'I went back to teaching for one year but found it too stressful. I then got a post at a local government office. It soon became obvious that some of my work colleagues found me smelly. I have

very bad wind problems which I cannot always control. Some people with very sensitive noses seemed to find me offensive all the time – my bowel doesn't empty properly and this may be the problem here. They would make remarks which I tried to ignore. The office employed more than 500 people, and as the months passed, I became an office joke with one or two little references in notes and even snide remarks in the office newsletter.

'I sought medical help but this only seemed to make matters worse. I didn't want to be beaten by the problem, but in the end, after 18 months, I had to give up the job for my own sanity.

'I then found a job doing individual coaching with children at a private school. I enjoyed the work, but there were only two staff loos in the school and this caused me problems as they were often both engaged. There was also one member of staff with a particularly sensitive nose – there always is! – and she made sure everyone knew of my problem. The stress, of course, made the problem even worse and I started to avoid contact with the other staff as much as possible. After three-and-a-half years, I finally gave up and left. I now am back at home!'

Many readers will feel sympathy with Lorna about what she went through. The general public need educating about IBS so that sufferers are treated more sensitively.

Having IBS can prevent people from taking up jobs they would like. Louise wanted to take up nursing but realized her guts would never cope with the shift system and the stress of the job. IBS kept Rosemary at home once her children grew up when she would have liked to return to work. Claudia had hoped to study at university and go on to get a good job, but IBS put paid to her plans and she had to leave school early.

'I worked in a shop for about a year. I eventually plucked up the courage to get a better job, but I had to be very choosy. It had to be one where there was always noise to hide my tummy noises, and where I was free to go to the loo without being too obvious. I worked in a building society. This was fine until I progressed to being a cashier. I was caught in the trap again: as soon as I had a customer and thousands of pounds waiting to be counted, I was churning inside again and physically almost sick trying to get through to the end of the transaction. I eventually left the building society with "nerves" again.

'I had a year off work hoping relaxation might help. I was very frustrated. I knew I was capable of using my mind but my body wouldn't let me.

'After my year off, I got a job in an office (carefully planned for noise and escape routes). This was fine, but as I was promoted, I had to attend meetings and that was impossible, so I managed to coincide that with being able to start a family and escaped that one.'

Time off from work, not only due to the symptoms but also visits to the doctor, hospital and other health professionals, can mount up. Sean agrees:

'Fortunately, I am self-employed; the scores of working hours I have lost, in the recent past, is distressing and frustrating to me, but would presumably have been more so to an employer!'

It is very important that employers recognize IBS as a debilitating illness. As there is still much ignorance surrounding the condition, you are lucky if those you work with are understanding. Bernard has twice suffered at the hands of unsympathetic employers.

'The stomach problems in 1987 were probably the result of stress caused by marital problems which have considerably worsened since then. It was from 1987 that my health worsened to such a degree that it necessitated me having sick leave. My situation was not helped by a very unsympathetic employer who was apparently suggesting that I was malingering by my absence.'

Eventually, after having worked for this firm for a number of years, Bernard was made redundant, although he considers that he was sacked. Next, after passing the examination and declaring he had IBS, he found work with the Inland Revenue. By this time his health had considerably worsened.

> 'I had had little in the way of sick leave, but certain members of management were keeping check of my visits to the toilet. I was finding it difficult to give of my best with all of these pressures.'

Finally, the Inland Revenue terminated his employment. Since then, Bernard has been registered as disabled with anxiety and depression.

Domestic life

Tiredness, lethargy and pain can affect housework as they do other activities. Tasks are made slower and more difficult or they may not be possible at all. Joyce worries that she neglects her children because she spends so much time on the toilet.

Shopping can be difficult for those of us who need to be near a toilet. Some people only shop during pub opening hours so that their facilities can be used; others stick to one shop. Some people cannot go shopping at all. Queueing can often be a problem; several sufferers mention having to leave the queue to go to the toilet quickly.

Travel

A vast number of IBS sufferers say that travelling is restricted – nearly 70 per cent in our study. Both long-distance and short everyday journeys can cause all sorts of problems for the IBS sufferer. As Malcolm says: 'I need to find out where the toilets are before I travel anywhere.'

Motorway travel and traffic jams can be a source of anxiety, and some people can never travel by public transport – although those who need toilets nearby often feel better on trains or planes.

The daily journey to work can be quite harrowing for some people. Rita goes by car:

'Travel puts the fear into me, even the 15-minute journey to work – what could happen if the car breaks down or an accident causes delay, etc.? I try not to think too much about it but I have been caught out once too often.'

Julie's IBS restricts her travel greatly. She lives in London and usually travels by bus.

'After a couple of narrow escapes on the Underground, when I had to ask to use the staff loos, I am now scared stiff to go on the tube. The thought of getting stuck between stations acts as an instant enema, yet before I got IBS I travelled everywhere by Underground without giving it a second thought.'

Travelling abroad may be impossible or only undertaken with difficulty. Brenda says that for her:

'Travel abroad is out – my gut keeps Greenwich Mean Time! I can only visit where there is more than one loo. No journey can start before 10 am.'

Sheila says:

'I've been abroad this year and it was horrendous, being cramped in an aircraft with a stomach like a balloon and pressure in the cabin making the symptoms worse. I could have gone mad.'

Social life

Dealing with the effects of long-term IBS becomes a way of life. It is not unusual for all a sufferer's activities to be arranged around her or his symptoms. This can seriously restrict people's lives.
Rita describes how it has affected her:

'For nearly eight months last year, I only went to work, to the village or stayed at home, and it was not much of a life. In desperation, I even asked for my gut to be removed and a bag attached to let me live a better form of life, but that was greeted with horror by my doctor.

'I no longer go on holiday, out for the day, on theatre trips, etc. My husband has been long-suffering – we do disagree about the way it affects our lives, but he has also been very understanding. Our social life has been greatly reduced, as sickness, diarrhoea and pain have a disastrous effect on it.'

As Rita says, IBS restricts where she is able to go. It can sometimes cause a sufferer to be unable to leave the house at all. Amy is almost a recluse because of the wind she suffers. Andrea has been agoraphobic for five years, since she was 21:

'It began when I started to suffer constantly from severe pain and nausea. I am working on it but I don't go far from home at present. Shopping is very difficult. My life is severely restricted. IBS has caused the agoraphobia and compounded the problem. But I'm resourceful and I'm not going to give up trying to improve the situation.'

Claudia finds that every part of her life is affected.

'Everyday life is ruined. I can't even sleep without being troubled. We have to have the TV on at meal times to disguise my stomach noises or I am dashing to the loo. I make excuses not to go to friends' houses for coffee, not to join any groups or societies, not to go to any meetings. Even going to the library is an ordeal. I dread being a passenger in a car and having to wait for someone to stop talking or get out before the engine starts again. I dread being caught in a conversation in a corridor or a shop. I always have to keep myself busy dashing around so that I have an excuse not to be caught. And underneath, I am so tired and would love to do all the things I am running away from.'

Invariably people with IBS say they cope by taking each day at a time. Forward planning is often impossible, as Megan explains:

'I don't like letting people down, but being constantly unwell you have to keep cancelling arrangements.'

The tiredness that sometimes accompanies IBS can prevent people from doing what they want, and other symptoms can also be restrictive. Fiona, a 23-year-old student, says:

'Sometimes, if my stomach is bloated, I don't feel able to do my exercise class or go swimming – it makes me too self-conscious.'

And Judy says:

'Most leisure activities take part in the evening and I don't usually feel very good then so I don't go out.'
   'IBS has really dominated my life to such an extent that I have given up on going to the theatre, given up on evening classes and as for exams, well, forget it! I spent more time in the loo than in the exam hall, an experience I would not like to repeat!'

says Audrey, who suffers particularly from severe bloating after a meal and often an urgent need to go to the toilet. Because she has to dash to the toilet before breakfast it makes staying in a hotel or with friends unbearable for her.
   Ruby, who has had IBS for five years, says:

'I cannot go on holiday easily now as I'm always afraid of soiling clothes or bedclothes.'

Sheila feels that because of her symptoms she is 'totally unacceptable socially.'
   Ida is 76, and has been discouraged by other people's attitudes:

'I have been very active and gone dancing for years, but the past years I have felt a nuisance. People don't understand. I felt they thought I was making a mountain out of a molehill, so I have given up dancing.'

Ingrid is 77. Some days she spends two hours making frequent visits to the lavatory. She finds it usually occurs when she is active in the garden or doing the heavier housework and it has meant that she cannot enjoy her hobby of walking.

'The distressing time occurs when I'm out walking or shopping. I have only a few minutes' warning and must find a toilet. On several occasions I have not arrived in time, much to my distress. I have coped with this by cutting out walking in the country and trying at all times to be within easy reach of a toilet.'

IBS can even affect the clothes a person wears. Maisie, who suffers from severe abdominal pain, says:

'I can't wear any fitted clothing, not even loose elastic, because it makes my symptoms worse. I can't therefore wear skirts or trousers, nor even tights or some swimsuits. This breaks my heart because I love clothes and it makes me feel good to look good. However, with some careful shopping, I've come up with some good alternatives – dress suits, hold-up stockings, cat suits, etc.'

And Sarah explains how it has affected what she has been able to wear over the 17 years she has had IBS.

'When I first began to suffer from it really severely I would go to work in the jeans I had been accustomed to wearing for years, but would find that by about lunchtime I was having to go home and change into skirts with baggy tops to try to hide my huge distended stomach. Eventually I had to more or less change my style of clothing and the size of my wardrobe to cope with the fact that I could no longer tolerate anything around my stomach and waist that was even slightly fitting. It profoundly shook my self-esteem and sense of self-identity as my body image completely changed. I also stopped being able to exercise as much as I had been accustomed to and this added to my increasing size. Fortunately, after about a couple of years, baggy trousers became fashionable and I was able to go back to wearing pants again which restored some of my old sense of identity.

'It has taken years for me to begin to feel really comfortable with my body again. And it's only in the last three to four years, since I have learned to control my IBS, by taking care about my diet, that I have felt comfortable to start exercising again. It was just too painful before.'

Some people may also be restricted in eating out, socializing and travelling because of the diet they are following. Some of the diets thought to help IBS symptoms, such as gluten-free and anti-candida diets and those that avoid potential allergens, can drastically reduce the foods and drinks a person is able to consume. You may also suffer from loss of appetite or only be able to tolerate small meals. You may be in pain after eating. You may need to go to the toilet after eating, or during a meal, which can be restrictive and embarrassing. In fact, your enjoyment of food can be thoroughly ruined. Julie describes her diet as 'gluten-free, caffeine-free, dairy-free, red meat-free, fun-free!'

Not everyone, however, leads a limited life. Maria, who is 58 and has had IBS for two years, says:

'I don't let it affect my work or my leisure. I get on with my life and carry on regardless.'

A study done in London discovered that over 40 per cent of the patients who took part were affected by their IBS in the areas of work, travel, socializing, sexual intercourse, domestic and leisure activities, food and eating with others. Women were more likely to be disabled by their symptoms and their sex lives were more likely to be affected. The study found that women, on the whole, were more seriously affected by their IBS than men. The question remains as to whether women are more easily incapacitated by their symptoms or whether their symptoms are actually worse than men's – or even, are women more ready to admit to symptoms, especially psychological ones?

The above study is the only one we have come across in our research that looks at how the lives of people with IBS are affected, and even this one does not go into much detail. While there are many studies that examine the possible causes of IBS and the psychological make-up of the sufferer, here the physical and psychological consequences of living with the condition are looked at in depth.

IBS can have various other physical effects in addition to the well-known symptoms. Janet, a 48-year-old credit control clerk who has suffered from the condition for 22 years, has a deep pain in the left groin that affects the muscle and has made walking difficult, at times impossible. Osteopathy has made the muscle more supple and has helped her to walk more easily, but she still has attacks when she needs to use a stick.

Living with IBS

It must be said that, although the consequences of living with IBS that are described in this chapter make depressing reading, most people do not experience such a severe effect on their lives. This chapter is, in part, a reflection of our sample of sufferers. Those people with IBS whose lives are not seriously affected were much less likely to write to us about their experiences.

When one of the authors (Susan Backhouse) was first diagnosed as having a 'spastic colon' 22 years ago, few people had heard of it. She suspected then that the term didn't mean much, but was simply describing a symptom. Even today, IBS needs to be more fully recognized by those in the medical profession and the general public. More acknowledgement needs to be given to the pain and distress that those with IBS may suffer, and more information needs to be made available about self-help methods while the medical profession can offer us so little. People with IBS need to get together and talk to each other. Finding ways that have helped someone else may help you. Talking to others with the condition, especially if you've been newly diagnosed or have spent years not knowing of anyone else with IBS, can be a liberating experience! Reassurance and affirmation can work a lot better than anti-spasmodics and bulking agents, although perhaps you will want the lot! Most importantly, sufferers should be taken seriously and not be dismissed casually.

Andrea says:

'Having IBS makes me angry and resentful. I am frustrated by the restriction and angry about people's attitude to it. Anger is very bad for your health and it doesn't help your guts! Society should not blame people for becoming ill. It is not something that happens by "incorrect thinking" or subconscious choice.'

The final word goes to Maisie.

'IBS is one long nightmare. To me, it is like being stuck in a tunnel. All the lights have gone out and the communication system is not working. You do not know why the train has stopped and what is wrong with it and nobody can tell you because the intercom system has failed. You are sitting in darkness and can see no light at the end of the tunnel. However, deep down, however frightened you are, you know that you will eventually get out. It's just a matter of when.'

Chapter 3

Coming to Terms with IBS: Sufferers Speak Out

Christine P. Dancey and Susan Backhouse

'Nothing has helped my IBS except my own attempts to remain calm and not let tension build up. I try to make contact with as many people as I can and help them in whatever way I can. When I start to feel I am being creative and fulfilling my potential in some way, I feel altogether different.'

IBS sufferers often feel out of control of their bodies and out of control of their lives. Probably the most crucial aspect of coping with it is regaining that feeling of control. This chapter looks at the many different ways that people with IBS are attempting to do just that.

Coping with IBS as a child

Some people don't realize that they have IBS until they have suffered its symptoms for a long time, either because the medical professionals haven't diagnosed it as such or because they haven't sought medical help at all. For some sufferers, symptoms begin during childhood.

One of the authors (Susan Backhouse) recalls:

'For many years I was unaware that other people suffered in the way that I did. I first remember the symptoms occurring when I was 12, but I didn't go to the doctor until I was 15. By then, I was affected every day and my life was very much tied up with coping with the symptoms. As a girl and young woman who didn't talk to anyone at all about it, the coping option open to me was mainly trying to avoid situations where I couldn't go to the toilet whenever I needed to – not easy, as children's lives are usually controlled by various adults. I would "skive off", pretend to be ill, dose myself up with kaolin and morphine (I never got constipated!), try not to let people know I was going to the toilet in case I needed to go again soon and they commented on it. I consciously avoided people and situations that made me feel restricted and out of control. I developed, in all other aspects of my life, an attitude that nothing was worth worrying about; if it happened, then I'd cope. All my energies were, instead, devoted to the anxiety about not being able to get to the toilet in time!'

Coping with IBS is hard for anyone who doesn't know that others have it, but it is especially hard for children and young adults because they have less control over their lives.

Like many aspects of our behaviour, the feelings that will affect our ability to cope with a condition such as IBS can often be traced back to our very early years. A lot of damage can be done to a child who is made to feel ashamed about his or her natural bodily functions. It is extraordinary how something so universal and so essential as having a bowel movement has been distorted. We know of one child who was very surprised to find out that the Queen had them! Psychologist Dorothy Rowe believes that the way children are toilet trained can have a great effect on their future bowel health:

'For many small children the most stressful, frightening time of their life is the months, or even years, of toilet training. Many parents get extremely distressed and angry when their child fails to be continent according to the parents' wishes . . . The most common letter I get is from mothers and grandmothers who are greatly distressed by the child's failure to be toilet trained. They describe scenes which, from the toddler's point of view, must be extremely frightening. They say things like, "I'm at my wits' end" and "I've tried bribing him and slapping him, but nothing works." "When will he learn to be clean?" they ask, without realizing that the toddler is learning something very well and that is that anything to do with his bowels is associated with fear, anger and punishment.

'Toddlers are often shown that their parents, indeed everyone, rejects them because they have made a mess. The whole point of toilet training is to be clean, which is control and organization, as against dirty, which is uncontrolled and chaotic. No wonder most of us grow up with many anxieties about being acceptable and being clean.

'For many people with IBS the worst part is not the painful physical symptoms but the fear of being rejected and being dirty. Thus their worry about being rejected and being dirty create the stress which initiates and maintains the physical symptoms.'

How can it have happened that a normal, natural bodily function can arouse so many ambivalent feelings? It is an indication of the 'dis-ease' from which our society suffers. Gastroenterologist Ken Heaton of the Bristol Royal Infirmary says that as a culture we have 'demonized defecation': it cannot be discussed in polite company, it isn't mentioned on television (except in cheap jokes), very few books have characters in them who go to the toilet or have bowel movements (though Raymond Briggs's books for children and adults are a welcome exception!). This all makes it very difficult for anyone who has a problem with defecation to discuss it without fear of ridicule or embarrassment. Heaton points out how this can make it extremely difficult for a doctor to find out exactly what a patient's problem is. Many people have trouble just finding the words to describe what their bowels are up to and misunderstandings can arise. He remembers:

'A retired headmaster, who should have been a model of precise speech, once said to me, "Doctor, I have great difficulty doing anything serious with my insides." After several questions, he admitted that what he meant was that he had to strain to defecate! Another patient, who was asked to write down his complaints, put down "uncooperative activities of alimentary canal" when he meant diarrhoea!'

Coping with the medical profession

Sarah, who has suffered for 17 years, feels optimistic that her IBS will improve. She can go for long pain-free periods now, though she used to be permanently in pain. She believes it is necessary to stop looking to the medical profession and says it would help if there were a more open attitude from doctors, who should be prepared to accept their ignorance of many things instead of implying that their patients are hypochondriacs.

Many of us have been brought up to have a lot of faith in the mainstream medical profession. Doctors are often looked up to and few of us question their competence. After all, they are the experts. They have the knowledge and the power. One of the problems with this is that we don't learn to take responsibility for our own health; we are too dependent on doctors and the prescriptions they give us. Another problem is that, as patients, we can be made to feel IBS is 'our fault' and that we're wasting the doctors' time asking for help with this condition. Some doctors may hide their ignorance by treating the complaint as unimportant. You may find that you know more about IBS than your GP!

Sarah says:

'The bowel specialist said I should be ashamed of wasting everybody's valuable time and ... I was obsessed with my bowels. I never was told I had IBS in those early years. I went to a medical library and started taking responsibility for my own health.'

She felt what she needed most when she first sought help was someone consistent who would have 'stayed with her' until the problem was discovered and treated instead of being sent from one person to another and having to start all over again each time.

Sometimes doctors can trivialize the patient's problem. Connie is in her twenties and has been unable to work for 15 months because of her IBS. She says:

'I truly believe that my condition has been made worse by local doctors and specialists I have seen, as their general attitude has been: "Go away and forget about it and it will go away." One doctor told me to have a baby and that would clear me out – I wonder if anyone else has tried this!?'

It is because, at present, the mainstream medical profession seems to offer so little to people with IBS that sufferers have to find their own ways of coping with it. Many sufferers want to be able to take responsibility for themselves because, as one put it, 'it makes me feel less of a victim.' The need for self-help groups is especially apparent (see Chapter 13 and Appendix III). Reading as much as possible about the condition is one way of finding out more information and attempting to take control again. However, until recently there has been little available to the layperson on the subject. (See Appendix I for a book list.)

A large number of people try complementary (or alternative) medicine, in spite of this often being very expensive. The range of disciplines that are tried includes homoeopathy, acupuncture, herbalism, osteopathy, naturopathy, reflexology, autogenics, massage, colonic irrigation, Alexander technique, hypnotherapy, aromatherapy and iridology. There doesn't appear to be any one particular technique that is especially beneficial to IBS and people often try several before they find one that helps, if indeed any do. However, some types of complementary medicine do seem to significantly reduce certain symptoms and, of course, there is less worry about side-effects and dependency. (See Chapter 10).

Sarah, whose main symptoms are pain and bloating, together with constipation alternating with diarrhoea, explains how she copes:

'For a long time I tried to get help from the medical profession but was so appalled with the attitudes I came across that I started to seek help from the "alternative" health care movement. I tried acupuncture, massage and so forth, which were some help, but eventually I found that a combination of therapy and reading widely to develop my own dietary regime were the things that have most reduced the stress of it. However, if I have an attack before or around social events, I still find it very stressful, although I can usually reduce the attack considerably by drinking lots of camomile tea and live goat's-milk yoghurt. Knowing that this really does work for me has been a big help in reducing the related stress and anxiety.'

Coping with pain

Abdominal pain is the most commonly reported symptom and it is believed to be the one that is most likely to cause people to seek help from the medical profession. A study conducted in London among hospital outpatients with IBS found that half of those taking part were in pain for more than three hours a day, over half for 21 or more days in a month and just under half experienced 'marked or severe' pain. It is no wonder people seek help!

Sean is in his forties with two teenage sons. He has been suffering from painful IBS attacks for five years.

'When in severe pain – I judge that it's severe, because I know from experience that my pain toleration is quite high – I supplement the anti-spasmodic drugs with soluble aspirin, which seems, anyway, more quick-acting and effective than anything!'

He goes on to describe the pain he experiences.

'It varies in intensity from a mere niggling and persistent discomfort, sometimes felt in the stomach, sometimes in the back and sometimes even in the shoulder blades, to a grand series of contraction-like pains which reduce me to lying flat on the floor – and this position sometimes helps the attack to pass. During the attacks I feel slightly faint and nauseous, and

I find it virtually impossible to concentrate on anything until the worst is over, which transpires after taking an anti-spasmodic or aspirin (or both) but sometimes spontaneously, the pain going as quickly as it came.'

Ingrid suffers from severe abdominal swelling 'to the size of a football', wind and pain.

'I've had so many tablets and none of them has been any help at all. The only way to relieve the pain and swelling is for me to lie down with a hot-water bottle on the area and stay there overnight. By morning I am usually back to my normal size again and the pain has gone.'

Felicity has found that the pain she suffers has become particularly vicious since she had an operation to have her spleen removed. She has found that massage helps.

'When in the middle of the pain I get my husband to massage my back from the hips upwards. It seems to alleviate the pain. He does that about twice a day. I haven't yet found any of the tablets I've been prescribed to be of any use.'

If you have ever been told that your complaints about your pains were due to your having a 'low tolerance' of pain (meaning that your pains are probably not that bad, it's just that you complain of them more!), it may be encouraging to know that a study done in 1987 found that IBS sufferers were able to tolerate pain a lot better than people without IBS. IBS and non-IBS people had to undergo various painful tests. The former reported less pain than the latter, and reported the pain a lot later.

Pain should not be ignored – it is the way our bodies tell us that something is wrong. If you have an injured knee, for instance, you may relieve the pain by taking painkillers, but there may then be a temptation to treat it as you would a normal knee while it still needs a chance to heal. Similarly, with abdominal pain. If possible, give your body a chance to deal with pain itself. The more you use drugs as painkillers the more the production of the body's natural painkillers, endorphins, will be reduced and they will become less effective. You are more likely to feel pain if you are tense, so learning to relax your mind and body will help. A hot-water bottle wrapped in a towel and held on the abdomen is a good way to ease pain; rubbing, stroking and gently pressing the painful area may also help by inhibiting the passage of nerve impulses and triggering the production of pain-relieving hormones.

Marie Langley runs an organization called Unwind – a non-profit-making self-help group for people who suffer from pain in all its forms: physical, mental and emotional (see p. 353 for address). Through her own experiences of pain and her studies into pain control techniques, she has developed several self-help programmes on tape to help people deal with their pain.

She tells us that helplessness makes pain more overwhelming. Her programmes are aimed at achieving a feeling of control over the pain. Because the way we think has such an influence over the perception of pain, positive thinking is very important.

Keeping morale up

Sometimes coping is an attitude of mind. Many people with IBS report that they keep busy to put it out of their minds, and they feel dwelling on it too much makes it worse. For Maisie, it is important that she tries to remain optimistic that things will change for the better.

'My symptoms have got steadily worse. I'm an optimistic person by nature; I only hope I don't run out of optimism before I'm better. I think mental attitude is very important, but if that's the case, I can't understand how I have not been successful in willing myself better! I cope by being positive, optimistic and never giving up the battle. Occasionally, I allow myself a good cry, but then I feel better for it and ready to fight another day.

'I socialize with friends regularly. The way I look at it is I'd rather be in pain in a restaurant with friends than in pain looking at the four walls at home. A sense of humour is a great asset to have if you're suffering from IBS. Unfortunately, cinema, theatre, concerts, etc. are things of the past. So is travel. I just can't bear the discomfort of sitting through it. Having said that, I do put up with it in restaurants and in friends' houses, but the mental effort I have to put in knocks me out.'

Julie copes by

'not forcing myself to do things I really don't want to do and not feeling guilty about it.

'I suffered terrible IBS only 12 months ago, but now I have learned to control the symptoms considerably by calming down and cutting out the anxiety which is my main problem. Now I can feel an attack coming on and can control it so that my symptoms do not get too distressing.'

Lily, a 47-year-old farmer's wife, says:

'I try not to get angry and upset about things that don't matter that much. I try not to lose my temper. I try to take each day as it comes. If I were calmer I think my IBS would go.'

Chrystal believes that she would have coped better in a past generation when life wasn't so hectic. Maureen, a 40-year-old shop assistant and housewife, says: 'I've taken time to be me and to be quiet.' Sarah says 'I think having a strong, positive personality has helped me to survive IBS.' And Louise states: 'I have to get up early to deal with my two to three trips to the loo, then I try to forget about it for the rest of the day.'

Brenda makes it clear to colleagues that she may have to break appointments or be late for them. Almost invariably, people with IBS say the way they cope is to take one day at a time. George says: 'I know if I only go to the loo once in the morning it's going to be a "good" day.'

Tricia tells her story and how she copes:

'I have suffered from IBS for the past seven years and know what utter misery it can bring.

'Mine started innocently enough after a meal out with friends. Half an hour after leaving the restaurant I developed violent diarrhoea and had to ask them to stop the car several times on the journey home so that I could dash into a field. This was dreadfully embarrassing, but luckily I knew them well.

'At first, I never really gave it another thought, presuming it was a touch of food poisoning, but later I began to be concerned about it happening again. This fear grew and grew over the following months until, after about a year, I was terrified to leave the house. I couldn't even walk to the post office, five minutes away. The only journey I could manage was to work and back – four miles. Anything more than that and I would break out into a cold sweat, have palpitations, violent stomach cramps and instant diarrhoea. Shopping at the weekend had to be accomplished within pub hours so that I could use their facilities.

'Eventually I knew I had to seek professional help before I became completely housebound. A pharmacist friend suggested I try an anti-diarrhoeal drug, and to my intense relief, I found it worked perfectly. At first I would take six a day, then stop for a couple of days as I found I would become constipated. I talked over the problem with my doctor, who was quite understanding and gave me the drug on prescription. He also suggested a psychologist might help. I was a bit wary of this, but it turned out to be the first step on the road to recovery.

'The lady he sent me to was wonderful. She explained what was happening to my body and why and made me keep a graph of my stress levels. She also taught me the art of relaxation. After a dozen or so appointments, I felt I was able to cope on my own. The only time I reach for the anti-diarrhoeal drug now is if I am going on a journey of any length. I even manage to go on foreign holidays without too much anguish. I never leave the house without a few capsules in my handbag, but I find that a pack of 12 will last me three months or more.

'Relaxation tapes played through headphones at night just

before you go to sleep are wonderfully soothing. I also leave affirmations around the house and in the car, such as "Do the thing you fear and death of fear is certain" and "My stomach muscles are smooth and soft." Anything really that reminds me to relax my tummy muscles.

'I am fine until someone suggests a sudden journey and I haven't had time to prepare with my anti-diarrhoeal drug – I take two capsules two hours before I need to leave and that keeps me loo-free for 24 hours. It's almost as if someone kicks me in the stomach and I can feel the message whiz down my bowel, my heart thumps and I begin to panic. If I can get out of the situation, I will, and I've made some bizarre excuses, knowing that people are thinking I've gone completely off my head.

'I am quite sure that no one thing cures IBS. It has to be a combination of sensible eating, self-awareness, exercise and relaxation, and understanding relatives and friends.'

Nicola recounts her story:

'I was first diagnosed as being an IBS sufferer seven years ago by what I now realize was a surprisingly sympathetic and knowledgeable doctor who took a very matter-of-fact approach to my symptoms. Having just experienced the most excruciating stomach cramps that left me doubled up in pain and breathless, I was amazed to be told, "Spastic colon, not surprising given what you've been through, let's try you on an anti-spasmodic." So from being totally ignorant of the existence of IBS, I was suddenly pitched into a new period of my life as an "IBS sufferer". I remember feeling an overwhelming sense of relief: at least now I had a name for the pain, and I wasn't dying of cancer – in fact I wasn't dying at all! I consider myself to be very lucky. My doctor's manner was so pragmatic – briefly explaining the possible causes and treatments, recommending certain diets – that I instinctively adopted the same approach. This, coupled with the fact that few of my friends and relatives had even heard of the disease, led me to treat it with a degree of indifference that I still advocate today.

'On a practical level, I know that I may well experience the symptoms, so I carry my survival kit with me (anti-spasmodics and a high-fibre biscuit), but by doing that, I feel that I have some control over my life, which seems to reduce the likelihood of an attack. Furthermore, I've learnt to identify what might be called "risky" times – stressful situations that are, at first glance, uncontrollable (the obnoxious colleague at work who makes your life miserable, the boyfriend who's too demanding, the next job interview), but which, when I think about them, can be broken down into more manageable and therefore controllable chunks. In addition, for the last five years, I've been meditating, a practice I thoroughly recommend – somehow it puts everything into perspective, reduces my feelings of anxiety and, increasingly, the frequency of my attacks/symptoms.

'Over the last few years, I have become increasingly aware of, and surprised by, the number of friends who have developed IBS. Often their stories have elements in common with mine – a traumatic life event (in my case, the loss of my partner) followed a few weeks later by spiralling anxiety and the dreaded stomach cramps. Unlike me, however, most fellow-sufferers that I know still have violent and debilitating symptoms that don't seem to respond to any of the treatments. I see myself as one of the IBS survivors. Perhaps my experiences will give others some hope? My life isn't all pain, doom and gloom, ruled by this mythical beast. In fact, I thoroughly enjoy my life and feel I have control over my IBS and not the other way round. It's not all pain, and it's not fatal, there are practical ways of dealing with it.'

Lucy, who has had IBS for 14 years, has recently returned from a year travelling abroad during which she surprised herself with what she was able to do.

'It took me a long time to agree to give up my security of a flat, a job, family and friends and to go travelling in Central America and Mexico for a year.

'There were so many other things to worry about that I didn't spend too much time worrying about the problems of having IBS while on the other side of the world. One fact comforted me – the guide books told me that everyone who visits Mexico is troubled by the dreaded "Montezuma's Revenge", so I wouldn't be the only one dashing to the toilet.

'To be honest, if I'd known exactly what was in store for me I either wouldn't have gone or else I'd have worried so much I'd have made myself quite ill. What I hadn't anticipated were the bus journeys (the only way for people on our budget to get around). Generally these were between 7 and 14 hours and sometimes up to 24 hours. Toilets on board were almost unheard of and almost always locked when they did feature. I never once checked if one was open in case I found it locked and ended up panicking. The buses would generally stop every four or five hours (less often if it was a night bus) for half an hour. The worry here would be being able to go to the toilet once if necessary and not set my bowels off so they would want to go ten more times. The other worry was that the bus would take off, leaving me stranded without my luggage, or my boyfriend, in the middle of nowhere. I won't say much about the toilets other than: if you've gotta go, you've gotta go – no seats, often no doors, no water, no paper, lots of cockroaches, spiders and lizards.

'The routine prior to a bus journey was to eat very little for 24 hours beforehand, to go to the toilet as much as possible before leaving the hotel, then to take one or two codeine phosphate tablets or anti-diarrhoeal capsules one hour before the journey. The difficulty is taking the right dose so that the bowel is stopped for 24 hours but not much longer, especially if there was a series of journeys to be taken over a period of time. For one period of three weeks, we took buses every other day – I didn't relish the idea of not going to the toilet ever again!

'Sometimes I felt very panicky on the buses – I would always try to sit next to a window that would open and to keep my face and neck cool with water, do deep breathing, look out of the window and listen to mellow songs on the Walkman to calm down and distract myself from what once would have been the worse nightmare imaginable.

'One aspect that really helped was that everyone really did get diarrhoea so I wasn't alone. All the travellers we met would talk about their bowel habits just after meeting them. Suddenly diarrhoea was not a taboo subject – the whole world understood if anyone had to disappear in mid-sentence to find a toilet. Even a nasty accident was not uncommon among "normal" people and was treated with sympathy and humour.

'I firmly believe, after my experiences, that it is important to face up to whatever the worst fears are – little by little. Being able to cope with them gives new confidence to push yourself further. It wasn't very long ago that I had to break a 40-minute Underground journey to go to the toilet on many occasions. Before that there was a time when I couldn't leave the house for more than half an hour without panicking. Now I've just had the best year ever, something which would have been unimaginable a couple of years ago. I hope this will give some of you hope because things can get better. My problems haven't left me but I feel I am running my life now and it is not my bowels that are making the rules.'

Martin had an equally positive outcome:

'My first experience with IBS, as far as I can remember, was about seventeen years ago, while having my hair cut. I vividly remember the nauseous feeling and panic that set in. I was sure I was going to be sick. All I could do was to suddenly remember an urgent appointment as an excuse to get out and rush home to the toilet. I wasn't sick but the pain and spasms frightened me. I didn't dwell on it, until it happened again on the train on the way to work.

'I visited my GP who prescribed liquorice tablets. And later, I had my first barium meal.

'Things seemed to settle down and it was a couple of years later that my tummy decided to rebel. I had been promoted at work and had moved to London. It was wonderful. I had a whole new life, new friends, my own flat. Although I was used to travelling everywhere on the tube, one day I suddenly felt that feeling, my tummy turned, I became drenched in sweat and I needed the toilet. I was desperately gasping for air, not knowing whether I was going to die, have a heart attack, be sick or have diarrhoea! After leaping off at the next station, I calmed myself down and very shakily returned home.

'I was alternating between constipation and diarrhoea, and the frequency of my attacks was increasing. I was walking four miles to work to avoid tubes, and long journeys were a nightmare. I was told that I was suffering from anxiety. I was then put on tranquillizers – for the next four years! I remember very little, except that my world had got smaller and I was, by this time, being treated for agoraphobia. I had three weeks off work, sitting on the floor for days on end, until I snapped. I realized that only I could help myself. I felt that the psychiatrists were more stupid that I was. I knew I was sensible, but had become out of control through drugs and, unfortunately, alcohol. The latter was the only thing that could relieve my depression, temporarily, but it only made things worse the next day. I screamed (inwardly, fortunately for my neighbours!) and sat by the toilet throwing away all the hundreds – I mean hundreds – of tranquillizers that I had been prescribed, which I had accumulated by cleverly ordering repeat prescriptions very regularly.

'Learning to cope with IBS was not easy, but some time later I discovered the IBS Network, put everything into perspective and started to take control of my life. I do have a medical condition. It is IBS. It comes and goes. I am not mentally unstable, although I have "learned" symptoms of agoraphobia and did have panic attacks, anxiety and depression brought on by the medical profession's lack of knowledge and understanding. The anti-depressants helped both ways, especially with the sedative side, allowing me to be rational in awkward situations.

'Several trips to the toilet, plenty of water and other fluids, and keeping very busy doing things around the house and garden are my way of coping. It is fatal to sit down, mope and get depressed – put on a favourite happy record and dance around the house until tomorrow, when you know you'll be OK again – until the next time!'

Coping with IBS in the long term

IBS is rarely a short-lived problem, and although some people do recover from it, you may reach a point where you need to adjust to the realization that it isn't going to go away easily.

Judith Brice is a psychiatrist who has struggled with IBS herself. She says that people with chronic intestinal illnesses have to cope with psychological aspects that often go unacknowledged. You may feel the loss of the healthy person you once were. Your self-image may change, and there may be a feeling that the illness is somehow your fault. People who suffer from IBS also have to live with the unpredictability it brings – they don't always know when the symptoms will occur.

Dr Brice says,

'A certain amount of predictability is vital for planning and controlling one's life. When you can't plan from one month to the next, or even from one week to the next, because you can't say how your health will be, that unreliability tends to eat away at your mood, your psyche, your self-esteem, and finally at the very relationships that have the power to make you feel good about your life.'

We also have to cope with embarrassing and 'socially unaccep- table' symptoms. Frightening symptoms, confusing symptoms, too. Dr Brice says that good care of oneself doesn't guarantee that the condition will go away, and there is often confusing advice about what constitutes good self-care so that sufferers find themselves on an endless search for the best way to handle the symptoms.

Because IBS often has a psychosomatic label attached, there is also the implication that intestinal illness is caused by the sufferers themselves because of their lack of control over their emotional state. Sufferers often feel guilty for being somehow less emotionally mature than others because they cannot handle the stresses of daily life without becoming ill. If your self-esteem is low anyway because of the condition, self-blame can only worsen it. As Dr Brice says, 'Don't let anyone convince you that the solution lies solely with you and your will power.'

Nearest and dearest

Support from family and friends can make all the difference to how we are able to cope. Here is what some sufferers say on the subject. Tricia, who told her story earlier, writes:

'I think it's terribly important to get the support of your family and friends. Their attitude can make or break you. My partner of ten years is only now beginning to appreciate that I have a problem, thanks mainly to wider public awareness. At first, he would get really angry with me if we were out in the car and I asked to stop so I could go to the loo. I think he felt I was being terribly weak and pathetic and imagining everything, and he couldn't understand how a normally sane person turned into a gibbering wreck because she wanted to go to the loo. Eventually, anticipating his reaction, I found I was dashing to the loo umpteen times before we even got in the car. In contrast, my mother knew exactly how I felt and was terribly patient with me and never complained no matter how many times we had to stop; I found I never needed to go so often when I was with her. Books on IBS, left open at strategic places, seemed to convince my partner that I wasn't subnormal and that there were other people in the world who had the same crippling problem, and he is now more tolerant.'

Some people don't feel able to talk to relatives and friends about their suffering at all. Daisy says:

'I have not told anyone, even the man I've lived with for 15 years. I grit my teeth and pray. I feel *stupid* for being so oversensitive and over-reactive.'

Natalie is lucky in that, although none of her immediate friends have IBS, she has plenty of helpful support from them. She says:

'Some friends have helped with the practical things like taking the children to school on the (fortunately rare) mornings that I can't escape from the bathroom for more than 60 seconds. Others have provided newspaper articles related to the problem or recommended books, and as a result I've learnt quite a lot about IBS.'

Says Victoria, another sufferer:

'I sometimes marvel that I've still got a husband and a son, it's been so bad for them. They should have permanent halos above their heads, as they make every allowance possible and support me through every gut-churning episode. It has been known for my son to be sitting outside the toilet door, talking me through the pain, rather than let me suffer alone.'

Try to make sure you have people around who are sympathetic and will offer you practical and emotional support when you need it. Research has shown that 'social support' can have a positive impact on not only mental health but physical health as well. Social support can include the support of partner, family and friends, as well as membership of self-help groups.

Why does such support help? Researchers believe that it is because it can bring about changes in behaviour. For instance, people in self-help groups can be encouraged to make changes in their lifestyle which will promote improved health. Emotional support provided during stressful episodes may reduce the severity of the illness, as well as helping the sufferer to cope better and even recover.

Psychological factors are at work in the benefits offered by social support. For instance, stress and low self-esteem lead to depression and increased susceptibility to disease. On the other hand, the knowledge that support is there if a sufferer needs it can increase self-esteem and give a sense of personal control, both of which are related to successful coping. Social support gives sufferers greater resilience in the face of adversity.

Health-care workers can provide information and advice.

Friends and relatives can assist in practical ways by giving the sufferer lifts, or helping with other chores.

Non-supportive relationships can have a bad effect on a patient's well-being. In another study, depressed rheumatoid arthritis patients who reported minimal support and bad relationships experienced the highest level of symptoms. Close relationships can serve as a potential source of stress as well as a source of support for individuals coping with chronic illness. Ill-health is more pronounced for those who lack support.

Judy says:

> 'Lots of people haven't heard of IBS and don't know how much it affects your life. Most of my friends and relatives haven't the faintest idea what IBS is, and even though I have described my symptoms, because it's not life-threatening or even something well known, I feel they don't really think there's anything the matter.
>
> 'If we had visual signs like a broken leg we would get much more sympathy from those around us, instead of the same old phrase, "Oh, not another bad stomach. It must be something you've eaten." If only it was that simple.'

Try to surround yourself with people who are able and willing to validate you. If you don't get the support you need from your family, look outside it to friends or perhaps a self-help group.

Self-help groups

Self-help groups can be a good source of support. Maisie writes:

> 'Self-help groups can have advantages and disadvantages. It can be very disheartening to discover that some people have been suffering from IBS for up to 20 years, but they can reassure you that you are not suffering alone, they can provide an outlet to vent your emotions and to gain a sympathetic ear or two and they are a way of exchanging ideas on how to help each other.

Talking about bowels all evening can be very amusing and is sure to give you a damn good bellyache. After all, laughter is the best medicine.'

All the people to whom we have talked about IBS self-help groups have said much the same thing: that they discussed their symptoms and how they had been in the time since they last met, as well as particular issues of concern to IBS sufferers and treatments that have been found helpful. Most groups have occasional speakers – gastroenterologists, aromatherapists, dietitians and homoeopaths, for example. The size of the groups varies from five people to as many as 37, although most groups seem to contain a core of about eight people.

Self-help groups are discussed in more detail in Chapter 13, but in the meantime, here are some people's experiences of how such groups have helped them.

'I find the self-help group interesting: it's good to know how others have suffered and sometimes found solutions. I feel the group is supportive. I live alone – fortunately, as my symptoms are very anti-social. I haven't any other support – my employers are not sympathetic, and neither is the doctor. Friends don't understand.'

'I decided to join a group just to have someone to talk to who understands what I am going through – it helps knowing my fellow sufferers. I can count on my friends to be sympathetic, and my employers, but I'm afraid my doctor isn't really concerned.'

'I joined to get more information about IBS and to listen to other sufferers' problems and see whether any treatments have been of help to them. I think on the whole that I have had quite a lot of help in understanding how other people have dealt with the complaint. At the group, we are treated with understanding and know that everything is done in confidence. All the members are friendly and cooperative. I can't count on anyone else for support – so many people seem unaware of the problem and are not all that interested in something that does not affect them. The doctor has not discussed this with me either.'

It can be seen that meeting other IBS sufferers can provide a source of support which is missing from other relationships. So many sufferers feel that they cannot discuss their IBS problems with their partners and colleagues, and being able to relax and talk to others who understand can be a great boost. The majority of people who wrote to us found self-help groups beneficial, although a few were sceptical:

'The doctors couldn't help me, so I felt I was on my own and had to help myself. The only way I could think of was to talk to other people with IBS to see if we could establish what causes it and how we can get better. I've been five times, but it hasn't helped me at all. It has just rubbed in how hopeless it all is. The sort of people who attend are desperate, so it is one desperate person trying to help another. It didn't make me feel any better knowing that most people in the group had had it for 10 to 15 years and I had a long way to go. Unfortunately, nobody has the same symptoms as me so I might as well be sitting in the same room with someone suffering from another illness. We all want a doctor with IBS to attend! Some of my friends and colleagues are sympathetic to my IBS, and that's one reason I don't feel desperate to talk to people in a self-help group. With all the good will in the world, no one can really understand what I am going through. I don't know anyone who has my symptoms and who is in dreadful pain every single minute of the day, and has been for the last three years. If there is someone out there, then I'd like to have a very long chat with them, please!'

Lifting the taboo

'IBS and its symptoms are thought to be funny or "not quite nice" by many people, so we have to suffer silently and attempt to feel like attractive, acceptable human beings in spite of it.' (Glenda)

Half of the people taking part in our survey said that they didn't know anyone else with IBS, and a further 25 per cent knew only one other person. This makes the condition something that often has to be coped with alone in spite of it affecting such a large percentage of the population. However, even if you do know someone else who has been diagnosed as having IBS, they may have completely different symptoms and cope quite differently.

Although IBS is so common, there is a taboo, certainly in our society, about anything to do with bowel functions. They are supposed to be private and personal and the message is – keep it to yourself! This taboo can lead to problems for the individual sufferer. Not only can she or he remain isolated and lonely (quite unnecessarily so, given the prevalence of IBS), but she or he may feel unable to tell her or his family or even the doctor about it, so support and treatment will not be forthcoming. A large number of people with IBS do not talk about it at all to anyone except perhaps close family members, and *nearly half* the people in our survey talked to no one at all. It is quite possible you know several people who also suffer, but if everyone thinks they shouldn't mention it, sufferers will continue to be isolated.

Nicky, a 31-year-old single mother, says:

'I think it would be better if things like IBS could be talked about more openly, and that it wasn't such a taboo subject because it involves a normal bodily function such as going to the toilet.'

Hattie, who has had IBS for nine years, says:

'I talk to people now about it, but it was the biggest hurdle to be able to admit that I had such a personal problem.'

Coping through diet

As IBS is a condition affecting the gut, a common way of coping is regulating what you eat. This topic will be discussed in greater detail in Chapter 7, but here are examples of the experiences with food and drink of some IBS sufferers.

Judy, a 31-year-old who has had the condition for ten years

and suffers from pain, constipation, bloating and wind, says: 'I find that, if I keep my meals small, the symptoms aren't so bad. I don't go out for meals.' And another sufferer, Malcolm, a bus driver, states: 'I only have one small meal a day, in the evening, and the symptoms have improved.'

Madeleine recommends:

'The best thing probably is to eat little and often, never to go too long without food and to eat a small, nourishing breakfast (which I don't always do) and certainly to avoid eating late in the evening, particularly anything strong or indigestible.'

Siobhan has found that foods containing vinegar, as well as tomato sauce, chutneys, pickled beetroot, meat pastes and wine, and acid oranges and lemons, bran and stodgy foods don't suit her.

Some have found help simply through giving up tea and coffee, alcohol, citrus fruits, fatty foods, wheat or milk. Others have to stick to rigid diets. A wide range of diets may help IBS, but they are often extremely restrictive, expensive and time-consuming. Says Fran:

'For the last three-and-a-half years, I have based my diet on the Hay System as described by Doris Grant and Jean Joice in their very readable book, *Food Combining for Health*. The basic principle is that one should not eat protein and starch foods at the same meal, but you will have to read the book to understand that better. Because I also cook for a growing family and have a full social life, I do not follow it strictly, but enough to have cut out most of the pain, the exhaustion of "illness", the constipation, heartburn, sleeplessness and build-up of tooth plaque! If I could only follow this fairly difficult regime perfectly, maybe it would be even better!

'Then I cut down on sugar, milk and wheat products. This eliminated all the nausea and, provided I don't eat wheat products after tea-time, the nocturnal churning of the stomach.

'Finally, I take a personal homoeopathic remedy, which sends me to sleep in the event of over-indulgence in alcohol or a churning stomach caused by after-hours wheat intake or just plain overeating late in the evening.'

It is important to weigh up the pros and cons of restrictive diets. If one works for you, it may offer great relief from your symptoms and therefore be of value. On the other hand, you might feel your life is limited enough already! This is how Zoe feels about giving up wheat:

'I don't think the improvement sufficient to give up wheat totally. Besides, I'm sure it would be near impossible, as bread forms the major part of my diet. IBS has deprived me of so many of the things in life which I used to enjoy doing that to have to give up something which I like eating and gives me pleasure is a depressing prospect!'

Not everyone finds a 'healthy' diet helps. For Pat, it's just the opposite:

'This sounds very unhealthy, but I'm OK with crisps, packet food, sweets, meat, nothing green, no pulses, cabbage, spicy foods. "Natural" food seems to be worse for me.'

Cindy attended a clinic specializing in detecting food intolerances.

'I attended the clinic a few years ago and followed the exclusion diet. It was through this that I discovered I have an intolerance to milk and dairy products. They are really helpful and supportive there, and I did feel that at last someone was trying to help. My doctor at that time insisted that it was "nerves" and that I was a bored housewife who needed to find something to occupy her mind and stop worrying about her stomach.'

Food intolerance does have significant implications for IBS sufferers and is discussed in more detail in Chapter 4.

Other tips

'At present I am taking concentrated slippery elm capsules, and did feel a soothing of my stomach at first, with less wind, but reverted to the usual condition after a few days. This happened to me with linseed oil – initial improvement only.'

'Slippery elm is very helpful internally where inflammatory irritation exists as diarrhoea, dysentery, etc. You can buy slippery elm powder from a herbalist – the health stores mainly sell a commercial drink called slippery elm but containing other ingredients, though they also sell slippery elm tablets if the drink proves unpalatable.'

Ursula has had IBS for over 30 years:

'However, before Christmas I went into my health store and got two lots of tablets – peppermint oil tablets and New Era Combination E Tissue Salts – and I am pleased to be able to tell you that I have been much better and feel I am more able to cope.'

Others have tried a wide variety of remedies:

'For years I was on codeine phosphate until I changed to a new doctor who took me off that and has since been trying various prescriptions. I have a permanent one for loperamide capsules, which I take if travelling or on an outing. My doctor advised me to use them only as a back-up for confidence, as did the hospital specialist.'

'At present I am trying Colpermin capsules, which are peppermint. They are definitely helping with the bloated feeling.'

'I have found that mashed potato often calms the seething turbulence within. It doesn't always work, but sometimes has a soothing effect on both wind and pain.'

'I have tried an elimination diet and found I was much better giving up red meats, rich foods, jams and, strangely, vinegar.'

'Walking after meals helps to reduce gas.'

'Since I stopped drinking cow's milk about six months ago, I believe my IBS has improved considerably. I read about lactose intolerance and decided to give it a whirl, on the "nothing ventured, nothing gained" principle, known only too well by IBS folk.'

'The most beneficial thing I have found is yoga taught with relaxation. It is excellent and I combine my lessons with a daily workout at home.'

'My problems began seven years ago after a holiday in Kenya. Things have definitely improved over the years, but I can still remember with clarity the times when I didn't quite make it to the loo in time. I now never go anywhere without my "shit kit"' – a small cosmetic bag with wet wipes, toilet paper, clean panties and a plastic bag and also my codeine phosphate. Just knowing I carry those items with me gives me peace of mind and makes me feel calmer.'

'After two years of diarrhoea, flatulence, nausea and losing two stone in weight and utter misery, I thought, at 80 years of age, this is it. With the aid of an anti-spasmodic and codeine phosphate, also careful watch of diet, I feel so much better.'

'Some divine intervention led, for reasons not connected with IBS, to taking lecithin capsules, and within three to four days, the symptoms of IBS became considerably lessened and controllable. By taking three to four capsules daily, I have found not a total cure but an amazing improvement in my condition.'

The range of things that people with IBS try in order to help themselves is vast. Some people live constantly in the hope that this or that will be the cure at last. It can be very dispiriting when, time and time again, you are disappointed. In the 20 years that Susan Backhouse had IBS, she tried traditional drugs, peppermint capsules, garlic capsules, slippery elm, a wide selection of herbs, Bach flower remedies, acupuncture, homoeopathy, exclusion diets, dairy-free diets, gluten-free diets, high-fibre diets, giving up tea and coffee, eating lots of yoghurt, relaxation, yoga – the list goes on. And she realizes she is not atypical. As she wrote five years ago, when she still had IBS symptoms:

'I know the hope and the disappointment when things are tried but don't help. In fact, the best thing I have done is co-found the IBS Network with Christine, because suddenly there were letters from a great number of people with similar, and different, stories to mine. I found it easier to talk about my IBS and no longer felt anywhere near so isolated. My way of coping now is to work with others towards improving things for all of us who have IBS.'

Chapter 4

Lifestyle and IBS: The Experience of Sufferers

Susan Backhouse and Christine P. Dancey

> '*My IBS is affected by pressure at work, very little support and the lack of someone "there for me". I do get anxious and I'm not good at sharing my problems. I'm trying to rectify this.*'

IBS affects a wide range of people living a wide range of lifestyles. It used to be thought that it was a specifically Western condition, but it is now known to occur in developing countries. Both men and women suffer from it. It is suffered by all age groups, and some people feel they have always had it. There is no typical kind of lifestyle that makes IBS more likely, and there is no lifestyle formula that will guarantee an IBS-free existence. However, in this chapter we will look at the ways in which IBS sufferers themselves have tried to improve their way of life through dealing with stress, adopting better eating habits and increasing exercise. Much of this is also discussed in greater detail later in this book.

Can stress cause or aggravate IBS?

The professionals tend to believe that stress plays a large part in IBS, and people with the condition are often advised to reduce the stress in their lives. But how easy is it to control stress?

It does not seem to be simply a matter of taking up meditation, learning relaxation techniques or even finding out what causes your stress and then removing it from your life. In our survey, we found that many IBS sufferers have made changes to their lifestyle in order to reduce stress; some have taken drastic measures such as taking early retirement, changing their job or getting divorced, only to find that, although they were experiencing a lot less stress, their IBS was no better.

We live in a world that can cause us to suffer extreme stress and anxiety. We may not be able to remove the source of stress from our lives, and it may not always be easy to deal with the stress in a way that doesn't do any harm to ourselves or others.

Stress is much discussed and written about these days. People were once said to be suffering from 'nerves', with the implication that they were weak and unable to cope with life. Now there seems to be some acknowledgement that stress is something we all have to deal with and that people cope in different ways.

When researchers study IBS patients, they find that many say that their symptoms are made worse by stress, and one study found that half the patients recalled an acute episode of stress before their first symptoms. Sometimes the beginning of IBS can be traced back to a time of emotional turmoil such as a bereavement, an accident or an operation (although there is evidence that certain operations can cause *physiological* changes that give rise to IBS symptoms). This is, apparently, very common among diarrhoea-predominant IBS sufferers. Another study carried out in 1982 concluded that some people have a biological predisposition to respond to any stressful situation with increased movements in the colon. In a large study of 800 IBS sufferers, three quarters of them found that stress affected their IBS symptoms, and half of them said that stress led to abdominal pain.

A study done by gastroenterologists Kumar, Pfeffer and Wingate found that their IBS patients were more anxious and obsessive than other people, but not more depressive. Kumar and his colleagues say that the idea that IBS is primarily a psychopathological condition has been attractive to the medical profession because of the lack of evidence, until recently, of something organically wrong. They say that some researchers suggest that it is a symptom of depression, others that IBS patients have 'pain-prone personalities' and that pain represents a means of emotional expression. There are even some who believe that IBS is a manifestation of 'illness behaviour'. Consequently, psychotherapy or anti-depressants have been advocated.

More recently, however, studies have indicated that IBS could be an organic disorder. What then, asked Kumar and his fellow researchers, of the anxiety associated with the condition? Could it be the consequence rather than the cause of IBS? And have the psychopathological aspects of IBS been over-emphasized, due to flaws in some of the studies? Comparing IBS sufferers with healthy controls might reveal more about the differences between the well and the unwell rather than IBS specifically, for instance. In the Kumar study, they compared IBS sufferers with people suffering from benign organic gastrointestinal disorders such as duodenal ulcer, gallstones and inflammatory bowel disease as well as with healthy people. They found that the IBS patients were more anxious and obsessional than healthy people but there was no difference for depression or phobic tendencies. Those suffering from the other gastrointestinal disorders were in between the other two groups. They say that these results are 'consistent with the state of mind of a patient who is still searching for some rational explanation – and some effective therapy – for his or her symptoms' and that 'IBS patients are not helped by being told that "there's nothing wrong", when this is manifestly at odds with their own experience.'

They go on to say that, when effective treatment is found, it is likely that there will be no greater levels of anxiety and other neuroses than you would expect in any group of people suffering from a chronic gastrointestinal disorder.

Is stress responsible for your IBS?

'If I hear the word *stress* again from my doctor, I shall scream.'

When IBS sufferers are told their condition is due to stress, it can be very frustrating and can seem too simplistic.

'Stress makes me dash to the loo more, but I still have problems on calm days.'

'Severe symptoms can often occur even when my life is going well.'

'If I have symptoms due to stress, they tend to be mild and easy to cope with by comparison with other times. Stress will aggravate a problem if it's already there – i.e. if I feel queasy anyway and then get upset, it tends to get worse. But stress is not the cause – the symptoms are too severe and the stress too little. The most stressful thing in my life is constant nausea and continual pain. Everything else seems to pale in comparison.'

So says Andrea, and her feelings that it is IBS that causes the stress in her life are echoed by many.

'I honestly feel that the only stress I have difficulty coping with is my painful gut, which adversely affects the quality of my life far more than the cancer which I have lived with for the past number of years.'

'Many people who are suffering from diarrhoea for just a few days are very stressed and fed up – so people like us are going to be very stressed as the condition lasts for so long and it is too embarrassing to discuss with others.'

'The anxiousness over IBS symptoms causes stress, which worsens the symptoms, hence creating a vicious circle.'

The contradictions experienced by many of us are voiced by Maxine:

'For myself, I have yet to understand if stress can be such a large part of suffering with IBS. Over the past few years, I have had traumas – buying a house, becoming a single parent, money worries, housing worries, etc. – and yet I can say that IBS never presented itself, unless IBS triggers quite some time after the events.'

Mo also feels there is no straightforward answer to the IBS-and-stress dilemma.

'The past few years have been difficult ones for a number of reasons, so it would be easy to put the symptoms down to this. But I am not satisfied that this is the only reason. I have had plenty of other stressful incidents in the past, and have not suffered in this way. Equally, I have been on holiday and enjoying myself, and still had the symptoms. The trouble is, if no true cause is known, then if you are not careful you can get paranoid about food and become stressed about the possible stress!'

Annette says:

'The usual answer from the medical profession is "stress". This suggests my problem is psychosomatic, not biological. I firmly believe it is the latter, and doctors haven't got the answer so stress is a good word to pacify patients.

'One of my worst bouts last year was walking over Welsh hills with my family – about ten of us, aged between 2 and 80. A happy band, enjoying the walk. We were coming back and *wham!* It was that familiar gut problem. I asked my son for his house keys and ran like hell, shouting, "Don't follow me!" But I didn't make it. Luckily, I was washed and changed before they arrived home.'

It is not uncommon to find that IBS strikes when we at last have a chance to relax and enjoy ourselves. Sean doesn't feel he has much stress in his life.

'My doctor seems to favour the stress theory, and talks of "taking it more easy", "getting away from it all", and what he cryptically refers to as "taking the edge off things". Of course, I realize that stress is a relative term and that all of us have some stress in our lives; and while I definitely belong to the "nervy and fastidious" brigade, rather than the "laid back and easy-going", I can't pretend that I have a huge amount of stress in my life.'

There are some who feel stress is not a factor in their IBS. Ruby is one:

'I have not been able to identify stress as a cause of aggravation of my condition. As I now have little stress, almost none at all really, I cannot include it as something which affects my IBS.'

And Maisie agrees:

'In my opinion, stress had nothing to do with my onset of IBS. I get very angry when anyone suggests otherwise. I was off work for seven months solely to concentrate on me – to get better – but it didn't work. I got worse.'

In spite of this, over 70 per cent of those taking part in our study said that stress aggravated their IBS. For Hazel, stress is a direct trigger of her symptoms. She says:

'I'm sure stress makes my IBS much worse. I'm rather a perfectionist and get very strung up if things don't go the way they should.'

Fiona, having made significant changes in the food she eats, found that this has helped her symptoms:

'It seems to be something that I can exert a positive control over, unlike stress, with which I still find myself constantly battling. Any stress attack brings on the symptoms. I become stressful with myself when I don't achieve the high standards I set, and I also worry about events before they happen. My symptoms have decreased over the last few months. I think that, if I were calmer as a person, they may even disappear totally.'

And for Lucy, the relationship between stress and IBS is very closely linked:

'The difference between me and people without IBS is that I find certain things stressful or anxiety-causing that a "normal" person wouldn't. I feel anxious about the possibility of having to go to the toilet too frequently (I don't care how often I have to have a wee – weird!) or having to have a crap at a time of day or a place where no one else would (e.g. a party, someone's house for dinner, etc.). It does take away the anxiety a bit if I'm with people who are open about bowel habits. For some reason, I can't admit to having IBS symptoms when a "normal" person would admit to getting the shits before an interview, exam, scary meeting, etc. Because I feel stressed because I have IBS, it's impossible to tell whether I caused the IBS by handling the stress badly or whether I am more stressed because of IBS. What came first, the stress or the IBS?'

When we asked people with IBS what they thought the cause was, several cited reasons such as stressful jobs, family problems, being involved in an accident, bereavement, depression and general stress and worry. It is known that specific hormonal changes can occur when a person is under stress and that they in turn can affect the bowels. In a discussion on IBS and stress in 1991, Dr K. W. Heaton wrote:

There have been some remarkable experiments on the effects of stress on sigmoid colon [last part of the large intestine] motility. The point which came out was that it was not the pain inflicted on the volunteers that caused the sigmoid colon to become active but the hostile reaction when the volunteers decided that they could not tolerate it any more.

This has interesting implications for sufferers of pain: it means that it may be possible to reduce colonic activity by using pain-control techniques. (See Chapter 3 for more on pain control.)

Does personality make a difference?

In our study, we found that a high proportion of sufferers described themselves as 'worriers'. Is this the cause of their IBS, or does living with the condition turn them into anxious people? Worrying about IBS will very likely make it worse.

Lucy feels she generally worries more than other people

might, although most of what she worries about is related to IBS.

'I find it hard to stop thinking about something that has annoyed me. I tend to brood on things and keep coming back to them even though I try not to. I worry about some things happening that might never occur – for example, running out of petrol or breaking down on the motorway. This way of thinking applies to IBS-related worries as well – I constantly worry about "what if something happens" rather than solving the problem when it arises.

'Because I have IBS, I spend a lot of time worrying about whether or not it will affect me during each day. Whenever there is anything major to worry about, I will spend a lot of time going over and over the possibilities in my mind. I have been told that I always need something to worry about – as if I enjoy it!

'Having said this, no one other than my boyfriend would ever know I was worrying. Everyone else believes I'm incredibly calm and unruffled by life. I think this calm exterior can be dangerous and means that there is a lot of suppressed anxiety which I believe manifests itself in IBS.'

We asked people if they thought that aspects of their character made IBS more difficult to deal with. Common themes were: setting very high standards for oneself, having difficulty relaxing, caring too much what people think, finding it difficult to talk about IBS, insecurity, and lack of confidence and self-esteem.

Not surprisingly, it was clear that our sample of sufferers had a wide range of personalities, lifestyles and ways of coping with IBS and life in general. Living with pain and the other symptoms for any length of time can certainly cause a person to change their behaviour, and even, say some, their personality.

'It has made me less confident, more introverted, less tolerant, more impatient.'

'My personality, that's changed dramatically. I'm nasty, vicious and aggressive and can't tolerate much of anything.'

What causes stress?

There are some things that most people would find stressful – an important relationship going wrong, harassment or victimization, financial problems, homelessness, for example. It is believed that change can cause stress, even change for the better. Stress is also caused by feeling out of control. However, it can be a very individual thing. The list of stressful life events has divorce as highly stressful, but if the divorce is wanted, it could mean that a person's worry and anxiety levels are reduced. A lifestyle that to one person is peaceful and relaxing can be very boring for the next person – and even boredom is stressful.

Here are some explanations of what causes some sufferers stress, starting with Lucy, who works as a graphic designer:

'I feel stressful if I have to do things I don't feel comfortable doing, things which I know will cause my IBS to get worse – for example, travelling with people I don't know well (or who don't know I've got IBS), working on location where I can't go to the toilet inconspicuously, eating with people I don't feel comfortable with, travelling somewhere just after eating (the list goes on!).'

'The things that cause me stress include early morning appointments, going to church in the morning, being invited out for meals or to stay with anybody at their home.'

'I suffer stress if I feel under constant pressure at work and also if I am underemployed. Other people's tantrums and distress upset me. Stress builds up if I am subjected to incessant noise.'

'I think any stress was due to isolation on account of my husband's 24-hour-a-day job (as a doctor) and no extended family.'

'My husband being in the army and him going away a lot.'

'I live in a neighbourhood where there is a lot of vandalism, glue sniffing and young people forever tormenting older people. Life today causes stress unless you are someone who doesn't care.'

'Meeting deadlines on VDU work.'

'Being a single parent to three children, low pay, an ageing parent, harassment at work, threats of job loss through cuts recession, loneliness because not in a relationship at present.'

'Tubes, crowded transport, car travel in the morning. Awkward people. Crowds pushing and shoving, being squashed in a crowd. Not being treated fairly at work, too much work, too little time to do it and boss being unreasonable.'

'People saying nasty things or my boss on my back for any reason, or a heavy workload. I panic.'

'I worry over work, not fulfilling my potential, money problems, not knowing how to use my talents and fighting fatigue.'

In addition, family and relations were frequently cited in our study as the cause of stress.

How stress affects us

Dorothy explains what happens when she is under stress and how it aggravates her IBS symptoms:

'Under stress I tend to neglect my own needs. I also get very angry that I seem unable to switch off and put myself first. When stressed, I breathe shallowly, never seem to relax, have disordered eating (binge eating), all of which worsens my IBS. I feel stressed when I feel powerless to change any part of my life – e.g. work, accommodation. I freeze in response to any threat or change (real or perceived) rather than act/try something/ask for help or advice. I isolate myself in a sort of psychological straitjacket.'

And Susie, who is 42 and has had the condition for over seven years, describes the link for her between IBS and stress:

'Knowing I have to go out – e.g. for an appointment – causes me stress because of the agoraphobia I suffer from. This causes me to go to the toilet frequently, up to nine or ten times in the previous 18 to 24 hours. The pain caused by wind can also be worse. Fear of disapproval and rejection is probably the major factor in my agoraphobia, and the feeling that my body will let me down by diarrhoea or nausea increases the stress.'

When sufferers experience traumas, the way they relate to their IBS can alter, as Lucy describes:

'Important life-changing events (e.g. the breakdown of a relationship) have made my IBS much worse and the feeling of anxiety is raised to the forefront of my consciousness. Because of this, it has been easier to talk about the anxiety and express it, come to terms with it and cope with it. Probably because it is socially acceptable to feel anxious, get stomach cramps, feel nauseous and have diarrhoea during a major trauma like this, it is possible to admit to these feelings and be comforted by friends. Other than a major trauma bringing on these symptoms, I would never let anyone know about IBS symptoms normally.'

Panic

Sixty per cent of the people taking part in our study said that they had experienced panic attacks at some time. There is a specifically named condition called 'panic disorder', and an American study, published in 1984, tried to find out if people with IBS symptoms were really suffering from this problem. IBS sufferers who had experienced panic attacks were treated with anti-panic medication. The result was a quick improvement in their gastrointestinal symptoms. It concluded that there are strong links between gastrointestinal complaints and panic disorder.

The authors of the study considered it worth mentioning whether the subjects' families had a history of agoraphobia, depression, alcoholism and so on, but there was no mention of how the symptoms might be caused by non-inherited factors, such as the sufferers being under a lot of pressure.

However, later studies found that it is unlikely that there is a relationship between panic attacks and IBS. The association between the two was the result of the tendency for those who suffer from panic attacks to report many different symptoms (including irritable bowel symptoms), and the tendency for high levels of anxiety to cause diarrhoea and abdominal pain.

What can be done about stress?

Many of those who feel that stress is significant to their IBS realize that they need to make changes in their lives but often feel unable to do so. May is 60, a housewife, and has had IBS for eight years.

'I think my stress is caused by loneliness. I have three lovely daughters who are marvellous to me, they help me in all sorts of ways, but they have their own lives to lead. I need to change my life, but I don't know how.'

Anita is 21, and explains:

'I suffer stress from the inability to do things I'm fully capable of, physically and mentally. Living with parents is a major problem, but I can't afford to move out. I also suffer from situations I want to change but can't from low self-esteem.'

Even getting out of a stressful situation doesn't necessarily result in instant recovery. Frances is 40. She was married to an alcoholic who was violent, and she is now trying to rebuild her life with another partner. However, she still suffers from the stress that she endured during her marriage.

Hannah's main cause of distress is wind, and the embarrassment is turning her into a hermit. It has been developing over the last 12 years.

'My life is very curtailed by this condition, which is a great pity as after a very stressful life I have now reached much calmer waters. It seems very perverse that I coped with the stress and then I develop this stressful condition when my life has become so much freer. I now happily live on my own in a lovely area surrounded by kind and friendly people.'

Hannah is 70 and her general health is very good. She feels she could lead a much fuller and outgoing life were it not for her condition. She goes on to say:

'If I did not fret so much about the possibility of being embarrassed or maybe embarrassing others by my wind problem, perhaps it would not be such a problem.'

Coping with stress is fraught with contradictions, as Holly writes:

'It is right when they say avoid things that really upset you, but you can't hide for ever.'

Ruby feels she has done a lot to try to improve her lifestyle but to no avail.

'I have tried to change my way of life by taking more exercise and changing my diet, but my life is probably as stress-free as it could possibly be. I have been unable to find the trigger which sets off the intense pain I suffer.'

Ruth has found practical ways to deal with stress:

'I have developed various ways to minimize the detrimental effect of stress. Vitamin supplements, especially B vitamins (which are yeast/sugar/lactose free as I am on an anti-candida diet), help but it has been very difficult when all the GP can do is say, "It's your nerves," and push anti-depressants at you. These do not help the fatigue/depression or the constipation.'

The two ways of dealing with stress are to change your exposure to it or your mental response. If you feel your IBS is caused or aggravated by the tension and pressure in your life, you may decide to take a long, fresh look at your situation and your attitudes.

Like pain, signs of stress are warnings to be heeded. Be aware of how you, as an individual, respond to pressure, frustration and feelings of impotence or guilt. Do you find it difficult to let go and to express emotions, whether happiness, fear, anger, sadness? Emotions kept inside often result in a churning stomach. Have you tried eating when you're upset? Your body rebels against you 'swallowing your anger' down with your potatoes. You soon end up with stomach ache.

Imagine this scene: you are out with some friends. It's a lovely day and you are enjoying yourself. Then into your mind comes the thought: 'There isn't a toilet nearby. What if I need to go?' And in no time, your body starts working and you do need to go – and quick! The feeling may pass, or it may not. At best, it's on your mind and clouds your enjoyment of the day. At worst, you feel panicky and overwhelmed.

Does this sound familiar to some of you? If it has happened to you, you will be aware of the power of your mind and how your imagination can work against you.

It is also worth remembering that this power can be used for your benefit. It can be hard, though, to change your mindset and you need to open up to a new way of thinking. Try not to expect and fear the worst: concentrate on visualizing a pleasant or successful outcome instead of your feared one. When you wake up in the morning, and throughout the day when you remember, try saying positive affirmations to yourself. For instance:

- I feel love for myself and my body.
- I am not responsible for anyone else's feelings, only my own.
- No one else is responsible for my feelings.
- I am in harmony with my body.
- I have nothing to fear but my fear.

Dr Vernon Coleman, in his book *Bodypower*, writes of the value of daydreaming to relax the mind from tensions and pressures. He suggests focusing on a happy memory – a holiday, a beautiful place you've been to, for instance – and transporting yourself there. If you picture the place vividly, you will be able to involve all your senses – smelling, hearing, feeling, tasting even, as well as seeing your surroundings. Keep the action peaceful and calm. You may want to lie down to daydream at first, especially if it is a long time since you have done it. With practice, however, you will be able to do it anywhere, any time. Use it to escape to your own private, calm place when you need to. Many of us have been brought up to think that daydreaming is undesirable; parents and teachers often stop children from doing it. But Dr Coleman believes it has benefits over meditation. With the latter, the mind is cleared of all images and you concentrate on emptiness or perhaps one image. Daydreaming focuses on a loving, happy memory and will fill the daydreamer with loving, happy feelings. Daydreaming is, he says, a natural process whereby the mind can 'cut out' for our own protection.

Treating IBS and stress

In 1990, a study was completed by Dr Steve Wilkinson and Dr Nicky Rumsey, consultant gastroenterologist and research psychologist respectively at the Gloucester Royal Hospital. It compared conventional drug treatment of severe IBS with a programme of six 90-minute sessions designed to teach groups of six to eight patients stress management and relaxation techniques. In this psychological programme, a typical session would comprise a 15-minute talk, followed by a discussion and coffee. A second talk would be followed by a relaxation session and a summary. Topics covered were:

- What is IBS?
- The role of stress in IBS
- Progressive muscle relaxation
- Using relaxation constructively
- Diet and fitness
- Problem-solving
- Long-term management of IBS

The results of the study were encouraging. At the end of the treatment period, improvements in IBS symptoms and in measures of anxiety, depression and stress were evident for the majority of patients (26 out of a total of 37) no matter whether they had received drug treatment or had taken part in the psychological programme. However, six months after the end of the treatment period, patients in the psychological management group reported significantly fewer IBS symptoms and lower levels of anxiety, depression and stress than those patients who had received only drug treatment.

The conclusion was that group stress management is a viable, and even preferable, alternative to drugs for the treatment of IBS. When looking at why the treatment worked, the researchers say that, although it may be only speculation, the patients clearly liked the approach. Some felt more in control of their condition, some were pleased with the information on how to deal with it and others felt their self-confidence had increased. Overall satisfaction was very high. (This may well be because of the general lack of support and information available to IBS sufferers until recently.)

The researchers report that this approach is much cheaper than conventional drug treatment. For instance, from August to October 1989, the 277 GPs who make up the Cleveland Family Practitioner Committee wrote nearly 6000 prescriptions for anti-spasmodics. This averaged out at seven prescriptions per GP per month, at a total cost of £34,062! Dr Rumsey believes that patients should be given an explanation of both the psychological and drug approach and allowed to choose which they would prefer.

It is to be hoped that the results of this study and of future research will encourage doctors and psychologists to consider setting up similar programmes on a more permanent basis. There is scope, too, for this kind of approach to be explored by self-help groups.

Other studies back up the findings of Drs Wilkinson and Rumsey. One found that when IBS patients were treated psychologically as opposed to medically and where anxiety levels were high beforehand, the anxiety decreased. Psychological intervention alone was shown to reduce distress by the reduction of both anxiety and IBS symptoms.

Psychotherapy has also been used with success on patients in Manchester. Dr Else Guthrie has found that specific techniques in which the importance of the developing relationship between doctor and patient is a fundamental part of the treatment, have helped many long-term sufferers. Dr Guthrie reports a reduction in symptoms, less pain and a decrease in the limiting effect the bowel symptoms have on the sufferers' lives. It seems that this method works well with people who believe that their pain is exacerbated by stress. Those who suffer constant pain don't seem to benefit. Those who have psychiatric symptoms such as anxiety and depression are likely to do well, according to Dr Guthrie. You will find more about psychotherapy and IBS in Chapter 8.

Hypnotherapy can also be very effective in treating IBS where stress is a factor. At Dr Whorwell's clinic, also in Manchester, patients say that they can cope better with various other stresses in their lives by using the techniques learned during hypnosis. They are encouraged to see hypnotherapy as giving them a way to control their symptoms, rather than offering a magic cure. (See Chapter 9 for more on hypnotherapy.)

Therapies such as massage and aromatherapy work well, too. Because they are such relaxing and pleasurable experiences, they have an indirect effect on the IBS symptoms, making them easier to cope with.

All complementary therapies have a holistic approach to treatment and therefore look at the patient's lifestyle and state of mind as well as physical symptoms.

Does exercise help IBS?

On the whole, our study found that, although most people took regular exercise, it wasn't felt to bring about a direct improvement in the symptoms. Some people are unable to exercise at all when having a bad patch. However, many agreed that it has a general uplifting effect.

Here are some sufferers' views on exercise:

'Exercise makes me feel worse physically, better mentally.'
'Good for settling the gut and improving mental outlook.'
Brenda, who swims, does fitness sessions and hill walking.
'Swimming can help me pass trapped wind, or helps to lessen the pain – or makes it worse!'
'I have tried aerobics and keep fit. They seemed to aggravate IBS – in particular, upper abdominal pain.'
'Intense physical activity, like cycling, gardening or even walking (I would no longer even attempt sports) tends to encourage attacks on subsequent days.'
'I cope mainly with the stress of IBS by playing tennis. It is very therapeutic whacking a tennis ball as hard as I can. It helps get rid of my frustration and gives me a sense of well-being. It's also great fun and laughter, after all, is the best medicine. The endorphins (natural painkillers) which the body produces during exercise also help. But the exercise has to be very vigorous and sustained to help me in any way. At least my tennis has improved!'

Diet

The connection between food and digestive function is an obvious one; many people with IBS feel that the food they eat has an effect on their symptoms, for better or worse. We found that two out of three people said that some foods aggravated them. Our study also showed that a high proportion of the sufferers taking part took great care with their food, many of them eating what is considered to be a healthy diet – low fat, little or no meat, plenty of fresh fruit and vegetables, unrefined carbohydrates. Many said they were eating these foods in order to help their IBS.

A change in diet is often one of the first steps IBS sufferers take, in the hope that it may ease or eradicate the symptoms. It is important to check with your doctor first before undertaking restrictive diets and, ideally, you should get the help of a dietitian to ensure you get the required nutrients. You will find more about diet in Chapter 7.

General dietary advice

It will almost certainly help you if you are able to follow the guidelines below:

- Eat a varied diet, full of food that you enjoy.
- Eat little and often – big meals are notoriously troublesome.
- Eat when relaxed, take your time and don't rush your meals. Consciously taste the food you eat. Listen to your body and stop eating when you have had enough.
- Eat when you feel hungry – not when the clock says it's time for food.
- Ensure a good intake of fruit and vegetables, especially green leafy ones which contain rich supplies of the vitamins and minerals that are most commonly found to be lacking in many ill or elderly people. A daily intake of raw or lightly cooked green vegetables or salad may also help protect against some of the more common and more serious diseases in Western society.
- Eat good-quality fresh food, preferably organic if this is available. The medical effects of insecticides and fertilizers sprayed on crops haven't been fully studied. Although organic fruit and vegetables are often expensive and hard to obtain, consumer demand may change this. More supermarkets are now providing organic produce. There is also a move towards the setting up of organic food co-ops modelled on the Seikatsu Club in Japan, where those joining pay a small amount each month and their groceries are delivered to the door each week. The co-ops are able to buy in bulk direct from the suppliers, thus reducing the costs. They are especially beneficial to those living in rural areas.
- Fibre is important, especially if you suffer from constipation. However, do not rely on only one source of food for your fibre – for example, wheat bran. Fibre is contained in beans, fruits (including dried fruit), vegetables, whole grains (such as oats, rice, barley, wheat and corn).
- Avoid highly processed food with additives and preservatives. Check the E numbers, as many of them are believed to cause digestive disturbances.

- Include in your diet small amounts of good-quality, unrefined, cold-pressed oils such as sunflower, safflower or walnut oil (buy in small amounts and keep in the fridge because they can go rancid). There is no such thing as a completely cold-pressed oil because the pressing of the seed generates heat, but most commercial oils are pressed with extra heat. This may cause damage to the essential fatty acids, thus greatly reducing the nutritional value of the oil. Refined oils are treated with a variety of chemicals, including bleach, deodorizer and petroleum-derived antioxidant. Olive oil is a good oil to cook with. In general, avoid frying as heat will destroy essential fatty acids. Avoid, as much as possible, hydrogenated and partially hydrogenated oils; the process of hydrogenation converts unsaturated fats into saturated fats in order to prolong shelf life. In other words, a perfectly good product such as soya oil is turned into saturated fat which may clog up your arteries and interfere with your body's ability to use essential fatty acids. If you regularly read the lists of ingredients on packets, you will know it is very hard to find any processed food that doesn't contain these oils. From a health point of view, you are better eating small amounts of butter than normal amounts of margarine or low-fat spreads that contain hydrogenated oils.
- Keep your intake of sugar, salt, caffeine and alcohol to a minimum.
- Avoid any foods you know don't agree with you. It may sound obvious, but it's worth mentioning.

High fibre or low fibre?

Doctors will often recommend that someone with IBS increase the fibre in their diet, no matter what the particular symptoms may be. In fact, if you suffer predominantly from diarrhoea, flatulence or bloating, a high-fibre diet can make things worse.

What is the evidence on high-fibre diets, and why are doctors still recommending them? McCloy and McCloy, in their book *The IBS: Clinical Perspectives* (Meditext, 1988), state that a report from the Royal College of Physicians failed to establish a link between dietary fibre and gastrointestinal disorders. Also, there seems to be no difference in the amount of fibre ingested by IBS and non-IBS people. Bran may not be a good idea for people with IBS as it has other effects on the bowel apart from acting as a bulking agent. It prevents the absorption of calcium and bile, and increases the levels of prostaglandins (chemicals that produce pain). We do not know what effects this has on gut motility, but many IBS sufferers find bran aggravates their symptoms. Some people simply put coarse wheat bran on their food and continue to eat a low-fibre diet otherwise. It is more advisable to increase the amount of fresh fruit and vegetables, particularly raw ones, and to eat as much unrefined, unprocessed food as possible. If this is very different from your usual diet, it should be done gradually to give your digestive system a chance to adjust.

There are two types of fibre: soluble (found in oats, pulses, bananas) and insoluble (found in wheat bran, cereal grains, apple and pear peel). Many people find that soluble fibre produces less bloating and is easier to digest than insoluble fibre.

Some people may find that a low-fibre diet suits them best. This means reducing or cutting out fruit and vegetables, nuts and wholegrain cereals. It allows fruit juices and includes highly refined products such as white flour. Such a diet may tend to be high in fat and sugar and is best worked out with the help of a dietician to ensure that you get all the nutrients you need.

High protein and low fat
Two researchers stated in 1988 that a diet low in fat and high in protein may help IBS. Foods that fit that description include chicken and turkey without the skin, white fish, tofu and low-fat dairy products such as skimmed milk and low-fat cheeses.

Food intolerance
Some people with IBS find that they cannot tolerate certain foods. Dairy products, wheat, citrus fruits and tea and coffee are common offenders. It may be worth cutting these out of your diet for a time to see if your symptoms improve and then reintroducing them one by one, every three days or so, to see if symptoms return.

You may decide that you want to try an exclusion diet to see if there are other foods that are aggravating you. The idea is that, for a week or two, you eat only two or three foods, preferably ones you rarely consume, and if your symptoms improve, you can be pretty sure that food intolerance is your problem. Reintroduce other foods gradually, and if all goes well, you should notice your symptoms return soon after you eat an offending food. However, exclusion diets can be difficult and the results confusing; if they are done incorrectly, they may result in multi-nutrient deficiencies, so it is important to undertake such a step with the guidance of a dietitian. An added factor is the effect of additives and pesticides on the individual, which can cause a reaction quite apart from an intolerance to the food itself.

Susan Backhouse went on two exclusion diets, carefully following advice from a book on the subject, but she wasn't sure if her symptoms improved during the exclusion period. Then, after she began to reintroduce foods, she would find that one day wheat seemed fine but another day appeared to give her diarrhoea. In the end, she had to conclude that the results were inconclusive!

Ida has had bowel problems ever since she was a child. She eventually discovered that she cannot tolerate certain foods:

'I had always found that I was better without coffee or carrots in my diet but was convinced that something else was causing the problem. I went to a homoeopathic doctor to have an allergy test. He diagnosed me as being sensitive to gluten, chocolate, monosodium glutamate and demerara sugar.

'This all happened five years ago and I have since followed this diet very carefully. I read every contents label in the supermarkets and am very aware of additives in our food. My friends and relations are all very understanding and we discuss the menu when I am visiting. I always take my own bread and my own gravy thickened with corn-flour.

'I do still have the problem, but it is not nearly as bad as it was.'

We found that one person in seven is on a restricted diet because of their IBS. Below we look at some of these diets.

Wheat-free Wheat-free means, of course, cutting out wheat – no ordinary bread, pasta (although you can get pasta made out of buckwheat, which isn't wheat in spite of its name: read the ingredients to make sure it doesn't have extra wheat added), anything made out of wheat flour (watch out for things such as thickeners in soups, some vending machine drinks, Ovaltine and Horlicks, baking powder and Mars bars, for example), no wheat bran or wheatgerm. Wheat can also be found in some sausages, condiments, puddings, tinned foods, stuffing and many other foods. Avoid ingredients described as edible starch, modified starch, cereal filler, cereal binder and cereal protein.

Gluten-free diet No gluten means not eating wheat, barley, oats, and rye. Rice, maize and soya products are all gluten-free. You can't eat ordinary bread, but you can get gluten-free flour loaves, biscuits and cakes if you are able and willing to pay the earth! Rice cakes are a substitute for crackers, although they may take some getting used to (some say that they taste of polystyrene). Cornflour, potato flour, rice flour, soya flour and arrowroot are gluten-free. Rice flour is great for cakes and biscuits; although it is hard to work with for pastry (it doesn't roll very easily), its nutty flavour is great for quiches. It is impossible to make pancakes with rice flour – try buckwheat flour instead. For thickening, use cornflour or potato flour. The latter is pretty awful in cakes, pastry and so on – the resulting product is like a stone. Fresh meats and bacon are gluten-free, but many sausages are not. Most ready-made dishes have gluten in them, as do most cheap ice cream, liquorice and many inexpensive confectionery items.

Starch-free diet A starch-free diet has been found by at least one sufferer to have helped her symptoms of distension and pain. This diet involves cutting out starch in all its forms including all grains, soya beans, potatoes and all cooked vegetables (starch is released in cooking but raw vegetables can be tolerated). The diet is then made up of fresh vegetables and fruit, dairy products, meat and fish. This diet may well reduce the amount of bloating and therefore, pain, as it is undigested carbohydrates that ferment in the bowel and cause wind. However, this diet is extremely restricted, tends to be high in saturated fat and could lead to nutritional deficiencies. It should only be undertaken with the help of a qualified dietitian.

Dairy-free diet A dairy-free diet means cutting out milk, cheese, yoghurt and all products that contain them. As above, reading the list of ingredients on processed food is essential. Avoid non-fat milk solids, caseinates, whey and lactalbumen, and note that many margarines contain cow's milk derivatives. You may find goat's and sheep's milk products an alternative, but some people are aggravated by them, too. Eggs may also cause a problem.

There is now a good range of soya products available, although some people are not able to tolerate them. Soya milk, unsweetened or sweetened with apple juice, is often organic and may contain added calcium because soya milk is low in this mineral. The taste varies from brand to brand, but if you find one you like, it's a delicious, healthy (but more expensive) alternative to cow's milk. You can also buy soya yoghurt, soya cheese, soya custard (a good low-fat alternative to ordinary custard) and tofu. The latter is a traditional Japanese product made from soya beans. It is available plain, smoked and marinated and is very versatile. If you are not used to it, however, look for some recipes to give you ideas. (See Appendix I for booklist.)

With a dairy-free diet you need to make sure you get all the necessary nutrients from other sources. For example, milk contains vitamin B_{12}, which is hard to get if you don't eat meat, so vegetarians need another source. Cow's milk is also a major source of calcium and this must be obtained from elsewhere.

Candida and IBS

The yeast *Candida albicans* lives in our bowels, and as long as our bodies are able to keep it under control, it does not create a problem. However, there is a theory that, if it gets out of control, it causes the symptoms of IBS, particularly diarrhoea, constipation and bloating as well as the more usual vaginal or oral thrush. Both women and men can be affected by candida and you don't have to suffer with thrush to have the problems.

Taking antibiotics, anti-inflammatory drugs such as prednisone and hydrocortisone, the contraceptive pill, oestrogens and steroids encourages candida overgrowth in the large bowel, as does the consumption of refined carbohydrates. It has also been said that people coming off tranquillizers and sleeping pills after long-term use can have candida problems.

Angela says:

'After years of trying virtually everything, I was recommended to a naturopath. She told me that, from all the symptoms I was showing, she was absolutely certain I had candida, and asked if I'd be prepared to go on a very strict elimination diet. I was to eliminate all dairy products, all foods that tend to go mouldy – e.g. mushrooms – and wheat products. This left hardly anything – I was put on short-grain brown rice, all root vegetables and bottled water. This was for four weeks. Then I was able to introduce pulses and herb teas. I was on this diet for seven months, nothing else, and I had vitamin supplements. It was very, very difficult and I lost two stone in weight, but *I didn't have any pain*. My husband was very sceptical, and as it was costing a lot of money, he was convinced I was being conned; I didn't seem to be getting well because I had a lot of withdrawal symptoms. Then I was asked to give myself enemas once a week to clean the bowel, and all this was removing toxins from my body. It was a very strict and hard regime, but it has paid off for me. I now have less pain from the IBS with much longer periods pain-free, but it hasn't cured it completely.

'I began to reintroduce normal food, but I still don't eat white flour products as I seem to have problems with these. I can have wholemeal flour. I don't eat any red meat at all. All the drugs I had taken over a period of 18 years never solved the problem; in fact most of them made it worse.

'The thing with IBS is that no two people are alike, and I feel that everyone has to try and find their own way of coping with it.'

Chronic candidiasis can affect many parts of the body. The following symptoms, many of which can be long term, *may* indicate a candida problem:

- Irritable bowel syndrome.
- Fatigue, lethargy, irritability, headaches, migraines.
- Joint pains with or without swelling.
- Muscle pains.
- Nettle rash and hives.
- A history of oral thrush.
- Upper abdominal discomfort or burning.
- Worsening of symptoms after eating refined carbohydrates and heavily yeasted foods.
- Sensitivity to chemicals (petrol fumes, paint, cigarette smoke, etc.).
- Craving for refined carbohydrates and/or alcohol.
- Recurrent vaginal thrush/vaginal itching.
- Anal itching.
- Recurrent cystitis.
- Fungal nail or skin infections.
- Iron or zinc deficiency.
- Onset of IBS problems during, or shortly after, pregnancy.
- Sexual partner with candida problems.
- Symptoms precipitated by antibiotics (or a history of repeated or long-term use of antibiotics).
- Symptoms worse in low-lying or damp places, near new-mown lawns or raked-up leaves, or on days when the atmosphere is damp (all symptoms of mould allergy).

Much of the list above is rather non-specific, and the same symptoms could be ascribed to other conditions. Consequently, the above symptoms are meant as a guide only.

The role of candida in IBS is controversial and some medical practitioners do not believe it is important. However, it could be that a candida infection may sensitize certain parts of the body, or trigger certain symptoms in an already sensitive part. It could also be that somebody who is very anxious and has a tendency to have IBS also has a rather compromised immune system which allows some candida species to colonize.

So we have the situation where you do not know whether candida is there at all, and even if it is, you cannot be sure it is a cause of your IBS! All you can do is minimize the chances of candida colonizing your body – in other words, eat for optimal nutrition and minimize stress.

You can try eating garlic – Shirley Trickett, author of *Irritable Bowel and Diverticulosis: A self-help plan* (Thorsons, 1990), recommends eating three crushed cloves a day. They can be taken with yoghurt or milk and washed down with plenty of water, or taken on tomatoes with olive oil. She says that three cloves daily will be 'devastating' for the candida, but you may not feel able to take it raw, especially in view of the smell that will linger on your breath. If you want to try commercial preparations, they must contain allicin, which is the anti-fungal substance in the garlic. Sunflower oil, olive oil and food-grade linseed oil (not the sort that artists use; that is poisonous) also have natural anti-yeast and anti-fungal properties. Buy cold-pressed, unrefined oil in small amounts and keep it in the fridge as it can go rancid quickly. These oils are expensive but are really worth getting as they will benefit your immune system too; it is important to do all you can to strengthen this system, as only by doing that can you hope for good health. Cut out smoking, alcohol and caffeine, or reduce them if you can't stop all together. (See later in this chapter for more on boosting your immune system.)

Some people resort to a course of nystatin (Nystan), an anti-fungal drug available only on prescription. Nystatin must be taken for at least eight weeks to be effective. It is also thought to kill off the candida too quickly; the poisons from the dead cells can make you feel pretty ill. Some researchers feel that nystatin and other powerful anti-candida agents tend to increase problems rather than curing them.

Candida is 'fashionable' at the moment, and a lot is heard about how an anti-candida diet can help all sorts of disorders. Although there seems to be no medical evidence to suggest that such a diet is effective in IBS, some people believe it has helped them. Mary says:

'By sheer fluke, I tuned into the end of a TV interview where the miseries of the effects of candida overgrowth were being recounted. Among those mentioned was IBS. I hot-footed it to my nearest bookshop and examined every book mentioning candida. I settled for *Candida Albicans: Could Yeast Be Your Problem?* by Leon Chaitow. There, at last, were many pointers as to why I may have succumbed to IBS, and many hitherto unrelated minor medical problems became understandable – I wasn't a hypochondriac, after all! Hope (again!).

'I decided at this low ebb that I had nothing to lose in trying the candida diet – I had long suspected a food link but elimination diets had proved inconclusive. Once I started this diet, I realized why – there were so many seemingly innocent products that were riddled with additives, yeasts, etc. I couldn't stick rigidly to all the pills and potions recommended as, apart from the price being prohibitive, many were unavailable, but I cobbled together my own list of vitamin supplements, and after three very difficult and hungry months when my weight loss accelerated, I actually began to see an improvement. The discomfort didn't disappear at once. My confidence didn't reassert itself, but the diarrhoea ceased and my trips to the loo became far less frequent.

'I cannot pretend that everything is now perfect, but a year on, still adhering strictly to the diet and avoiding cereals which I personally cannot tolerate, I feel so much more in control. After trying so many remedies and feeling so disappointed when each failed, I really would recommend that you try the anti-candida diet. It's not an easy option – it's got to be a serious all-out attempt or it won't work. It takes a long time and it's a very severe diet. I still resent having to miss out on many of life's goodies, but when

I think of the alternative for me – fear of being embarrassed while in company, in formal meetings, travelling, etc. – I'd rather have my life back.'

The anti-candida diet

Just in case you want to try it, the anti-candida diet referred to above is included here.

This diet can be very limiting. It includes cutting out all bread with yeast in it, Marmite and other products containing yeast (such as brewers' yeast and various other supplements), alcohol, cheese (except cottage cheese), mushrooms, food that is not fresh, raisins, sultanas (in other words anything that is a fungus, is made with mould or may have mould on it); refined carbohydrates (anything with sugar in it, all white-flour products, including white bread, biscuits, cakes, white-flour pasta); chocolate; food with vinegar in it; citrus fruits or drinks, grapes and grape juice. Limit other fruit to two pieces a day and peel the skin, which can contain fungi.

There are different levels of diets, some even more strict, depending on how bad the problem is. Candida overgrowth is often characterized by cravings for the foods that feed the yeast, especially sugar. If you manage to clear up the problem, you can slowly go back to your usual diet, but candida will probably come back if you eat a lot of sugar.

It is important that, if you are underweight, you do not lose more than one or two pounds while on the anti-candida diet. Any problems should be discussed with your doctor. As the anti-candida diet is likely to lead to several nutrient deficiencies, it is essential to supplement your diet with vitamins, especially if you are vegetarian. Make sure, of course, that the supplements are yeast-free.

The Hay system

The theory behind the Hay system is that, because of the different digestive processes involved, starches and sugars should not be eaten at the same meal as proteins and acid fruits, and there should be four to four-and-a-half hours between each different meal. However, there is no scientific evidence to support the theory behind this system. Medically speaking, it is not logical – humans have evolved to eat a mixed diet, and it does not seem to make sense to separate starches and sugars from proteins and acid fruits. Nevertheless, the diet is a wholefood one, where vegetables, salads and fruits provide the major part and processed foods are avoided.

Doris Grant and Jean Joice have written *Food Combining for Health* (Thorsons, 1984), a helpful and thorough book about the Hay system which you should consult if you want to give it a go. It provides the theory behind the diet, lists of compatible foods, recipes and menu suggestions.

Dionne says the following about the Hay system diet:

'Because I cook for a growing family and have a full social life I do not follow it strictly, but enough to have cut out most of the pain, the exhaustion of illness, the constipation, heartburn, sleeplessness and build-up of tooth plaque!'

The practicalities of diets

Many supermarkets will provide lists of their products that are free from wheat, gluten, dairy produce, yeast, sugar, etc. You can write to the customer relations department of the supermarket chain to obtain these.

Food allergy associations (see Appendix II) will give details of suppliers of foods suitable for people who are intolerant of certain substances.

All of these diets are very restrictive and, in many cases, more expensive because of the need to buy products that are less readily available. There needs to be a move towards providing a better choice of, say, gluten-free products, at a reasonable price and more readily available. Restaurants and cafés also need to be more aware of the needs of those on restrictive diets. If, however, the example of vegetarian products is anything to go by, food that was once considered strange is now on all the supermarket shelves and on all the pub menus, so maybe the future is not too bleak.

The world we live in

Our way of life as part of society, as well as individuals, can have a direct negative effect on our IBS. There was a general feeling among many of the IBS sufferers in our study that there are aspects of the way we live that cause and aggravate IBS, and changes are needed to make the condition easier to deal with. This is, of course, true of any illness that is affected by stress in any way. Some of the sufferers' sentiments are expressed here:

'Less emphasis on the work-till-you-drop attitude.'

'Less pressure and urgency to keep achieving for success's sake. Healthier, greener environment. Less pollution, fewer chemicals in food, household and other products.'

'When I am in safe accommodation with a good financial base, in a job I find enjoyable and stimulating – i.e. when I am materially secure – it will help my IBS.'

'There need to be fewer expectations of the "perfect" mother/wife/daughter/teacher, etc. – we need to accept each other just as we are.'

Rachel describes what she thinks triggered her IBS:

'At 17, unemployed and with no dole, I had no food for months, just ate rarely, what I could get. I smoked and drank a lot.'

Many sufferers feel that more and better public toilets are important for them to be able to cope with their symptoms. According to Tony, an ex-headmaster:

'One becomes aware of the abysmal provision of public toilets and the disgusting habits of The Public! It amuses me when folk return from foreign holidays and complain about the facilities there. I direct them to the one down the road. Supervised lavatories must be provided as the public behave badly in other ones. I am surprised that more fuss is not made in the media about the situation. What a wonderful opportunity for the consumer programmes on TV!'

In some places, things are going downhill fast. In Sheffield, almost all suburban toilets have been closed, as well as several in the town centre. A statement from the City Cleansing Services said that this was due to necessary financial cutbacks and had not been taken lightly – they recognised the concern that the decision had caused.

The problem is not limited to Sheffield. Henry says that, on his daily drive to work through Manchester, he passes at least six or seven closed and boarded-up toilets.

'Suffering from IBS brings home very sharply the quiet scandal of Britain's disappearing public toilets. In tourist areas such as Cornwall or the Cotswolds, I have found provision of toilets generally reasonable, in terms of both number and cleanliness. However, in most of our big towns and cities, the opposite is true – toilets are being closed down all over the place for reasons of economy. Within the last couple of years, Manchester has closed most of its toilets, apart from those in a handful of shopping centres. My home town of Stockport has just followed suit and announced the closure of two thirds of the toilets in the borough, and from my travels around the country, this seems to be the pattern almost everywhere.

'There must have been a genuine demand for all these toilets when they were built, and with the rise in the number of elderly people, and the obviously large number of IBS sufferers, the overall need, if anything, must have grown. I have read of old people suffering from dehydration, as they are frightened of drinking anything in case they are unable to find a toilet when they are out. Local councillors are inflicting misery on millions of people for paltry savings, in the knowledge that toilets are a subject on which people are too embarrassed to speak out.'

The IBS Network (see p. 358) provides a 'Can't Wait' card to all its members. This can be shown in shops and other public places if you need to go to the toilet urgently. It can also be used to skip queues in public toilets without causing bad feeling from others in the queue.

Towards a better life – pushing IBS out of the way

'I'm optimistic that my IBS will improve. I believe continuing to identify foods to which I'm sensitive and eliminating them will help. When I feel confident and start making changes in my life, I think there could ultimately be improvements in my IBS.'

It is clear that there are no easy answers with IBS. Most of us know that there is no instant cure. Its many symptoms and combinations of symptoms in each of us makes it such a puzzle! How it started, what makes it worse, what part of it is hardest to deal with, what helps – every one of us can tell a different story. No doubt, in time, some people who have been diagnosed as having IBS may be found to be suffering from other conditions. Fifty years ago, what we now call irritable bowel syndrome would have included lactose intolerance, coeliac disease, colitis and bile acid deficiency. If this does happen, some of us may find we don't have IBS but another condition not yet identified and our symptoms may be easily cured. Gastroenterologist Professor Nick Read says, 'The many different presentations of this condition, the non-specific nature of many of the symptoms and the poor and variable response to treatment suggest that irritable bowel syndrome is not more than a convenient clinical category in which to place a large number of patients whose disease mechanisms are poorly understood. Therefore it seems likely that what we call irritable bowel syndrome is not a single disease but consists of many different conditions.'

However, even if this is true, what we have all got in common are:

- Symptoms that can be difficult to live with.

- A condition that is poorly understood by doctors and the general public alike.
- A condition that can cause embarrassment and which many people, sufferers and non-sufferers alike, find difficult to talk about.
- A condition that has a poor record of effective treatment.

Meanwhile, the way we live has a significant effect on the health of all of us. Below we look at what steps you can take towards creating optimum health.

Build up your immune system

The immune system is the body's defence against illness. It is made up of an army of special cells ready to go into action at a moment's notice. They attack and destroy anything foreign – from bacteria and viruses to cancers – that invades the body or threatens it from within. If we want good health, it is important to know what weakens the immune system and what strengthens it. A well-functioning immune system will help your body to heal itself.

Although science has conquered many serious diseases of the past, there are new threats that our bodies have to face. Chemicals in tap water, pesticides on food and other environmental pollutants weaken our immune systems. This has meant that allergies are on the increase, children especially are more prone to infections, and immunological diseases – such as Crohn's disease, multiple sclerosis and rheumatoid arthritis – are becoming more common among adolescents.

The health of the immune system is extremely important, and damage to it may provide the link with candida and other infections.

If you feel good about yourself and in control of your life, your physical health is likely to be strong and your body will be able to heal itself. If you feel that your outlook towards life is not helping your IBS symptoms, look for ways in which you can empower yourself to change. This may include joining a self-help group, undertaking individual counselling or simply taking a good, long look at yourself. The chapters later in this book may help you.

Important for a healthy immune system is optimal nutrition. Recent research seems to show that we need an adequate intake of essential fatty acids (EFAs). These are substances that the body cannot manufacture, so they must be obtained from food. It is believed that EFAs can reduce cholesterol levels in the blood, reduce the risk of heart disease and help sufferers of pre-menstrual syndrome and chronic fatigue syndrome (formerly known as ME). They are also crucial in the maintenance of the immune system. EFAs are found in food-grade linseed oil, soya, walnut and wheatgerm oil, but these must be from a cold climate, fresh, cold-pressed and not hydrogenated. They are also present in salmon, tuna, mackerel, herring and sardines (fresh fish is best as canning causes some loss of essential fatty acids, especially if vegetable oil is used), and dried beans.

Any deficiency of essential minerals and micro-nutrients will depress the immune system, which is why it is important to eat well. Seafood is a rich source of all the minerals, and fresh vegetables will provide the vitamins A and C. These vitamins, as well as zinc and iron, are important boosters of the immune system.

Remember that some drugs depress the immune system; these include steroids, anti-inflammatory drugs and some antibiotics. Stress also depresses the immune system.

Chapter 5

Testing Time: Medical Investigations

Christine P. Dancey and Susan Backhouse

'Doctors are not used to helping, just diagnosing.'

This chapter will discuss what to expect when you decide that you need help for your IBS symptoms, as well as the tests you may have to undergo. These tests, although not exactly pleasant, are not as bad as you may imagine. Our research shows that people who have information about medical investigations find them less stressful than do those who do not know what is going to happen.

Most people with symptoms of IBS go to their GP, although they may, of course, have already tried to treat themselves with laxatives, anti-diarrhoeal mixtures or indigestion remedies. As we have seen, the symptoms of IBS are common in the general population, almost a third of whom have experienced such symptoms at some time in their lives. In fact, one study found that one or more symptoms occurred frequently in nearly 50 per cent of women and 25 per cent of men! However, IBS as diagnosed by doctors is present in one in 10 women and one in 20 men.

People put up with these symptoms for, on average, four to five years before going to their doctor. Why do people wait so long? And why do some people seek help from the medical profession while others do not? Some researchers have suggested that the sufferers who go to the doctors with their symptoms are more psychologically disturbed than those who do not, although their symptoms may be the same as those who do not seek help. However, the researchers also found that the more symptoms people had, the more likely they were to consult their doctor (not surprisingly!). They were more likely to seek help for their abdominal pain rather than the other symptoms of IBS. The researchers concluded that IBS is very prevalent in the general population, especially in women, and that the factors that made some people consult their doctors, joining the ranks of the 'IBS patients', were the number and intensity of their symptoms.

We all know that there are wide-ranging symptoms involved in IBS. Some of us have many of them, others have fewer. All of the symptoms of IBS are hard to deal with, but, as in the study above, the people we talked to also stated that abdominal pain was the problem that made them seek help. People also mentioned that, as a consequence of IBS, they slept less, and were therefore more tired.

What happens when you go to the doctor?

Some GPs diagnose IBS without any tests at all. This is more likely to happen if the sufferer is young, and fit apart from the symptoms of IBS.

The GP is likely to feel your abdomen, and, if you are a woman, give you a gynaecological examination to make sure the problem really is to do with the gut. You will be asked to undress from the waist down and lie on the couch with your knees raised. A covering will probably be put over you, for the sake of modesty. The doctor will put on a pair of gloves and insert his or her fingers into the vagina in order to feel for abnormalities. A swab may be taken. This will be cultured in a laboratory to test for certain bacteria. The results are likely to show there is nothing abnormal.

The next test may be a rectal examination. This time you will lie on your left-hand side and bend your knees (the left-hand side is always used simply to ensure consistency in doctors' findings). The doctor will put on another pair of gloves and, using a lubricant, insert his or her fingers into the anus, feeling the rectum. You may find this unpleasant, but it should not be painful.

The doctor may take some blood or send you to hospital for a blood test and ask you for a urine sample and for a stool sample to send off for analysis. The blood tests will show whether you are anaemic or not, and whether inflammation is present. These results will be normal for most IBS patients. The stool sample will show whether you are bleeding, or whether there are parasites in the stools. Again, for most people these results will be normal. The doctor will then either send you for hospital tests, or make a diagnosis of IBS on the spot.

From our research, we can say that most of you will find your GP treats you fairly well, and with sympathy:

'My own GP was very sympathetic and he is pleased to discuss my problems with me any time.'

'He recommended a high-fibre diet, and experimenting with bran and medication, and added that it was very difficult to treat.'

'My doctor is always sympathetic and listens to me. She's very nice, although there's nothing she can do for the pain or the other symptoms. I've been going to her every few months for three years now. She may think I'm neurotic but she never shows it!'

However, about a quarter of the people who spoke to us felt that their GPs did not understand their problems and were not sympathetic.

'As if he thought I was making it all up to get out of going to school and didn't believe me.' (*Pauline, a schoolgirl at the time of diagnosis, has had IBS for 27 years.*)

'As if I were neurotic and needed a tranquilliser.' (*A 58-year-old woman, 38 at the time of diagnosis.*)

'He did his best, but he didn't really understand how devastatingly embarrassing it was for a girl just growing up. I felt unattractive because of it.' (*Andrea, 14 years old at the time.*)

'In 1966, GPs did not do so many tests. He said, "Go home and have a cup of coffee, it will calm you down."'

'The first doctor laughed – then advised bran.'

'I lost two stone in three weeks (reaching six stone) and he just gave me an anti-diarrhoeal drug and said he'd see me in another week.'

'I was given anti-depression tablets and told it was all in my mind and to go away and sort myself out.'

'They were patronizing – why don't you go and have a holiday? Didn't treat me with any urgency, as though just because I didn't have a recognized or terminal illness I couldn't be in much pain.'

'I was frightened to go back because he just dismissed me as neurotic, but recently I've had to go back because it's become so chronic. I'm signed off work for two months now.'

'I do find the doctors are not very sympathetic about this complaint and never seem to talk about it as an illness. They regard it as something we have to live with. I think if a few of them had it badly, they might go out of their way to find a cure.'

Diana was told by a specialist that her chronic diarrhoea was the result of eating a 'typical Western diet', low in fibre and with too many refined carbohydrates.

'He advised me to eat more wholemeal bread and cabbage. I was dumbfounded because he had come to this conclusion without asking me any questions about what I ate. As it happened, I'd been living on a smallholding. The large vegetable patch, soft-fruit garden, orchard and fields edged with blackberry bushes had given me ample supplies of fruit and vegetables, and I had regularly made my own bread with wholemeal or wheatmeal flour.

'Once [my GP] prescribed aspirin because it has a constipating effect. When I refused, he persisted and wrote out the prescription in spite of my protests. Tearfully, I tore up the prescription in front of him! I realized then that I had lost my faith in the medical profession.'

Indeed, some people may consider changing their GP because they do not feel they have been taken seriously. If you are one of these people, and you find your GP is not treating you as you would wish, then do not suffer in silence. Explain to your

GP just how your symptoms are affecting you. Ask to be taken seriously and perhaps show your doctor some literature on IBS – many doctors do not keep up with the latest research and still believe IBS reflects a neurotic personality. Even if this were the case, you still deserve to be treated properly!

If your doctor is really unhelpful, though, consider changing to another practice. Although this may be a bother for you, IBS can affect you over a fairly long period, and having a sympathetic doctor whom you can trust and talk to with confidence can really help you through this time. Although you cannot expect to be cured, you have a right to be treated with respect and sympathy. If you need to change your doctor, do so, but you must choose carefully – you do not want to change your doctor to one who is no more helpful.

Hospital tests

As there are no tests specific to IBS, investigations are done to reassure the patient and physician that the patient has no serious disease. Some say that tests should not be conducted without serious thought, because they quite often produce results which are contradictory and, if repeatedly done, may undermine the patient's confidence in the diagnosis of IBS.

The researchers McCloy and McCloy also feel that hospital investigations are not necessary to make the diagnosis of IBS. (However, they add that, since the onset of IBS is rare after the age of 60, any elderly patient who goes to their GP with IBS-like symptoms and weight loss should be investigated by hospital tests.) They feel that hospital investigations are distressing to the patient, who undergoes one negative test after another and feels more and more as if they are regarded as a fraud. They say that the approach of excluding all serious diseases leads to hospital doctors dismissing the patients as neurotic once all the tests have been found negative. Carol says:

'I have suffered considerable discomfort and pain for almost ten years now. I have had all manner of tests and X-rays, all with a negative result. This year I had a test under general anaesthetic to see if I have coeliac disease. However, again this proved negative, and the consultant I had been visiting discharged me, saying he could only put the problem down to IBS. I find all this really stressful.'

According to Deidre:

'When the results of barium X-rays indicate to the gastro-enterologist that there is an abnormality of the bowels, then he or she should be in a position to do something for you rather than saying that you have IBS and to go back and see your GP to prescribe you medicine. I had a barium meal and enema in 1989, followed by a further one recently as my pain had considerably worsened and my GP felt that a further test was well overdue. After my last visit to the gastroenterologist, I was no wiser, and actually felt it all to have been a waste of time. I feel, however, that the attitude of my GP is one of sympathy with this condition, and I have never been given the cold shoulder but have been prescribed with a variety of medicines. There is little else to suggest as the barium X-rays indicate IBS and at least a clean bill of health – there's no cancer or anything.'

McCloy and McCloy say that there are far too many tests, they cost the NHS vast amounts of money, and they mean both distress and risks to the patient. They want there to be positive criteria for diagnosing IBS, rather than diagnosis by exclusion. However, many doctors are cautious, knowing that if they do not send patients to hospital to exclude more serious diseases, IBS may be a misdiagnosis. McCloy and McCloy have shown that this is unlikely to happen, but it is still a possibility. Some people who are told that they probably have IBS no doubt want the tests, for they are themselves worried that they may have a more serious disease:

'I had a range of tests performed – these included a barium enema, a lactose tolerance test and a sigmoidoscopy. The tests were negative, but what really concerned me is that my father contracted rectal cancer when he was in his fifties and had to have a colostomy. Then the cancer spread to his liver and he died. My father's early symptoms were very similar to my own.'

'I have recently been diagnosed as having IBS, after lots of different tests – e.g. endoscopy, gall bladder tests, X-rays, dilation and curettage (a gynaecological procedure), laparoscopy, etc. These all proved negative. My GP told me it was all in the mind, but the hospital doctor said IBS is now being recognized as an illness. At times I thought there must be something seriously wrong with me, because my mother died of cancer; this was the first thing I thought of.'

The following is one woman's medical history since contracting IBS, consisting of many tests, all showing nothing seriously wrong. As you read it, you may feel that it is not worth going through all these tests, especially if you are young and, apart from IBS, healthy:

8.8.85   Codeine phosphate prescribed.
13.9.85   Consultant prescribes eight-day course of flagyl for suspected giardiasis [antibiotic for parasites thought to be in gut].
25.9.85   Radiodiagnosis washout and barium enema (no abnormalities).
4.11.85   Samples of stools over three days (for parasites).
18.11.85 Blood test and three more days of stool samples.
9.12.85   Blood test.
16.12.85 Gall bladder X-ray
18.12.85 Blood test for thyroid deficiency.
19.12.85 Further ultrasound (nothing shows up).
13.1.86   Barium meal X-ray (all clear).
11.2.86   Smear test (all clear).
16.4.86   More blood tests.
7.5.86   Thyroid uptake scan for thyrotoxicosis (all OK).
15.5.86   Stool samples over three days.
16.5.86   Barium enema.

21.5.86	Results of tests and scan all OK; no blood in stools. Diagnosis is giardiasis.
23.6.86	Still thinks it's giardiasis. Blood test and three more stool tests.
30.6.86	No sign of giardiasis in stools, but given eight more days of flagyl.
25.7.86	Gastroenterologist suggests it could be pancreas inefficiency: I have now lost two stone in weight, blood test for red cell folate.
31.7.86	X-ray – small bowel enema.
19.8.86	One swallow test. Tube and Crosby capsule X-rays and gastric juices test.
1.9.86	Endoscopy: all OK.
10.9.86	Not coeliac disease or giardiasis.
1.10.86	Diagnosis: body making too much bacteria. Four weeks antibiotics.
4.9.90	Overall blood test (result normal). Result: IBS.

This is another woman's experience of her symptoms and the tests that were conducted:

'I consulted my GP in February 1991 for lower abdominal pain, and pain on passing urine. The doctor said it could be appendicitis or a urine infection, and to send in a urine specimen, but to call her if the pain became worse. It did become worse; I couldn't walk; she did a home visit and I was referred to the hospital. I was sent up to a ward where the doctor examined my abdomen, took some blood and said there was nothing wrong and sent me straight home. Over the weeks the pain got worse – it felt as though something was going to burst inside me. When I had my period, the pain worsened. My husband had to call the GP, who saw me and referred me to the hospital, where I was admitted. I was told that I probably had a urine infection; a specimen was sent and came back negative. They said that, although it was negative, it was still probably a urine infection. I had blood taken and a scan was ordered, but this was clear. The pain was getting easier. Then one morning it was extremely severe, and the doctor who saw me ordered an injection of pethidine. Another doctor saw me and said they were referring me to a gynaecologist; I was discharged and told I would receive the appointment in the post.

'I was at home for a while, in pain but trying to tell myself there was nothing wrong. I then had to call the GP out again as the pain was unbearable. I was referred to a gynaecologist and admitted to the hospital, where I was told I probably had a pelvic infection. They took swabs. After this, I was put on two courses of antibiotics and discharged. Then I experienced unbearable pain. I was very frightened so went back to the ward I had been in. I was told it was appendicitis or an ectopic pregnancy. A specimen of urine was taken and I was given an injection for the pain. I was told that I would be going to theatre; then I was told it would be the following day. All I wanted was for somebody to find out what the pain was and to stop it. The next day came and I was prepared for theatre, but the morning went and the afternoon came and I still hadn't gone to theatre. The doctor eventually came to tell me that I would be going to theatre that evening for a laparoscopy. When I came out of the anaesthetic, I asked the nurse what was wrong. She said everything was clear. That was a relief, but what was causing my pain? The next day I was discharged.

'Days later the pain was still there, and my husband called the GP out. This GP said he thought it could be something to do with my bowel and referred me for an urgent appointment to a gastroenterologist. I saw this doctor within a week. He ordered a barium meal and told me to take Colofac. I had the barium meal, which was negative. I went to my GP for the results. He said everything was fine and that it was IBS. I asked what could be done; he said, "Nothing. It's due to stress," and that was that. I felt then that I had wasted everybody's time, and that some GPs' attitude is that it is stress and so you as the individual can control it. I don't think that people who have never suffered from this realize how it can affect your life. I know it's not a disease and is only a condition, but I think that GPs should start to recognize it and not just dismiss it or the individual. I have never been back to my doctor about my IBS; I just keep getting repeat prescriptions of Colofac. I want to be able to relax and to control my condition, but on occasions the pain is unbearable still.'

Should you take the tests?

Whether you undergo tests or not depends on the circumstances. If you are at all worried that you might have cancer or some other serious disorder, the tests will put your mind at rest. Dr Chris Mallinson, consultant at Lewisham Hospital, London, says: 'If you have a patient whose symptoms have lasted a long time and who is still in their early twenties, who has the typical IBS picture and who obeys the doctors' ideas of the Manning criteria, it's perfectly reasonable not to do the tests. However, if you've got someone who is over 40, and whose symptoms are new and rather well localized, then there's no getting away from the tests, however convinced you may be [that it's IBS].'

Dr Mallinson says that, if people start having IBS-type symptoms when they are, say, 50, a doctor would be taking substantial risks not to recommend taking some tests. Although it is possible for IBS to start at this age, it is unusual, and it is at this age that the risk of other diseases increases. Cancer is the big worry, of course, although it is much more likely that the person has diverticulosis. (This happens when the muscles of the colon wall become weakened, and lose their elasticity. Pouches called diverticula are then formed, which may become infected.) Tests would normally eliminate these possibilities. Despite the advice from experts, some of our older members who were in their sixties and seventies at the time of diagnosis were told that they had IBS without any tests at all. We suggest that, if you are over 50 and your doctor does not refer you for tests, you should ask for them just for safety's sake.

What the tests look for

Tests can detect ulcers (persistent breaches in the lining of the stomach or duodenum) and patches of inflammation as in Crohn's disease. The latter causes inflammation of the intestines which gives rise to symptoms similar to those of IBS; sometimes the affected part of the intestine has to be removed surgically. Polyps (benign tumours which can lead to cancer), malignant tumours and diverticula can also be detected.

Which tests are conducted depends on the symptoms. If the patient has lower abdominal pains, erratic bowel movements and tenderness of the left side, the first test indicated is a barium enema because this investigation examines the lower part of the guts. If the pain is higher up and there is not much bowel upset, the doctor may suspect something is wrong with the small intestine, in which case, a barium meal and follow-through (see pp. 125–6) may be indicated as this shows the upper part of the gut. If the patient has symptoms very high up in the gut, an endoscopy may be performed, which shows the doctor if there is any abnormality from the throat to the stomach and a little way into the duodenum. If there are many different symptoms, as in IBS, the doctor may recommend several checks for certain patients to be on the safe side – for example, a barium enema, a barium meal and a scan. If a patient has sharp pains in the chest area which get worse with exercise, the doctor may even want to check the heart with an electrocardiograph (ECG). If the patient complains of pains in the back, sides and abdomen, a kidney X-ray may be recommended.

Why do people worry about tests?
Quite often IBS sufferers feel that there must be something seriously wrong. This is a natural fear when you are in a lot of pain, have disturbed bowel habits and may have lost weight. Doctors, of course, find that most people who have tests have nothing seriously wrong with them, so they are sometimes indifferent to your fears. However, some IBS patients may have had relatives with bowel cancer, or they may have had serious medical problems before IBS symptoms began, so it is understandable that they worry. It is important to remember that, for the vast majority of people with IBS symptoms, the tests will be straightforward and there will be nothing seriously wrong.

Some people may be worried because they fear pain or embarrassment, or think they will feel undignified. However, if you are well informed about the tests, you will be prepared for them; your anxiety level will be lessened, and the tests should not then cause much discomfort. Most tests do not hurt, but anxiety can cause you to tense all your muscles, which makes investigations like barium enemas painful. If you can relax, you will be all right.

Routine tests

The first thing the doctor is likely to do is to feel the abdominal area, and then carry out a sigmoidoscopy. A very straight, narrow tube is inserted into the rectum and pushed as far as possible (different people can tolerate different lengths). The doctor looks through the instrument to detect cancer of the rectum, piles, fissures and cracks in the rectal wall. With the sigmoidoscope, the doctor can examine the lowest part of the bowel; it reaches the parts that the barium enema cannot reach. The patient lies on the left side, with the knees up. Although it can be painful, the pain passes as soon as the instrument is withdrawn.

'It was like having your ears pierced – by the time you realized it was painful, the pain was gone.'

'It was a bit unnerving to have to lie there with doctors looking at my backside, but I was pleased to have the test because I wanted to make sure nothing serious was wrong.'

You can be told the results of this test immediately. The usual result is that nothing abnormal was found.

Barium meal and follow-through Barium is a thick liquid consisting of barium sulphate, which is either swallowed or injected into the rectum. The liquid is radiopaque (opaque to X-rays) and casts shadows on a film. X-ray pictures can show any abnormalities. The 'meal' that is swallowed is insoluble, which means that none of the substance will be absorbed from the intestine.

You will have to do without food for some hours before the barium meal. Swallowing barium (a thick white drink which doctors jocularly refer to as a 'milk shake') makes the digestive tract become opaque. The barium (which has not got an unpleasant taste) moves down the digestive system and is recorded. The X-ray pictures detect ulcers and tumours in the upper part of the digestive tract.

'The doctors and nurses were very nice – joking and laughing with me. They asked me to drink a white milkshake, quite a lot of it. It didn't really taste of anything, but the texture was sort of gooey and chalky. Then I had to lie down on a stretcher for a while. They fetched me into the X-ray room and took a few pictures. Then I had to drink another pint or so of the liquid, wait a while, and then have more pictures taken. It went on for ages. There was nothing painful or embarrassing about this test – it was all quite boring. It took about an hour and a half, and they told me there and then that there was nothing wrong.'

Barium enema The colon must be empty before the barium enema is carried out. This usually means drinking only fluids for a set time before the enema, and taking laxatives the day before. A tube-like instrument is inserted into the rectum (this should not hurt if you relax), and barium flows into the large bowel; air is also pumped into the bowel, which you may find uncomfortable. The pictures of the bowel are transferred on to a monitor – often you can watch what is happening on the screen. The barium enema can detect tumours or inflammation. Most people find the test unpleasant but not particularly painful. Shirley, aged 37 at the time of the test, remembers:

'I was given a sheet telling me what to do before the test. About two days before I could only eat a low-residue diet – fish, eggs, I can't remember what else. Then the day before, just fluids or clear soup. Also the night before I had to take some sort of laxative to clear out the bowel. I was having so much diarrhoea at the time, going to the toilet up to 15 times a day, that the laxatives didn't make any difference anyway. When I went to the hospital, the doctor asked me if the laxatives had given me diarrhoea. He didn't look as if he believed me when I said they had made no difference. Then I had to lie on the bed while an instrument was inserted into the rectum. This didn't hurt at all, but when they started pumping air into me, I found it quite painful, rather like having bad wind. The white fluid was also pumped up inside, and I could see the fluid flowing through the bowel on the screen. It was quite interesting. Pictures were taken while I was lying down and standing up. The tests were negative. The whole procedure was quite quick. Afterwards, the doctor said to drink plenty of water because the barium would make me constipated. After six months of diarrhoea, I was looking forward to a change!'

Afterwards, you can expect to have flatulence and to keep feeling as if you need to go to the toilet – but it's only air and barium. It can take up to three days to get rid of the barium, during which time your stools are white and don't flush away very easily.

Colonoscopy This is a more comprehensive test and is conducted in hospital under general anaesthetic. The colonoscope (a tube-like instrument) is inserted into the back passage. The doctor looks through a viewer attached to the colonoscope. This test will show up patches of inflammation, as in Crohn's disease, and is the most sensitive way of finding polyps. It also discovers tumours and diverticula. The colonoscope does everything a barium enema can do, and can discover certain things an enema can miss such as small polyps. If polyps are found, they can be removed at the time.

For this test, the bowel must be empty. It is not the test of first choice, as it takes longer and is more expensive than a barium meal and enema. As it is usually done under general anaesthetic, no one wrote to us with an account of their colonoscopy!

Endoscopy An endoscope is used to relay pictures from the upper part of the digestive tract. An instrument is placed in the throat and the patient swallows it, along with the attached cables. (The throat is first numbed by the use of a local anaesthetic spray or, alternatively the patient may be given a general anaesthetic; in either case, it is necessary to go without food and drink for some hours beforehand.) The doctor then injects air into the stomach, which inflates it, thus allowing the doctor to see more easily. A biopsy can be performed if necessary.

A 62-year-old woman wrote:

'The specialist came and told us that six of us were due to have the same test. He told us he would be inserting a tube about the size of a fountain pen down our throats and would then take it down into our stomachs and have a look around. He said not to worry that we would not be able to breathe – we would still breathe normally. We had two choices: we could have a general anaesthetic or we could opt to have it done without, in which case we would have our throats sprayed to make them numb and then swallow the tube. I asked how many people opted for it this way, and he said just over 50 per cent. It was explained to us that, if we had the general anaesthetic, we wouldn't know anything that was happening, but of course we would feel tired afterwards. Without the anaesthetic, there would be no after-effects, and if we found difficulty in swallowing the tube, we could then still have the anaesthetic. It sounded a bit gruesome, but we did not have to decide until the last minute.

'The first lady went in and came back about ten minutes later saying, "Look at me, I'm still alive! It wasn't so bad and I didn't have the anaesthetic." The second lady was away much longer as she had the anaesthetic and, when she came back, was still half asleep in the chair. Then came my turn. I said I'd be brave and not have a general anaesthetic. I was given a throat spray which tasted a little bitter and then a plastic gadget to keep my teeth apart. I was at this stage lying on my side – I did not have to undress. The doctor came in and gave my throat another spray, and took the tube and told me to feel it with my tongue. The next thing I was being asked to swallow, which I did and was given every encouragement. Then again I was asked to swallow, which made me retch a bit, and again a third time. I was then told the tube was in my stomach and they would now have a look around. The doctor said I could have a look on the video screen and see what was happening. I declined, but have been sorry ever since, as I am sure I would have been very interested. In no time at all, it was over, and apart from a slight numbness in the throat, it was no trouble at all. The numbness wore off after 20 minutes. We weren't pressurized at all in our choice. I think the doctor's chat to us together at the start was very helpful, as we all were able to talk to each other and give each other encouragement.'

Ultrasound scan This is the technique used on pregnant women. There are said to be no risks attached to it. Sound waves penetrate the body, casting shadows on the video screen. The scan will show up gallstones, fibroids, or any other abnormalities in the abdominal region. You must have a full bladder for this test. It is quite painless, as our respondents describe:

'It was interesting. I had to drink two pints of water before I went and nothing to eat after nine o'clock the previous evening. I was dying to go to the loo, but you have to have a full bladder, or the picture doesn't show up. Luckily they took me straight in! They rubbed a small box over me [a probe] which showed up pictures on the screen. I couldn't make sense of the pictures, but obviously they could. It didn't hurt a bit.'

'No, it didn't hurt, but it was a pain! I got there, full of fluids and feeling uncomfortable, and they were running about an hour late. I couldn't wait – rushed to the loo. What a relief. Then of course, when I went in they sent me out again, because the picture wasn't clear as I didn't have any water in my bladder. So I had to sit there for over an hour and a half drinking constantly. I had visions of them being late again, and having to go to the loo again, but it was OK. They didn't find anything abnormal.'

Intravenous urogram One female respondent had a kidney X-ray called an intravenous urogram. This is not a routine test for patients with IBS symptoms but it is carried out on some. Compounds of iodine are injected into the arm. These are also radiopaque, and cast shadows of the kidneys on to film. We give this account here just in case some of you are sent for it:

'The worse bit was all this purging of the bowel before the X-ray. I'd already done it for the barium enema, so I wasn't looking forward to it again. Two days before the X-ray, I had to take a bottle of laxative – it acted very quickly and very violently. I was on the loo most of the evening, and it was very painful. The strange thing is that the next day I was allowed to eat! I would rather have gone two days without eating than having to have this violent laxative. Anyway, the next day I had to take two Sennacot which didn't appear to do anything. On the day of the X-ray, I went in straight away, and the doctor introduced himself and his nurse. They were very pleasant. They explained what was going to happen in detail, in a reassuring manner. They injected a substance, which was a dye, into my arm, and about a minute after it was injected, I came over all hot as if I were going to faint, but luckily they had told me to expect this reaction, so I didn't mind. The feeling passed really quickly, then I just lay on the bed while they took the pictures. I had to get up and go to the loo, and then come back for more pictures. They had told me to expect to be there for over an hour, but because everything was normal, it only took half an hour. So I went to all that trouble of taking laxatives for nothing. Still, at least I knew I was OK.'

Test results

The staff at the hospital will normally tell you that they have found nothing seriously wrong. It is usually up to your GP to tell you what this means – that is, that you have irritable bowel syndrome. You are probably going to have mixed feelings about the results of the tests. If they are negative (and for a diagnosis of IBS, they will be), you may feel relieved on the one hand (thank goodness it's not cancer!) and annoyed on the other, because there is nothing to treat. Some people feel guilty, as though they are frauds and have wasted the doctors' time, because there was nothing wrong with them. However, remember: you have *not* wasted anyone's time. Most hospital tests performed are 'negative', and a good thing, too. If your doctor suspected IBS, he or she will be expecting the results to be negative, and both of you will feel relieved that they are. After all, although

IBS is very unpleasant it will probably improve, unlike more serious diseases. Also, in having excluded things like cancer and Crohn's disease, you now have a diagnosis of IBS, which is better than living with the uncertainty of not knowing what is the matter with you.

These are some of the responses you may have when you are told about the results:

'I suppose relieved but at the same time I would like to have been given some hope of anything to take away this pain and improve my way of life . . . I could not believe after six months of waiting that the best they could suggest was to take laxatives.'

'Initially relieved, but fed up as it got no better.'

'I expected it but I felt a sense of hopelessness at first, followed quite soon by a determination that it wouldn't defeat me.'

'Pleased, although I felt that was the end of the line and now there was no more treatment available that was likely to be effective.'

As you are reading this book, at least you know about IBS. Some people were totally perplexed when they were told that they had IBS as they had never heard of it. It is to be hoped that you will have more help than the following sufferer:

'I wanted to know more but could find no information anywhere. I sought help from a trained nurse, who hadn't heard of it either.'

If your GP is sympathetic, you should not have the problems of some sufferers who were informed that they should be able to cure themselves. Some people were told directly that IBS was self-induced, and that if only they could learn to deal with stress or food habits, their IBS would improve:

'In 1976, it was called spastic colon. I thought that, if I gave up work, I would be free of stress, so I retired. The IBS has not improved.'

'The doctor said it was "due to years of bad eating", which I consider impertinent and probably not true.'

'It was put down to exam nerves, then premarital nerves, then postmarital nerves . . . then change of water, etc. . . .'

'It wasn't explained to me . . . the doctor dismissed it and didn't recognize the problems it was causing me.'

'The tests were very worrying as I feared cancer – I was very relieved when told it was diverticulosis [later IBS was diagnosed] of which I'd never heard. The doctor said it was due to too much Devon cream, which I don't eat.'

'I was disappointed because I was told it was just my nerves and to go away and eat lots of fibre (with dire results).'

Keeping yourself – and your doctor – informed

If you go for any of these tests, make sure that you are kept informed about what is going on at every stage. You should know what the test is for, how long it is going to last, whether it will be painful or uncomfortable and so on.

Many IBS sufferers have told us that, when they were first diagnosed, they had never heard of IBS and they were not given enough information on it. They had no idea that it was a common condition and thus felt alone in their complaint.

The medical profession's track record of treating IBS patients is not a good one. We know of one 15-year-old girl who, in the mid-1970s, went to her doctor complaining of IBS symptoms. He felt her abdomen briefly and prescribed Valium! She was very worried about addiction and not being able to manage without the drug and, fortunately, took very few of the tablets. Nowadays, more than twenty years on, there is more awareness among doctors, and few of them, it is to be hoped, would blithely send a young woman down the tranquillizer road. There are, however, still many sufferers of IBS who are less than satisfied with the treatment received from their GPs and from specialists. We found that almost all of a sample of 148 sufferers said that medical treatment was inadequate.

When Mrs Collins began to suffer from feelings of fatigue and breathlessness, together with pains in her head and flutterings and bangings in her heart, she suspected that the cause was the codeine phosphate she had been prescribed for her IBS. She was sent for exhaustive testing which revealed no organic problem. The consultant, who had been sympathetic at first, became much less so and eventually sent her to a psychiatrist, thus, she felt, 'washing his hands of me'. She went on to say:

> 'During this time, several suggestions by my husband and myself to the consultant that the codeine phosphate might be to blame were brushed aside.'

Mrs Collins was sent, at her own request, to another hospital where she was pleased to find she was treated with understanding and courtesy.

> 'Almost immediately it was suggested to me that the codeine phosphate was the cause of my troubles, apart from the basic bowel problem, that is. I was told to stop taking it and ask my GP to prescribe a more up-to-date alternative. He prescribed Lomotil.
>
> 'My extreme tiredness vanished within a few days. My heart symptoms settled down and I discovered what it was like to feel well again. I feel that two years of my life have been wasted.'

It seems that many people, apart from coping with the stresses of a chronic illness, have to cope also with GPs and consultants who are unsympathetic, disbelieving of their symptoms and dismissive. In some cases, the patients are frightened to go back. IBS is not life-threatening and is not a 'serious' illness, but doctors should not underestimate the distress it causes to patients and their families. If you have an unsympathetic doctor, try to make him or her realize how distressing the syndrome is. Perhaps you could encourage him or her to read this book!

Chapter 6

Medical Treatment

Professor Nick Read

Our approach to the treatment of irritable bowel syndrome really depends on how we view it. Is it a disease like ulcerative colitis or cancer: something tangible that we can see and diagnose with confidence? Is it a syndrome, a collection of symptoms such as breathlessness or indigestion: a bodily discomfort and disturbance which can be caused by many different though specific conditions? Or is it a gut reaction to the vicissitudes of fortune: a disturbance that is neither all in the gut nor all in the mind but involves both? If IBS were a disease, treatment would be easy. It would be like treating a duodenal ulcer with tablets that block acid secretion or with combinations of specific antibiotics. But research over the last 50 years or more has not been able to identify a specific disease mechanism for irritable bowel syndrome. In the future, somebody may discover a specific virus or bacterium that is responsible for the condition, like helicobacter in duodenal ulcer disease, but so far, despite looking very hard, medical scientists have not come up with anything like that. So, because irritable bowel syndrome does not appear to be a specific disease, there is not a specific treatment for it.

Is IBS a syndrome?

What if IBS is indeed a syndrome, a well-defined cluster of symptoms, easily recognizable, that could be induced by several different conditions? The model here would be something like asthma, the combination of breathlessness, wheeziness and airway obstruction which can be brought on by infection, allergies to pollen, cold air and emotional factors. The fact that the condition is called irritable bowel *syndrome* indicates that this is the current view. Most doctors would regard it as a syndrome that comprises abdominal discomfort plus a disturbance of defecation which might be either diarrhoea or constipation, or a mixture of the two, and a few rather specific symptoms like a feeling of incomplete evacuation (wanting to go to the loo again after you have just been), lower abdominal pain relieved by defecation, passage of mucus and an urgent desire to defecate.

In recent years, there has been a determined effort on the part of some experts to define rigid criteria for the diagnosis, so that researchers throughout the world can be sure they are studying the same condition, and so that different treatments can be tested on a single well-defined entity instead of a hotch-potch of differing conditions which are collected together and called IBS. The problem with this approach is that everybody who has IBS is different. The combination of symptoms experienced by one person with irritable bowel syndrome may be quite distinct from those experienced by another patient. For example, the patient who suffers from frequent passage of sloppy stools associated with abdominal pain and the patient who suffers with abdominal bloating and constipation are both included under the category of irritable bowel syndrome. Furthermore, the condition encompasses a constellation of other symptoms such as headache, tiredness, breathlessness, frequent passage of urine, backache, leg pains, depression, anxiety and so on. In fact, some patients have so many bodily symptoms that it may be a matter of luck whether they come to a gastroenterologist and are diagnosed as having irritable bowel syndrome or whether they go to, for example, a cardiologist and are investigated for chest pain.

It is all very difficult; but perhaps it may be helpful to hold on to the notion that symptoms such as a frequent desire to defecate, pain relieved by defecation, feeling of incomplete evacuation, rectal mucus and recto-anal spasms imply an irritability of the lower end of the gut. This suggests that we should focus on what might be causing sensitivity or irritability in this region.

A complex of different diseases

I am often struck by the notion that, if we were puzzling over IBS 50 years ago, the whole portmanteau of conditions that cause abdominal discomfort plus a disturbance of defecation would include conditions such as coeliac disease, ulcerative colitis, Crohn's disease and cancer of the colon – distinct conditions that are easily recognized and diagnosed by doctors these days. So out of the large 'cake' that we call IBS, we have been able to cut slices which represent specific diseases and diagnoses. Perhaps if we pay sufficiently careful attention to what our patients are telling us, we may still be able to recognize specific subsets of irritable bowel syndrome that would respond to specific treatment. The following examples illustrate some of the possibilities for specific treatment.

Bile acid malabsorption
Ever since her husband had left her, Joyce had suffered with quite severe diarrhoea, needing to pass soft liquid motions up to 20 times a day. Joyce was not getting any maintenance from her husband and had had to take a part-time job to gain enough money to keep the family together. Going to work was a nightmare. Since Darren was born three years ago, Joyce had noticed that she could be incontinent of gas or liquid motions. Just to travel on the bus she had to wear pads and towels and always take two spare pairs of pants with her. Her boss had already complained about the time she spent out of the office in the loo. She was prescribed Questran (cholestyramine) as granules, which she mixed with a drink and took half an hour before each meal, adjusting the dose with the size of the meal (two before a big meal like dinner, and one before a small meal). Within two days, the diarrhoea and incontinence had gone – in fact, she was a bit constipated; but she experienced instead quite severe griping abdominal pains.

In recent years, some patients with frequent passage of sloppy or watery stools and abdominal pain have been treated quite successfully with resins that bind bile acids. Bile acids are normal constituents of digestive secretions. They act rather like detergents to disperse fat, making it much easier and faster to digest and absorb, and most are normally reabsorbed at the lower end of the small intestine. The overactive gut of irritable bowel syndrome can cause food and digestive secretions to pass down the small intestine much more rapidly than normal. As a result, a lot of the bile acids are not reabsorbed and go down into the colon where they cause irritation, resulting in diarrhoea. Treatment with the resin Questran can mop up the bile acids and stop this happening. Unfortunately, not very many people with IBS like Questran. Some dislike the texture and complain that it makes them feel sick; others, like Joyce, find that the cost of getting rid of the diarrhoea is the development of pain – as if her distress has to come out somewhere.

Urgency and faecal incontinence

Diarrhoea can be bad enough by itself, but when it is associated with incontinence, it is a disaster. Joyce has struggled on with difficulty. Other people tell me that they can only go out if they have a map of all the toilets in Sheffield just in case . . . and since the council has been closing 'conveniences' to save money, they live as recluses, confined to their houses.

This problem affects women in particular, and in most it is caused by damage to the muscles around the bottom during childbirth. Even if there is no actual tear into the anus, the stretching that occurs as the baby is born can damage the nerve going to the anal sphincter and cause weakness that can get worse with time. A lot of research is currently being directed at finding out whether changes in obstetric practice can prevent this distressing complication of childbirth. Pelvic floor or 'Kagel' exercises may help the pelvic muscles to recover some strength after childbirth, but will not be much use if the muscle is torn or badly stretched. The only recourse then is surgery: either direct repair of the torn muscle or a strengthing of the pelvic floor with the surgical equivalent of a 'darn' or, occasionally, a 'patch' or graft. Most surgeons, however, would try to subdue the irritable bowel first before contemplating pelvic surgery.

Lactose intolerance

This, like bile acid malabsorption and obstetric injury, does not actually cause IBS, but it can certainly make it much worse. Treatment is simple: a determined reduction in consumption of milk or milk products that contain lactose.

Lactose is milk sugar. In babies, it is normally digested in the small intestine by the enzyme lactase, which turns it into glucose and galactose, which can then be absorbed into the body. Most populations in the world lose their lactase enzyme around the time of weaning. This means that, when older children and adults drink milk, the lactose is not absorbed and goes down into the large intestine, where it is fermented by bacteria yielding large amounts of gas. Reputedly the gassiest person in the world, Mr Sutalf, who once passed wind 144 times a day, was deficient of lactase enzyme but drank milk.

Impaired digestion of lactose may not be too much of a problem for most people, but those with the sensitive and reactive bowels of IBS may suffer agonies of pain, bloating, gas and diarrhoea, and gain much relief from dietary restrictions.

Too much fibre

Sam is a fit, assertive 25-year-old. She believes in looking after her body. She attends aerobic classes five times a week, and she is very careful about what she eats, preferring cereals and vegetables and lots of fruit. Sam was well until she became engaged to John, who plays rugby and enjoys a drink with his mates. Sam developed abdominal cramps and became constipated; she felt like she was full of gas and worried about her protruding tummy. She began to step up her exercise programme and take more cereal in her diet. At first, she resisted the idea that she should cut down her fibre intake and eat a more balanced diet containing meat and eggs and cheese, but after a few weeks of trying this change in diet, her symptoms were not so severe. She expressed considerable anxiety about her engagement and asked if there was anybody she could discuss it with.

Like lactose intolerance, and for the same reasons, the enthusiastic consumption of dietary fibre often makes the symptoms of IBS much worse. Fibre contains polysaccharides that cannot be digested in the small intestine but are fermented producing a lot of gas when they reach the colon. Ideas regarding the use of fibre in IBS have changed. In the heady days of 'fibre for all' in the early 1970s, many doctors believed that IBS was a disease of fibre deficiency, condemning many patients to agonies of pain and bloating and the embarrassment of gas and diarrhoea. While it is true that fibre can be very helpful for some patients with constipation, it tends to make other symptoms worse. These days I tend to advise people with IBS to restrict their intake of fibre.

Bile acid malabsorption, lactase deficiency, obstetric injury and ingestion of too much fibre do not actually cause IBS, but they can make the symptoms much worse. At the moment, there does not seem to be any specific disease that can reliably be said to cause IBS, but there are a few candidates.

Candidiasis

Petra was cross. She announced her intentions as soon as she came in. 'I've got candida. I've eaten yoghurt until it's coming out of my ears. I've taken courses of antibiotics until they've made me puke. I've even had my colon washed out three times. You are my last hope!' We started to talk. Rather rapidly, as if what she was saying was of no consequence, she told me about her mother abandoning the family when she was two, the sequence of minders, raped by her uncle at 15, an abortion at 18, a failed marriage . . . 'And I don't want you to say it's all in my mind. I want you to look at the bacteria in my colon.' I said that I would be glad to work with her but I could only operate in a way that I believe was best for her. 'Oh, so unless I fit in with your mind set, you can't help me,' she retorted and stormed out.

The notion that a significant proportion of IBS may be caused by candida has received some public support but there is no good scientific evidence to support it. In any case, the large amounts of oral fungicides that need to be given to eradicate candida from the body can be quite toxic and cause other symptoms. I am inclined to think that, for most of the time, this organism lives in close harmony with us and only gets out of control in sites other than the vagina or the mouth if our immune system is severely compromised. There is no evidence to suggest the immune system is severely compromised in irritable bowel syndrome. I could be wrong, but I remain to be convinced that treatment regimes aimed at eradicating candida have any lasting benefit for IBS sufferers.

Rectal mucosal prolapse

Surgical treatment for IBS has received publicity recently with the news that Mr Bernard Palmer, a surgeon working in Stevenage, has been treating patients with IBS by taking tucks in the lining of the rectum to remove the superfluous 'skin' that may cause difficulty in defecation. At first, Mr Palmer selected his patients rather carefully – they were people who suffered feelings of 'rectal dissatisfaction', wanting to go to the loo but being unable to go – but he has since found that his operation can help even those people who have central abdominal pain or even indigestion. Mr Palmer reported that about 80 per cent of the patients he had treated were free of symptoms three months after their treatment.

The patients that Mr Palmer originally selected sound as if they might have had a mild form of rectal prolapse, where the lining of the rectum may actually come down and block the outlet, so frustrating defecation. Rectal mucosal prolapse or, as it is sometimes called, 'solitary rectal ulcer syndrome', can be recognized by the patch of inflammation or even ulceration in the rectum when doctors have a look inside with a sigmoidoscope. Long-term follow-up is necessary in order to assess the true efficacy of Mr Palmer's treatment. Until that is established, we have to keep an open mind, though I do find it hard to believe that something as simple as redundant rectal mucosa can be responsible for the multiplicity of symptoms that is IBS. Surgery, especially when conducted by a listening, caring and charismatic exponent, is a powerful placebo, but if it works, we should not knock it too much.

Diverticular disease

Some patients with IBS have undergone surgical excision (removal) of the sigmoid colon, on the grounds that this region of the colon can appear on X-rays or motility recordings to be in spasm. I cannot think of any patient with IBS who has been cured by such treatment. Sigmoid resection, however, has been quite successful in some patients with diverticular disease, a condition where the hypertrophied (enlarged) muscle of the colon results in high pressures and forces out little pouches at weak points in the wall.

Diverticular disease is a disease of ageing, but it has been suggested that patients with long-standing IBS may be more likely to get diverticular disease earlier than usual – on the grounds, I suppose, that a stressed-out colon is more likely to age more rapidly than one that has not been subject to the vicissitudes of life. I suspect that the association between the two may be that the presence of diverticular disease can produce many of the symptoms of IBS. IBS is not just a disease of the rectum or sigmoid colon; in most patients, it seems to involve most regions of the gut and many other organs as well. For most people, IBS is a disease of the whole body.

Post-gastroenteritis IBS

'I know exactly when it started. I had been fishing with some friends in Norfolk. We were coming back along the motorway and we stopped in this café for a meal. I chose the fish. I knew there was something wrong with it, but I was hungry and I ate it. The next day I came down with the most awful diarrhoea and vomiting. It lasted three days and I felt really awful. The funny thing was that the diarrhoea never really cleared up. It's now three years later and I can still go five times in the morning, but them ketotifen tablets you gave me certainly make it much more bearable. I can even play a game of football now.'

Ray had post-gastroenteritis IBS. A biopsy of his rectum showed a lot of inflammatory cells. Our recent research at Sheffield has shown that about 30 per cent of people who have an attack of gastroenteritis go on to develop IBS. We have been interested to find out whether there is any particular factor that distinguishes these 30 per cent from the rest who do not get IBS, and our preliminary results suggest that psychological factors may make some people particularly susceptible to IBS. It seems that we cannot escape the notion of the mind/gut link even for the IBS that is induced by an attack of gastroenteritis.

Nevertheless, despite the possible psychological link, some of these patients respond very well to anti-inflammatory drugs similar to those used to treat asthma or ulcerative colitis. I have a few patients in whom the condition has been controlled by the drugs ketotifen or Asacol (mesalazine) for several years now. Every time I try to take them off the medication, or even replace it with an identical placebo, the symptoms come back with a vengeance; but they go away when I recommence the treatment.

Food allergy and food intolerance
The popularity of food allergy as a cause of IBS has waxed and waned according to the fashions of time and society. The occasional patient with IBS may indeed have a true food allergy, but I can only think of two such patients in over 20 years' experience of trying to help people with IBS. In both, the ingestion of one particular food constituent – shellfish and nuts respectively in these particular cases – caused the most extreme symptoms of vomiting and diarrhoea and general malaise.

Food intolerance is much more common, to the extent that perhaps everybody with IBS has this to a lesser or greater extent. Food is an extremely important trigger for IBS. It is as if the gut has become sensitive to anything that goes into it or comes out of it. We all know that when we have been out in the sun and our skin has become burnt and sensitive, putting on a shirt will be quite painful. In the same way, if your gut has become sensitive, eating food will cause pain and perhaps make the gut try to reject the offending substance by diarrhoea and vomiting, or suppressed forms of these symptoms like a more frequent desire to defecate and indigestion.

Of course, some foods are worse than others. That is not surprising, because we all know that certain foods – spices, fats, onions perhaps, bran or beans – can upset the most tolerant guts. So, if you have guts that are particularly sensitive, such foods are likely to cause excruciating symptoms and are best avoided. It is important to understand, however, that it is not so much the foods that are at fault, more a question of how sensitive the gut is to food in general, and this may vary. Just because that spaghetti bolognaise caused you to go to bed with stomach upset that night your mother came round to dinner, you don't necessarily have to avoid bolognaise sauce for ever. It is easy to fall into the pattern of avoiding so many different foods that you could be at serious risk of malnutrition.

This sometimes leads me to question why eating, normally an activity that engenders happiness, comfort and friendship, can become so strongly associated with so much fear and distress. Is this related to a disease of the gut, or is it the result of psychological conditioning by painful associations with food or its provider?

IBS – a gut reaction

'I am just terrified of food,' sobbed Mandy. 'I just had a piece of toast last night and it seemed to stick in my stomach, just there, and it causes the most awful wind.' She made some popping noises with her mouth, finishing off with an impressive belch.

Mandy's symptoms had commenced when she was pregnant but got much worse after her little girl, Lindy, was born. Mandy had hardly eaten anything for six weeks and was now just six stone in weight. She had never felt wanted as a child. She didn't know her father and her mother had struggled to bring up three of them on her income from the factory. With Michael out of work, Mandy just didn't know how she would cope with her own children Lindy and Ryan.

In a recent IBS meeting, we asked patients to draw a circle on a sheet of paper and write inside the circle all of the things that made them feel secure and outside the circle all the things that made them feel insecure. They all put 'mother' and 'food' outside the circle. Hardly a scientific study, I acknowledge; nevertheless guilt, anxiety, fear, even terror of eating seems to be an important feature of IBS for so many patients. No, I am not blaming Mum for IBS; not entirely, that is – it's much more complicated than that; but perhaps these observations help us to view IBS from a slightly different perspective. Perhaps we (as doctors) have contributed to the current confusion over IBS by attempting to medicalize it, and treat it with diet, drugs and surgery. To be successful, these approaches must be seen in the context of the personality and life experience of the patient.

This brings us on to the concept of IBS as a reaction of the gut to life events. This would explain quite a lot of things. It would, for example, explain the way in which symptoms can vary from day to day. It would also explain their often symbolic nature. It is amazing how often some of my patients will complain of being unable to 'stomach' the things that are happening to them in their lives when they are suffering nausea or vomiting, whereas other patients may sometimes express a great deal of anger ('getting rid of all that shit!') when they have diarrhoea. The notion of IBS as a gut reaction would also help us to understand why the symptoms tend to be intermittent and episodic, why patients can have good days and bad days, and how frequently recurrence of symptoms is related to life events or emotional upsets, tension, anxiety, depression, anger and so on. The gut can appear to be such a sensitive barometer to what is going on in life that at times it seems as if there is a direct link between the gut and the emotional part of the brain.

I do not think I necessarily see an unusual group of patients with irritable bowel syndrome; but, having given myself time to listen to them and find out about their lives, I am surprised and saddened by the burden of difficulty, tension and tragedy that many of them seem to have to shoulder and by how many have had to cope with the most awful experiences even from the early stages of childhood. Would I hear the same catalogue of tragedy if I interviewed a random sample of people living in Sheffield? Has life for everybody really become like a script from *EastEnders*? I find that difficult to believe. Several studies have shown that patients with IBS have more anxiety and more depression, and have experienced more severe life events than patients with organic gastrointestinal disease or healthy people.

I do not mean to imply by this that IBS is totally a psychological disease. I think it is a condition that lies between the mind and the gut, and may be initiated by mental or gastrointestinal upset but always involves both. When we bear in mind the strong links between the gut and the emotional side of the brain, it is likely that psychological factors will have a greater effect on a gut that has already been sensitized by disease. After all, we are very familiar with the nausea that can accompany anxiety, the diarrhoea that can accompany apprehension, the choking and difficulty we may have in swallowing when we are upset, the constipation associated with depression. These are aspects of everyday life; they just seem to be much worse in people with irritable bowel syndrome.

If the most useful way of regarding IBS is as a gut reaction, then there seem to be two treatment strategies. The first is to use specific drugs to treat the individual symptoms; the second is to use psychotherapeutic methods to deal with the gut/mind complex. Psychotherapeutic methods are tackled in Chapter 8 of this book, so here I will confine myself to a consideration of symptomatic treatment.

The treatment of symptoms

'The pains I call "the gripes" catch me under the ribs on the right side and cause me to double up and take my breath away. Colofac helps these but has no effect on the soreness or what I call "wind pains".'

> 'The only thing I can do when the pain is bad is to lie curled up in bed with a hot water bottle against my tummy.'

There is no therapeutic trial that has ever convincingly demonstrated the efficacy of any drug in IBS.

Abdominal pain

Anti-spasmodics are currently the mainstay of treatment of irritable bowel syndrome. The pain of IBS is thought to be related to spasm of the colonic muscle, and anti-spasmodics, as the name suggests, reduce the strength of gut contraction. There are several anti-spasmodics available; they vary in their potency and side-effects. Those that are most commonly prescribed include Colofac (mebeverin), Spasmanol (alverine citrate) and Buscopan (hyoscine butylbromide). Some – in particular Buscopan – may have side-effects such as a dry mouth, a little blurring of vision or difficulty in passing urine. Unfortunately, although they may take the edge off the pain, many patients do not seem to find them helpful. In recent years, products containing peppermint oil (Colpermin or Mintec) have become available for treating IBS. Some patients like these, but in general, they do not seem to be particularly effective, although patients who suffer with flatulence may notice that their anal expulsions smell more sweetly of peppermint.

> 'The anti-spasmodic tablets helped a little, but I still knew that it was my own mind that could cure it and not tablets. I am trying to keep off any kind of treatment as I do not wish to be on tablets for the rest of my life, but if I'm bad one day, I will take an anti-spasmodic tablet, which aids me a little. I realize I have got to control my feelings.'
>
> 'I take one sachet of Regulan (bulk filler), two or three Spasmonal capsules (anti-spasmodic) and one Colpermin (peppermint) capsule a day. The treatment does not completely eliminate or alleviate the problems of IBS. I still have frequent pain, discomfort and feel very unwell.'

In Susan Backhouse and Christine Dancey's survey of IBS sufferers, most people did not feel that, on its own, anti-spasmodic medication helped them a great deal. According to Susan and Christine, this ties in with scientific studies showing that combined treatment (e.g. anti-spasmodic, bulk filler, tranquillizer) gives better results than any one medication alone. It is interesting that, although anti-spasmodic drugs are by far the most commonly prescribed drug, many sufferers seem to try to control their symptoms without the drugs, and prefer to resort to them when the symptoms are especially bad.

More general painkillers – such as paracetamol, codeine phosphate and Distalgesic and, particularly, the stronger ones such as morphine and Temgesic – have a constipating action. Constipation makes patients with IBS very uncomfortable, so taking these analgesics may create a particularly vicious cycle of pain and constipation.

Chronic pain is exhausting; it saps confidence and self-esteem and creates depression. Painkillers may help, but are best kept for emergencies only. Pain is a lot worse if you are anxious or tense. Taking time to relax and rest, maybe with a hot water bottle held close to the abdomen, can help. Relaxation and self-hypnosis tapes can be especially useful. Acupuncture and skin stimulation with TENS machines can also help some people.

Diarrhoea

Diarrhoea can be treated with substances such as loperamide (Imodium), Lomotil or codeine phosphate. These are quite powerful and can arrest the flow of the most severe diarrhoea. Unfortunately, patients with bad IBS often find that treatment of their diarrhoea with these agents is complicated by a very marked increase in abdominal pain, as if the diarrhoea had been responsible in some way for relieving the tension within the bowel. Too many anti-diarrhoeal tablets can lead to constipation, and alternating between diarrhoea and constipation is even less pleasant than having either symptom alone.

The most commonly taken drug for diarrhoea is Imodium (loperamide), which can also be bought over the counter as

Arrete. Imodium slows down the passage of waste through the system, increases absorption of water and can be very useful if you suffer from urgency or faecal incontinence. Imodium acts on the gut alone and is not absorbed into the system, so side-effects are unlikely. Lomotil and (particularly) codeine phosphate are absorbed and can cause side-effects of drowsiness or dizziness, and even dependency. All of these drugs are members of the opiate family, like morphine, and those that are absorbed into the system are potentially addictive, though not nearly to the same extent as morphine or heroin.

Questran, as indicated above, can be quite useful in treating frequent watery diarrhoea but is poorly tolerated by most patients with IBS. Bulking agents such as Fybogel, Regulan or Celevac have been advocated for use in diarrhoea as well as constipation on the grounds that they mop up excess fluid. My impression, however, is that they often tend to make the diarrhoea of IBS worse rather than better.

'I've got all the drugs, but I try not to take them. However, they're there if I need them. I don't like the effects of some, but I keep the anti-diarrhoeal tablets with me at all times. They always work.'

'I carry an anti-diarrhoeal drug wherever I go. I always feel safe with them, because they work like a dream.'

'I eat arrowroot thickened with juice – I read about it somewhere. It's really helped my diarrhoea.'

If you suffer from diarrhoea, consider whether you want to ask for an anti-diarrhoeal drug. Many of Susan and Christine's respondents said that they do not like taking drugs. However, many people find that, once they know they can take the tablets if they need to, they no longer need them!

Constipation

The constipation of IBS can usually be treated quite simply with extra fibre in the diet from cereals, fruit and vegetables, or by taking bulking agents. Regulan, Metamucil, Fybogel and Isogel are the most commonly taken; whichever is used, it is important to take it with plenty of water. Linseeds, which can be bought from health food shops, have the same effect. Tolerance to these various substances seems to vary. For some reason I do not understand, my patients seem to prefer Regulan to Fybogel.

Bulking agents ease the passage of waste matter through the system by retaining water and thus making the stools softer and easier to expel. Unfortunately, as explained above, they produce gas, causing distension and may make symptoms of abdominal pain, bloating, flatulence and diarrhoea much worse. Not surprisingly, the sensitive guts of IBS sufferers do not tolerate 'roughage' and gaseous distension very well. It is necessary to experiment with the dose of these agents to obtain the optimum benefit.

Irritant laxatives – such as Sennokot, Dulco-Lax and Normacol Plus – act by stimulating strong propulsive contractions in the colon. They may have to be given to get the really stubborn gut going, but because they can produce the most excruciating spasms in the sensitive colons of patients with IBS, it is best to avoid them if at all possible. Often anti-spasmodics have to be taken to relieve the discomfort of the laxatives.

Duphalac (lactulose) is an osmotic laxative: it encourages the secretion of fluid into the bowel and flushes out the obstruction. In the colon, it is fermented to produce a lot of gas. Patients with IBS do not tolerate lactulose very well. The sweet syrup often produces feelings of nausea, and the gas production causes cramping, flatulence and bloating.

The guts of people with IBS are often as sensitive to medications as they are to foods. Even a mild laxative agent such as lactulose or a bulk filler may tip them over into the most painful wind and diarrhoea. It is not just a mechanical problem of getting the dose right; it seems as if the sensitive and turbulent guts of IBS are not going to respond to a simple exercise in hydraulics.

Very few of Susan and Christine's respondents said they took laxatives. People who suffered from constipation tended to try to remedy it by eating high-fibre diets, taking bulk fillers and drinking plenty of fluids. Around 20 million laxatives are sold in Britain each year; about one in five of the population take them but many people keep quiet about their need for them.

Susan and Christine also report that the Eating Disorders Association are anxious that people do not abuse laxatives. They say that such abuse causes dehydration, which can have serious effects on the body – for instance, it can damage vital organs like the kidneys. What is more relevant to IBS sufferers, however, is that laxative abuse can cause permanent damage to the bowel, and prolonged use of laxatives has been linked with bowel tumours. In a survey conducted by the Eating Disorders Association among their members, nearly three-quarters had abused, or were currently abusing, laxatives. The survey also revealed many side-effects of laxative abuse including nausea, diarrhoea, constipation, flatulence and digestive difficulties. There were cases of IBS and anal bleeding which members felt were brought on or exacerbated by laxative abuse.

For constipation, quite a few of IBS Network members recommended eating linseed:

'You sprinkle it on cereal or on yoghurt. You can just swallow it. It doesn't help with the pain but it does help with the constipation. You're supposed to eat one tablespoon three times a day, but I find once a day is enough – it works gently, not like laxatives. This is the only thing I find that works, and I tried everything.'

'You buy it from a health shop. It certainly helps with the constipation, it makes you go naturally – not like some laxatives you can get.'

Gassy symptoms

These are often difficult to treat. There is no definitive treatment for bloating, distension and flatulence, although I often advise patients to cut down on gas-forming foods such as fruit, beans and other pulses, vegetables and cereal fibre (all the stuff that nutritionists have been telling us for 20 years is good!), and avoid bulk-forming laxatives such as Regulan. As explained above, some of the gassiest people in the world are intolerant of milk sugar or lactose: it is always important to enquire about the intake of milk or milk products since a reduction can alleviate this symptom quite remarkably.

Treatments for gas are more a matter of avoiding certain foods than taking medicines to absorb gases. Charcoal biscuits and simethicone are prescribed for excessive gas, though I have yet to meet anybody who has said these treatments are effective. But help may be on the way. Beano – no, not the comic – contains the enzyme alpha-galactosidase that breaks down vegetable fibre in the small intestine and leads to the absorption of sugars without the formation of gas. According to the *New York Times*:

> Studies sponsored by the manufacturer, anecdotal reports from scores of people who tried it on their own and personal experience strongly suggest that use of the product, aptly dubbed beano, can greatly reduce the gaseous legacy of many vegetable foods.

Beano is not available on prescription and is not to my knowledge marketed in the UK, but if experience in the United States continues to be so positive, it will certainly come here.

According to Susan Backhouse and Christine Dancey, there is research to show that excessive gas production associated with carbohydrate intolerance can contribute to symptoms in certain individuals. Carbohydrates and sugars cannot be digested in the small bowel and so they pass into the colon where they are readily fermented, yielding hydrogen and carbon dioxide (gas). Just in case this applies to you, try cutting down the amount of sugars you consume in drinks, cakes, biscuits, sweets, etc. However, the main culprit here could be wheat products. Cutting out wheat in the diet is fairly difficult to do, but might be worth a try. Rice products are a good substitute for wheat.

There are various home remedies that IBS Network members have experimented with, including peppermint tea and fennel tea – again, anything as innocuous as this is probably worth a try. If you ask your GP to prescribe something for flatulence, he or she may suggest peppermint oil. This comes in small capsules and can be bought without prescription at most health shops. Cinnamon, cloves and ginger also help bring up gas. The author

W. Grant Thompson warns that heartburn is sometimes worsened by taking peppermint. One GP suggested some yoga positions and exercises; this was also put forward in Shirley Trickett's book *IBS and Diverticulosis: A self-help plan*.

Thompson, in his book *Gut Reactions: Understanding symptoms of the digestive tract* (Plenum Press, 1989), devotes a whole chapter to 'burbulence' – wind, belching, gurgling and farting. He explains how these phenomena occur, and how we can help ourselves become less 'burbulent'. For instance, he recommends leaving out fizzy drinks, soufflés and whipped desserts – anything to reduce swallowing air. Susan and Christine suggest that IBS sufferers don't chew gum, smoke, or talk too much when eating. They should also try to minimize the gastric trapping of air, and avoid foods which lead to flatulence, such as beans. A high-fibre diet may make flatulence worse.

Some patients report that wind is their most difficult symptom:

'The main symptom is wind. I do get a lot of pain, but the wind is not only painful, it's embarrassing. In shops and in other people's houses, I frequently have to go to the toilet or go outside. In public, where sometimes I haven't been able to help myself, I see people looking at me as if I'm disgusting. But I can't help it. I just can't. And the doctors can't seem to do anything for wind. They think I'm over-exaggerating it, that I'm neurotic. After all, wind isn't life-threatening – when people have cancer and road accidents, what's a bit of wind? But they don't have to live with it day after day.'

Balancing symptomatic treatment

Symptomatic treatment is very much a question of balance: fibre improves constipation but makes distension worse, loperamide helps diarrhoea but may worsen pain, painkillers help pain but worsen constipation. This causes frustration for both the patient and the doctor. The patient feels that the doctor has really not understood the condition, while the doctor is frustrated by the inability of the conventional medical model, in which he or she has trained, to deal with the large numbers of patients that seem to suffer from gut reactions.

The placebo problem

One of the most striking phenomena associated with IBS is its high placebo reactivity. This is the problem that has bedevilled most therapeutic trials in IBS. How can you demonstrate that the new wonder drug, Polodium, is effective against the abdominal pain of irritable bowel syndrome when a so-called 'inactive' placebo relieves pain in up to 60 per cent of sufferers? The wonder drug would have to relieve more than 80 per cent of patients before we could be sure it was effective, and there is no anti-spasmodic or analgesic as good as that. It is said, on not terribly good evidence, that the 'placebo effect' wears off after about three months. That seems to correspond with my own experience.

> 'You know them tablets, that you gave me last time, doctor? Well, I thought we'd cracked it. I were marvellous the first week, then the pain came back a bit and now I feel just as bad as I did when I first came to see you.'

This is so soul-destroying, not only for the patient but for the doctor as well. What does he or she do? Try another tablet with the almost certain knowledge that the same thing will happen? Is it any wonder that both partners in this therapeutic interaction are frustrated? The most important thing is to avoid the spiral of care that can lead to surgical mutilation, extreme diets and colonic lavage. But that seems very negative and defensive. Is there a more positive approach?

Placebo responsiveness is linked to the power of suggestion, so perhaps it is possible to harness this suggestion to produce more prolonged relief. This is why hypnotherapy is such a powerful and useful method of managing IBS (*see* Chapter 9). It works, not by punitive dieting, invasive testing, traumatic surgery or poisonous drugs, but by quelling fear, establishing confidence and providing support. Whoever said that medicines had to be nasty anyway? Symptoms do not have to be tortured into submission. Their fear and anger can be quelled with kindness.

Treating the mind/gut axis

To date, the most effective means of managing irritable bowel syndrome have been psychotherapeutic techniques. In patients with mild forms of irritable bowel that come on in discrete attacks associated with life events, treatment may simply take the form of empathy, insight and advice. However, to undertake this effectively, doctors and other health workers need time to establish effective rapport with the patient, and unfortunately time is one commodity that is in very short supply in our current National Health Service. Other patients may be treated with tranquillizers or anti-depressants. Sleep disturbance is very common in patients with IBS, and many patients take sleeping tablets. Patients with particularly disturbing or chronic symptoms may benefit from more intensive forms of psychotherapy. These include bowel-directed hypnotherapy (*see* Chapter 9), exploratory dynamic psychotherapy and cognitive-behavioural therapy (*see* Chapter 8). The cost-effectiveness of these forms of therapy may be enhanced if they are carried out with groups of patients rather than on an individual basis.

Tranquillizers and anti-depressants
Tranquillizers are often prescribed for sufferers of IBS, and they can be helpful. Librium (chlordiazepoxide) and Valium (diazepam) are the most familiar – the 'mother's little helpers' of the Rolling Stones song. These drugs have come in for a good deal of adverse publicity in recent years, and rightly so. Some experts say that tranquillizers don't help with the stress that is often associated with IBS because they often reduce the capacity to deal with problems. They also induce dependence, and when somebody successfully stops taking them, the withdrawal symptoms can be extremely troublesome. They should therefore only be prescribed in short-term treatments. Side-effects include drowsiness, confusion, unsteadiness, visual disturbances,

alterations in sex drive and retention of urine. More benefit is obtained by relaxation or stress-management techniques and the opportunity to discuss problems and stresses with a trained counsellor. Adult education classes in stress management and relaxation are quite common around the country.

Depression is very commonly associated with IBS, and anti-depressant medication can be very useful, especially when combined with practical help to sort out problems and deal with stresses. Anti-depressant medicines are particularly useful in patients with severe chronic pain, as they seem to have a rather specific effect on pain perception. Anti-depressant drugs differ in their strength and side-effects, but they do not seem to be blighted by the same degree of dependency and withdrawal problems as tranquillizers. The drugs commonly prescribed to IBS patients include Prothiaden (dothiepin), Tofranil (imipramine) and Tryptizol (amitryptiline). They all cause side-effects of dry mouth, constipation, blurred vision, drowsiness, dizziness, weight change and loss of sex drive. Bolvidon is a new type of drug with fewer side-effects, though drowsiness can still be a problem.

Many IBS sufferers, report Susan Backhouse and Christine Dancey, will not want to take anti-depressants or tranquillizers because this confirms their fear that IBS is 'all in the mind'. Such medication, however, may be useful in the short term if only because they help you cope with the anxiety you are bound to feel with a disorder such as IBS, although they also have a direct relaxing effect on the gut itself. Nevertheless, the worry about dependency and side-effects may mean you don't want to risk taking them. Tranquillizers and/or anti-depressants were prescribed to a third of the people that Susan and Christine talked to during the course of their research.

It is important that you do not feel pressurized into taking tranquillizers or anti-depressants. Remember you have a choice, and make sure you discuss any reservations you have about your treatments with your doctor.

According to a comparison of various treatments for IBS, reported in the *British Medical Journal* in 1980, a combined treatment programme works best – i.e. a tranquillizer or anti-depressant, smooth muscle relaxant and a bulking agent. However, not all people who receive this treatment experience a sustained improvement in their symptoms.

Hope for the future

Drugs for the mind/gut
Our knowledge about the way that the mind and brain may influence the gut is increasing very rapidly, and it is possible that, in the future, there may be drugs that act on the brain to calm down the irritable gut. In fact, some recent research has shown that a substance called leuprolide, which acts on the hypothalamus at the base of the brain to influence the release of sex steroids, can calm down gut reactions in women. This discovery may help to explain why irritable bowel syndrome and other gut reactions appear to be more common in women than they are in men. Other substances currently being investigated act on the gut to reduce sensitivity, rather like anaesthetics. Ondansetron is one of these substances, but is currently only available for the treatment of vomiting induced by chemotherapy; fedotizine is another. By reducing gut feelings, these agents may also reduce gut reactions, including emotional consequences.

The link between the gut and emotions goes both ways: emotional upsets appear to be able to make the gut more sensitive and reactive, and gut sensations can influence our emotions, pain inducing anxiety and satiety being associated with a feeling of sleepiness and calm. I feel that there will be some exciting developments in our understanding of the relationship between the brain and the gut in the near future.

'Breaking the mould'
The major difficulty in managing irritable bowel syndrome is the sheer number of patients with the condition. It has been estimated that about 50 per cent of referrals to gastroenterologists suffer from 'gut reactions' such as IBS, non-specific indigestion, chronic

abdominal pain, chronic constipation, chronic diarrhoea and so on. Bearing in mind how difficult it is to treat these conditions by a medical model, this is an enormous burden on the health services. No wonder doctors and patients become frustrated. Is there another way of dealing with the problem? I think there is – namely, to work with groups to educate and provide insights into the management of IBS.

There is no standard way of conducting group management of IBS. The model we have developed in our department at Sheffield incorporates between eight and ten evening meetings, each lasting about two to two-and-a-half hours. The first two meetings are educational and use visual aids as well as discussion to explore areas such as: what is IBS? when should you be worried that this is not IBS and something that needs further investigation? the role of diet in IBS; the role of stress; medical management; stress management and relaxation. These educational sessions are aimed at enabling patients to manage the disease themselves. In the remaining sessions, they are encouraged to think about their symptoms in relation to their life experiences. We have used a number of devices to encourage this. The circle of security, described above in relation to 'mother' and 'food', is one. In another exercise, patients draw an outline of themselves and, within each part of the body, put a diagrammatic representation of what that part feels like. These simple techniques often generate discussion of the symbolic significance of the symptoms in relation to previous life events. At the end of each group session, there is a period of relaxation; it is possible that simple hypnotic techniques could be used to enhance this.

These groups need not be run by consultants or medical experts in IBS; they could be run by members of the health team who have had some training in counselling and group skills. After a time, they could be facilitated by patients who have been members of previous groups. The idea is that the groups would be seeded by the team and would then propagate throughout the region. This is an area where health workers and patient self-help groups could work together very successfully. Our initial results are encouraging.

Conclusion

I feel that the way in which diseases such as irritable bowel syndrome are regarded by patients and doctors alike is undergoing a quiet revolution. There is a growing realization that the conventional and traditional management of IBS according to a medical model does not really work. Doctors, therapists and other health workers need to work with patient self-help groups to bring about a change in the management of the condition. Self-help groups such as the IBS Network are in the vanguard of this movement, and can help to bring about this change. It is very important, however, that they work in collaboration with health workers. The medical model may be criticized for being patriarchal and closed-minded, but self-help without training and guidance can lead to confusion.

To my mind, we are more certain now of what IBS is and how to manage it than we have ever been. Over the last 30 years or so, IBS has been regarded as a disease of fibre deficiency, a motility disorder and a disturbance of gastrointestinal sensitivity; but now it is being increasingly regarded as a psychosomatic condition: either the gastrointestinal expression of psychic conflict, in which mental torment is focused on the gut because it is intolerable to accept it in the mind; or a gut sensitized by disease to the gut-wrenching influence of psychological factors. In my experience, the former seems more likely, but this is the one that is rejected by many IBS sufferers. Indeed, it would have to be: somebody who has subconsciously converted suppressed traumatic experience into gut symptoms to avoid intense anxiety or depression is likely to resist strenuously attempts to unmask any psychological mechanism that may lie behind the symptoms. Talking to patients with IBS can be like opening Pandora's box; the most awful tragedies and problems lie buried in there. Would the same problems exist in representative samples of healthy people or patients with other gastrointestinal disorders such as Crohn's disease? Is this just what our life is in post-industrial societies? I do not think so. Studies have shown that patients with IBS seem to have experienced more traumatic life events than patients with other gastrointestinal disease or healthy subjects.

The management of IBS can appear to be in a state of confusion because health workers and patients shy away from seeing it for what it is – a disease at the interaction of the mind and the gut. Such conditions have long been regarded as not being 'proper diseases', and patients dismissed with the admonition that they should 'pull themselves together'. It is time that IBS is treated seriously without fear or prejudice. It is not the patient that is the failure; it is the medical model that is inappropriate. Acknowledgement of this must pave the way for more sympathetic and effective treatment.

Chapter 7

Dietary Treatment of IBS

Alan Stewart and Maryon Stewart

Irritable bowel syndrome is a very common condition that, though not life-threatening, can have a profound effect on the quality of life. There are numerous ideas as to its causes. Many experts, however, are of the opinion that IBS is commonly influenced by two main external factors: stress, and what we eat. Both these factors have the potential to influence the normal functioning of the muscles in the bowel and thereby influence the symptoms of IBS.

The evidence that IBS or the symptoms of IBS are influenced by what you eat comes essentially from three different types of studies: studies that look at the effect of fibre-rich foods on the gut in healthy people and those with IBS; studies of diets that initially exclude a large number of foods and try to determine the influence of individual foods or food groups when they are reintroduced into the diet; and studies that look at the effect of individual foods on gut function, either in the normal population or in those with a bowel problem (but not always IBS). These rather mixed sources of information now allow us to have some idea of the role that diet can play in IBS.

An important and sometimes confusing issue is that of food intolerance and food allergy. There is much controversy as to how common genuine adverse reactions to food are. The word 'allergy' is reserved for those reactions that involve the person's immune system, such as those that occur in asthma, eczema and nettle-rash, and sometimes with bowel-related problems. True food allergy can be immediate, as in reactions to peanuts causing lip swelling and asthma, or delayed, taking perhaps several days before there is a discernible reaction to cow's milk protein or wheat. This can sometimes be the case in IBS. More common, though, are food 'intolerances', where eating or drinking the item in question can result in bowel or other symptoms. The immune system is not involved and the adverse reaction involves a chemical effect of the food – as, for example, when the caffeine in tea and coffee aggravates anxiety, causes palpitations or influences some bowel symptoms. The cow's milk sugar, lactose, is not digested by some and consequently stimulates diarrhoea because it chemically attracts water into the gut. This is an example of an inability to tolerate a certain chemical component of a food. Intolerances can occur to a number of dietary items, and these may be factors in an unknown proportion of those with IBS.

In an ideal world, there would be some simple test that would provide us with a quick and accurate assessment of food allergies and intolerances. This is not the case, nor is it likely to be so in the near future. Very often an assessment of these problems is first made by the person following a 'few foods' diet or an exclusion diet for two or three weeks. Such diets are typically composed of some meats, a few fruits and vegetables, rice instead of wheat and bread, soya milk instead of cow's, and water instead of tea and coffee. If benefit is obtained, after a short while the careful introduction of specific excluded foods at three- to four-day intervals may allow the sufferer to identify those dietary elements that aggravate their symptoms. Certain food allergies can be assessed by use of blood and skin tests, but these are not frequently undertaken.

It would seem from published research that this type of approach has achieved significant success in treating IBS. Such diets are best followed under the supervision of an experienced doctor or dietetic adviser, though more simple versions may not always require this. They should not be undertaken without medical assessment and guidance by those who are underweight, children, pregnant or breastfeeding women, the elderly, those with a history of eating disorders or serious depression, diabetics or anyone with any serious current illness. Additionally, those who have lost weight, have been eating poorly, are already on a restricted diet or have symptoms suggestive of nutritional deficiencies such as fatigue, depression, recurrent mouth ulcers, cracking of the lips or muscle pains may well need nutritional supplementation. The need for this should be assessed before an exclusion diet is undertaken and medical involvement is again necessary.

To make sense of the use of dietary manipulation in treating IBS, we need to look at the symptoms of irritable bowel and how they are caused. However, before leaving the topic of allergy and intolerance we must point out an important guiding principle. There is an enormous amount of individual variation in reactions to foods. This means that two people with IBS, even two who have the same symptoms, may respond to quite different dietary measures. One may respond to one kind of dietary change and the other may respond to a different diet, or may not benefit at all from dietary manipulation but may gain from some other type of approach. It is individual assessment that seems to produce the best results.

Diet and the symptoms of IBS

By understanding how the symptoms of IBS can be caused, we can gain some insight as to how our diet – and, in particular, how some particular foods and beverages – may cause or contribute to their production.

The symptoms of IBS have been described in Chapter 1 of this book. To summarize, the common features of the condition are: abdominal pain; a change in frequency of bowel movement, either diarrhoea or constipation; a change in stool consistency; a change in how it feels to pass stools; passage of mucus in stools; slime in the stool; and abominal bloating (usually with wind).

Looking at these one by one, we can suggest likely explanations.

Pain

The pain felt in IBS can be anything from a mild ache to a severe cramp and can be felt almost anywhere in the abdomen or it can be felt as low back or pelvic pain. This pain seems to be mainly due to an excessive build-up in pressure in the gut when the muscles of the gut fail to contract in a smooth and regular fashion. A wave of contraction passing down the gut reaches a segment which is already in spasm. There is then a substantial rise in pressure inside the gut as the 'unstoppable force' meets the 'immovable object'. A high level of pressure inside the gut itself tenses the wall and this causes pain.

This explanation as to the cause of the pain has been confirmed by experiments in which volunteers have swallowed a fine tube with a balloon on the end. When this is inflated, it presses on the walls of the intestine and causes pain. Often a point somewhere in the small bowel can be found where inflation of the balloon exactly reproduces the pain that that person experiences as part of his or her IBS. So pain can be due to a rise in pressure inside the gut.

In those with true food allergy, there can be a release of chemicals from the wall of the bowel that produce inflammation. These chemicals are the same as those that are produced in arthritis and other situations where the tissues are irritated and trying to heal. They could certainly contribute to or aggravate the pain of IBS.

Diarrhoea

The term 'diarrhoea' is used to describe excessively frequent or loose bowel movements. 'Frequent' means more than three stools per day, and 'loose' means anything from the consistency of soft putty to watery. Diarrhoea mainly comes about because food has moved too quickly through the gut so that there has not been time for the water in the bowel to be absorbed. Though you might think that diarrhoea would often be accompanied by an increase in the activity of the muscles of the gut, this does not appear always to be the case: the gut muscles may be *less* active as food passes through unimpeded by gut contractions.

Diarrhoea can certainly be due to dietary factors, including:

- true food allergy, where there is a reaction to a food involving the immune system as in reaction to wheat protein or cow's milk protein.
- food intolerance, where the food may irritate the gut without involving the immune system, perhaps because of an inability to digest and absorb the food or part of it, as in lactose (cow's milk sugar) intolerance or fruit sugar intolerance.
- a direct chemical or drug-like effect on the gut, as with tea or coffee.

Diarrhoea, if prolonged, could lead to a lack of some nutrients, but this rarely occurs in IBS.

Constipation

Constipation is defined as infrequent passage of stools, usually three times a week or fewer, but may also refer to difficult or incomplete evacuation of the bowels. It is a common problem for those living in industrialized countries. Modern lifestyles, with a relatively poor intake of fibre-rich foods and a low level of physical activity, are thought by many to be important in the development of constipation, with or without the other features of IBS.

Constipation is due not to lack of muscle activity but rather to the wrong kind. There would appear to be a lack of regular coordinated waves of relaxation and contraction passing along the gut. Instead, there may be areas of heightened activity resulting in spasm, which may then impede the regular gut action. Furthermore, the muscles at the lower end of the bowel that you use to help push when you open your bowels may not be very strong, or conversely may be in spasm, too. So constipation in IBS may signify disturbance in muscle function.

Constipation can result from a variety of dietary factors, including:

- a lack of fibre-rich foods, the bulk of which in the large bowel helps to stimulate normal waves of muscle activity.

- food allergy, when irritation of the bowel might induce localized spasm that interferes with normal bowel muscle activity.
- possibly a lack of other factors in our diet, such as foods that are natural laxatives and vegetables that are rich not only in fibre but also in magnesium, a traditional and simple laxative.

There is another aspect to severe constipation, especially in women, that deserves consideration. A number of studies have revealed that this symptom can be associated with other health problems, including breast lumps and precancerous changes in breast tissue; hormonal abnormalities (e.g. low oestrogen level); more painful and irregular periods; a greater chance of hysterectomy or operation for a cyst on the ovary; pain on intercourse and difficulty achieving orgasm; infertility; hesitancy in starting to pass water; cold hands and a tendency to faint. Curiously, the group of women who suffer with these problems do not tend to eat less fibre than other women. These diverse health problems can be explained by the important part that the bowel plays in the metabolism (breaking down) of the female sex hormone, oestrogen. Many of the women who suffer from these conditions appear to have poorly coordinated and excessive contraction of the muscles around the lower end of the bowel, vagina and bladder.

Wind and bloating
Excessive wind and abdominal bloating are common symptons that often go together. By wind is meant flatus, or gas passed through the back passage. Burping or, to give it its medical term, eructation, can also occur as part of IBS and is usually due to the swallowing of air.

Flatus comes from the breakdown of food residues in the colon and also from the residue of mucus or digestive slime and juices that our own intestines produce. Gases are produced by the billions of mainly friendly bacteria that inhabit our large colon. They are found only in very small amounts in the small bowel where the majority of digestion and absorption of nutrients takes place. They first appear in any quantity in the caecum, the first part of the large bowel. Here the bacteria are waiting to see what will turn up in the form of leftovers from the meal that you have eaten several hours before. This normally constitutes about 5–10 per cent of our intake of fat, protein and carbohydrate as well as all of the fibre. The bacteria break down the fibre and food residues, releasing a small amount of energy and some acids, and producing gases that our own cells are, for the most part, incapable of producing. These include hydrogen, methane and some carbon dioxide, all of which have no smell. In some people and under certain circumstances, the 'bad-eggs' gas, hydrogen sulphide, is produced – an event with which some of us are doubtless familiar. Also in the colon, a large amount of water and a small amount of some minerals are slowly absorbed.

There is quite a lot of activity in the normal colon, then. We all have some wind; the degree and type depend on:

- the type of food eaten, especially whether fibre-rich foods are included.
- how well the food is digested in the small bowel.
- how quickly food and food residues pass through the small bowel to reach the colon.
- the type of bacteria present in the colon.
- whether you have eaten foods to which you are allergic or intolerant.

The fibre question
Until the late 1970s, IBS was commonly considered to be best treated by a diet *low* in 'roughage' (vegetable fibre). Then came the observations of Dr Painter, a British naval surgeon, who noticed the association between a high-fibre intake and an absence of many of the diseases of civilization, of which IBS is one. Perhaps, it began to be thought, a lack of fibre might be the cause of irritable bowel? In recent years, a number of experts and expert committees have recommended that the British population as a whole should increase its fibre intake by about 40 per cent. This would mean eating on average about 40 per cent more fruit, vegetables and

cereals (bread and other foods containing wheat, oat, barley, rye and sweet corn/maize).

Several studies have also shown that the larger the intake of dietary fibre, the larger is the resultant output of stool; and the larger the output of stool, the quicker is the passage of food from one end of the body to the other, known as the 'gut transit time'. However, not everyone obeys these simple rules. Girls' bowels move more slowly than boys', and some girls have very slow bowels despite a reasonable fibre intake. So, though increasing fibre intake always increases the weight of the stool, the effect of this can be quite variable, and as you may already know, fibre is not always the answer to constipation and IBS.

Individual foods/drinks and IBS

Now we can look at how particular foods might be contributing to some of your IBS symptoms. In the sections that follow we will give you enough information to make what is essentially an informed guess about different foods and beverages. Remember that the biggest unknown factor in all of this is your particular, individual response to a particular food. So the acid test is: how does it affect *you* when you eat it?

Milk Milk can cause bowel problems – and, in particular, diarrhoea – in one of two ways. Some people, especially children and infants, may react to the protein in milk and this can cause abdominal pain (or colic in an infant), and sometimes diarrhoea. Other signs of allergy may be eczema, asthma or a blocked or runny nose.

Sometimes there can be a problem with milk sugar (lactose). If this cannot be digested, the sugar passes into the small bowel and colon, where it acts as a potent laxative. The severely affected sufferer is frequently troubled with diarrhoea, often with wind, within a hour of consuming milk or soft cheese. Hard cheese or small amounts of milk may be tolerated. This type of food intolerance is quite common in those of East European, Middle Eastern or Asian origin, and in others following an episode of acute gastroenteritis. Drinking skimmed or semi-skimmed milk makes no difference to either cow's milk protein or lactose intolerance as it is only the fat content that is reduced in these milks, not the protein or sugar content.

Constipation seems to be less of a problem but is certainly possible in those with cow's milk protein intolerance.

Wheat and other grains It now seems that wheat, together with the other grains, oats, barley and rye, which all contain a protein called gluten, is one of the foods that most aggravates the symptoms of IBS. This has been found in studies of food intolerance where an exclusion diet has been used, but has also been recorded as a cause of diarrhoea, especially in women. This situation is similar to, but distinct from, coeliac disease, in which gluten sensitivity is severe, resulting in damage to the lining of the intestine.

Together with diarrhoea, there is often weight loss, anaemia and nutritional deficiencies; constipation can also be a problem, or indeed there may be a combination of the two. Other studies have shown that there is a slowing in the rate at which the stomach empties when whole wheat is eaten, while the high-fibre content of whole wheat and wheat bran may speed passage through the colon (large bowel).

Although the first study of the use of wheat bran in treating IBS showed an improvement for most, it was not good for all: some in particular noticed an increase in pain. Subsequently other doctors have revealed a very mixed picture, with extra wheat bran likely to worsen abdominal bloating and wind but to ease constipation. Its only definite use is against simple constipation, but even here it may not suit everyone.

The fibre from fruit and vegetables is just as effective as grain fibre, comes with a good amount and variety of vitamins and minerals, and seems less likely to aggravate IBS symptoms in the majority of patients.

Finally, if you are very sensitive to these grains you may also need to be wary of 'modified starch', shown on the ingredients list of many prepared foods, which may be made from wheat and still cause problems in the very sensitive.

Sweet corn Maize or sweet corn can also cause problems. It may be tolerated by those who cannot take wheat, oat barley and rye as it does not contain gluten. However, some people do not get on well with it. It is hard to digest unless it is chewed well; indeed, a simple way of working out how long it takes for food to get from one end to the other is to eat sweet corn and not chew it – but watch out for the wind. Cornflakes are made from maize and are often a safe alternative for those who cannot take wheat or oats, but some will still have problems.

Tea Our favourite beverage does not escape without comment. A study by Scandinavian doctors showed that about half of a group of normal subjects experienced a change in the rate at which food moved through the gut when they replaced their intake of water with tea. For the other half, there was no difference. No wonder constipation is described as 'the English disease'. It is likely that, if you are a regular tea drinker and suffer from constipation as part of your IBS, cutting down on your tea intake and eating a high-fibre diet will be of some benefit. Remember to reduce your tea consumption gradually over a week or two, though, otherwise a caffeine withdrawal headache may well result.

Coffee This extremely popular beverage is also an excellent bowel stimulant. Both ordinary and decaffeinated coffee have effects on the gut, one of which is to stimulate a wave of contraction along the bowel. Many people use a cup of coffee as a way of helping them to go to the toilet. For some, however, it can actually be a cause of diarrhoea: so if you have diarrhoea and you drink coffee, you should cut down or stop completely – even decaffeinated coffee can affect the gut.

Hot drinks in general can also stimulate a wave of contraction through the bowel, so again it may be necessary to limit the number of such drinks that you have.

Alcohol Alcohol, too, can sometimes cause diarrhoea, though this is usually likely to happen only in those who drink very heavily. The safe limit for men is three units per day and for women it

Table 1: A summary of the possible influence of individual foods on the symptoms of IBS

Food/Beverage	Symptom		
	Constipation	**Diarrhoea**	**Wind**
Cow's milk	Rarely	Due to lactose intolerance	As for diarrhoea
Wheat, especially wholewheat and wheat bran	Surprisingly common	Certainly	With diarrhoea or constipation
Oats, barley and rye	As for wheat but usually less marked		
Sweet corn (maize)	–	Especially if not well chewed	As for diarrhoea
Tea	Definitely	–	–
Coffee	–	Definitely	Possibly
Alcohol	Unlikely	Definitely	Possible 'bad eggs'
Yeast-rich foods	Uncertain	Possible	–
Fruits generally	Unlikely	Too much fruit sugar (fructose)	As for diarrhoea
Citrus fruits	Unlikely	Possible	–
Honey	Unlikely	If you eat a lot	–
Sugar (sucrose)	–	Very rarely	–
Sorbitol (sweetener)	–	If you eat too much	–
Beans	Unlikely	Especially if not cooked thoroughly	Very possible
Onions	–	Possible	Possible 'bad eggs'
Green vegetables	Unlikely	Possible	Quite possible
Fatty foods	Unlikely	Possible if rapid gut transit	As for diarrhoea
Eggs	According to folklore	Possible but rare?	Quite possible
Anything else	Possible	Possible	Possible

Note: A dash indicates no known effect.

is two (a 'unit' is a half pint of beer, a glass of wine or a pub measure of spirits). Intakes higher than this are associated with a number of health problems from liver disease to an increased risk of cancer. Beer and cheaper wines contain quite a lot of the preservative sulphite which can contribute to the bad-eggs smell in those who are windy. So be warned.

Yeast Sometimes certain alcoholic beverages may aggravate IBS because of a sensitivity to yeast. This is possible with beer, especially yeasty-tasting real ales, and men are more likely to be so troubled than women. You may also find that other yeast-rich foods such as yeast extract, savoury snacks, packet soups and gravies as well as bread can also aggravate the symptoms of IBS.

Fruit and honey Though you might think that these foods are easy to digest, they may not suit everyone. Fruit, some vegetables and honey are all rich in fructose or fruit sugar, which is not absorbed into the body as quickly as some other sugars. Any remaining in the gut can act as a laxative. Many of us may have experienced problems of bloating, wind and diarrhoea after eating a lot of fruit, especially grapes, dates or other very sweet fruits. The same could happen with a lot of honey. The effect might be more noticeable if several pieces of fruit are eaten on an empty stomach.

About the only fruit consistently to cause problems seems to be oranges, and sometimes grapefruit and lemons. Why this is so is not clear. Certainly all other fruits can occasionally cause a disturbance in bowel function in some sensitive people. Stewing fruit can make it easier to digest, and this may be especially important for older folk.

Sugar Table sugar (sucrose) only very rarely causes problems. Diarrhoea can result in the few people who have difficulty digesting and absorbing it.

Artificial sweeteners One artificial sweetener, sorbitol, which is used in some sugar-free chewing gums and sweets (especially mints), as well as foods manufactured for diabetics, can cause diarrhoea if consumed excessively. Sorbitol is an 'artificial sugar' which tastes sweet but cannot be digested. It therefore passes through the small bowel intact, moving on to the large bowel where it can attract water in the same way that some mineral laxatives do. So eating too many low-calorie mints can be a cause of diarrhoea.

Beans, onions and green vegetables All of these foods have a reputation for causing wind. Alas, it is deserved, because they can for some susceptible individuals be hard to digest, and the remaining portion then serves as a food source for the gas-producing bacteria that are lurking in your large bowel. The following foods are all relatively likely to produce wind: vegetables of the Brassica family (cabbage, cauliflower, broccoli, and Brussels sprouts); Jerusalem artichokes; onions and other members of this family such as leeks and garlic.

These foods seem more likely to cause wind if they are not well cooked and are eaten in large amounts. Men may be more susceptible to the effect than women because of their faster rate of gut transport.

Fatty foods Too much fatty food can, if the digestion is poor, lead to diarrhoea. This is not normally a problem in those with IBS. However, any cause of diarrhoea that results in more than three stools a day can be associated with a small loss of nutrients in the stool, and a high intake of fatty foods could aggravate this. So take care, especially if your diarrhoea is worse a few hours after eating a large or rich meal.

Conversely, fat in more modest quantities actually slows down the rate at which the stomach empties and food moves along the small bowel. Nature knows that fat in a meal takes time to digest, and so the gut is sensitive to its presence. Certain fats seem particularly good at this 'braking' effect – for example, oleic acid, which is found in olive oil and rapeseed oil. It is thought that too low a fat intake may explain why low-fat diets in children can prolong toddler diarrhoea. If you have diarrhoea, try including small amounts of olive and rapeseed oils in your diet.

Eggs We know of no good evidence that eggs are 'binding', as some say; nor do we know why they have this reputation for causing constipation. They are, however, prohibited in most exclusion diets, and if you are allergic to them, they could as easily cause diarrhoea as constipation.

Anything else By now you should have the idea that virtually anything you eat could play a part in your IBS. Water seems safe; but there are some who feel that bottled water is better for them. The commonest chemical found in ordinary tap water is chlorine, which is added to kill off bacteria; and it is quickly lost if the water is boiled or left in the open air for an hour or so.

Overall you must trust your own judgement and do not rely too heavily upon the advice of others. Look at the information given here as suggestions; it may lead to an improvement, but equally, it may not.

Additional dietary factors that can influence the pattern of IBS symptoms

Size of meals Eating a large meal can trigger a reflex contraction of the colon muscles; this explains why you may have felt the need to open your bowels within an hour or so of your main meal of the day. It isn't that meal coming through already, but probably the day before's moving on. Some people with IBS are unduly sensitive in this respect.

Smoking Smoking a cigarette is known to increase the contraction of the colon muscles in those with IBS. If you smoke, or have been a smoker, you will know that a few puffs can cause a need to open the bowels. For many, a cup of coffee and a cigarette is their way of going to the toilet.

Drugs Certain drugs and nutritional supplements can cause

diarrhoea as a side-effect. The obvious clue is if the diarrhoea started shortly after you started taking the drug/supplement. Stopping it should result in improvement within a few days, though occasionally it may take longer. Anti-arthritic drugs and strong painkillers can irritate the upper or lower parts of the gut and produce severe indigestion or symptoms similar to IBS, usually with diarrhoea. Very large doses of vitamin C and magnesium can also cause diarrhoea, as can yeast tablets, which also cause bloating. Iron preparations and multivitamins with iron can irritate some people's digestion. Antibiotics, especially those of the penicillin family, can cause diarrhoea, almost certainly due to a change in the flora of the colon.

Candida A build-up in the bowel of the yeast *Candida albicans* can be a factor in IBS. This organism is well known as the cause of thrush, which commonly occurs in the vagina and sometimes in the mouth. It usually responds to treatment with anti-fungal agents and dietary change. Sometimes an episode of vaginal thrush or infection elsewhere triggers IBS in the first place. The part that this yeast organism may play in IBS has in our opinion been rather overstated in some of the popular press and understated in the mainstream medical journals. It can be found somewhere in the gut of some 20 per cent of the normal population and does not automatically cause bowel symptoms.

Certain factors can encourage a build-up of candida, such as use of antibiotics, treatment with steroids, diabetes, deficiencies of iron and the B vitamins, and possibly a diet high in refined foods and sugar and low in essential nutrients. This might then lead to bowel and other problems due to this organism. A few people are genuinely allergic to it; this had been reported in cases of urticaria (nettle-rash) and eczema. It would seem that some of those with IBS, where diarrhoea and bloating are the main problems, may benefit from certain 'anti-candida' measures. These include the use of antibiotic preparations that kill candida, eating a nutritious diet, cutting down on sugar-rich foods and avoiding yeast-rich foods such as bread, alcoholic beverages, vinegar, stock cubes and foods containing yeast extract. Improvement, if it is going to occur, should be evident within a few weeks. It may not be necessary to follow all of these measures indefinitely.

Gut bacteria Several non-prescription preparations containing friendly *Lactobacillus* bacteria are available. Their effectiveness is very much hit-and-miss and will remain so until scientific appraisal takes place. Similarly, there are some people whose food intolerances might be helped by taking enzyme preparations that increase the digestion of wind-producing foods.

Menstruation Many women notice that, in the week before their period, their abdomen bloats, they become constipated and they may have some generalized abdominal discomfort. The actual arrival of the period may be associated with diarrhoea. This may be due to the release of chemicals that stimulate the bowel to contract as well as the uterus. Constipation in association with premenstrual syndrome (PMS) may well respond to a change of diet, supplements of multivitamins and quite large doses of the mineral magnesium, which is known to help PMS symptoms, acts as a safe and effective laxative and can be lacking in some 50 per cent of women with PMS.

Evening primrose oil has also been used with some success in IBS, giving modest benefit to a group of women with known food intolerances who despite dietary restriction still experienced symptoms premenstrually and menstrually.

Diet and IBS: Can it help?

It would seem that there are many factors that can contribute to the symptoms of IBS. Dietary factors look like being the most common – and the most complicated. This probably explains why there seems to be little agreement about the best way to tackle IBS by diet except for the recommendation to increase fibre intake in those with constipation.

Very often the best way forward for the individual is some trial of dietary change which may or may not be supervised by a doctor or dietitian. The better-informed the therapist and patient are, the greater the likelihood of success. We hope that this chapter, together with the others in this book, will help achieve this.

Finally, it is very likely indeed that future research into the role of diet in IBS will allow better and more specific advice to be given to IBS sufferers – always, of course, remembering that it is the individual who makes the final judgement as to what foods or what factors suit his or her bowel function.

Three Case Histories

Diarrhoea: Jane

Jane was a 32-year-old veterinary assistant who for five years had experienced episodic and at times quite dramatic diarrhoea. She suspected that wine and dairy products aggravated her problems. However, it was not until she followed a quite strict exclusion diet for three weeks that her residual symptoms disappeared. They quickly returned when some foods were introduced into her diet. Milk resulted in diarrhoea and wind within an hour; cheese, citrus fruits, wine and milk chocolate resulted in diarrhoea and wind that built up over several hours. Being strict with her diet meant that she could stop her anti-diarrhoea drugs, and she also experienced a marked improvement in energy. It was likely that she had a true lactose (milk sugar) intolerance as well as other food intolerances, and it seemed that these had developed gradually over several years.

Constipation: Nicole

Nicole at the age of 30 was fed up with eight years of severe constipation and abdominal bloating. This had followed a bad road accident in which she had fractured her pelvis, after which she did not open her bowels for several weeks. Headaches, malaise and premenstrual problems were also problems for her. There was a surprising degree of improvement when she began a diet that excluded most grains, dairy products, yeast, tea, coffee and several other foods. There was even more improvement when she took supplements of magnesium and multivitamins to correct some mild nutritional deficiencies. Over the next seven years, she tried on many occasions to reintroduce these foods and always reacted badly to them. Indeed, her sensitivity to wheat became so great that even taking a small amount of biscuit or communion wafer caused mouth soreness within an hour which then developed into mouth ulceration. This pattern was strongly suggestive of a true food allergy. Her avoidance of all dairy products meant that she required a calcium and multivitamin supplement. Interestingly, her level of sensitivity to these foods increased over the years, though it would seem that it is more usual for such reactions to settle down.

Wind: Damien

Damien was a rather oversensitive 56-year-old theatre critic whose abdominal bloating, wind and diarrhoea could easily be put down to his nerves. This seemed likely, as two gastroenterologists had found no serious digestive disorder. However, it seemed worth him trying an exclusion diet, which he dutifully followed but without any significant benefit. The only time he seemed to improve was when he included a lot of milk and eggs in his diet. After several months, the only conclusion we could come to was that certain fibre-rich foods such as beans and wholemeal bread seemed to make his symptoms worse, though the effect was not dramatic. Further consultations with one of his specialists resulted in some advice to help control the build-up of gas-forming bacteria in the bowel. Taking a specialized preparation of healthy bacteria to reduce the concentration of the undesirable ones seemed to produce lasting and significant benefit after a few months. Damien was then able to tolerate foods that previously had aggravated his symptoms.

Meal ideas and recipes
(compiled by Susan Backhouse)

Avoiding those foods which are commonly thought to aggravate IBS symptoms sounds simple enough: you simply cut them out of your diet. However, embarking on a dairy- or gluten-free diet can be more difficult than this suggests, because these foods often make up a major part of our diet. Fortunately, there are many books available dedicated to gluten-free and dairy-free cooking: for suggestions, see the books section in the Appendix at the end of this book. (This list also contains a book that might be useful for people wishing to go on an anti-candida diet, which is out of our scope here.)

If you do want to undertake a restrictive diet, it is advisable to seek the help of a doctor or a nutritionally experienced health practitioner to make sure that you don't miss out on essential nutrients. However, there is much that you can do for yourself to ensure that you have a varied and interesting diet.

You can quickly get used to substituting dairy- and gluten-free alternatives for commonly used ingredients. For example:

- Instead of cow's milk, use goat's or sheep's milk soya or nut milk ($1/4$ cup ground nuts with $1 1/4$ cup water).
- Instead of cheese and yoghurt made with cow's milk, use equivalent made with goat's, sheep's or soya milk.
- Instead of butter and margarine, use dairy-free margarine (e.g. Whole Earth's 'Superspread', which does not contain hydrogenated fats) or cold-pressed oil.
- Instead of ordinary flours and cereals, use rice, millet, soya (usually mixed with other flours), buckwheat (though this is strong-tasting and is an acquired taste), potato, gram, sweet corn (maize), spelt (an old type of wheat), sago and tapioca (these last two tend to go 'glutinous' when used in sauces).
- Use gluten-free baking powder: many baking powders do contain gluten, but at the time of writing, Sainsbury's does not; also try wholefood shops for the gluten-free type.

Remember when you are buying ingredients and prepared foods to check labels carefully: there are often 'hidden' ingredients where you would not expect them. For example, monosodium glutamate contains gluten.

Many other useful ingredients are widely available, though

you may have to go to different shops for them – for example:

- Tahini (sesame paste) can be bought in Greek food shops, wholefood shops and some supermarkets.
- Tofu (soybean curd) can be bought in Chinese food shops and wholefood shops.
- Tamari (strong soya sauce that does not, as do many soya sauces, contain wheat) can be bought in oriental food shops and wholefood shops.
- Agar-agar (a vegetarian gelling agent) can be bought in wholefood shops.

You can also adapt your established cooking methods to incorporate the alternative ingredients. For example:

- Crumbles can be made with ground nuts, either on their own or mixed with brown rice flour, seeds, millet flakes and/or desiccated coconut (though check that this last is gluten-free).
- If you are avoiding milk or eggs, try mixing soya flour with a little water to make a glaze for pastry.
- It is a good idea to combine different types of gluten-free flours for baking – e.g. three-quarters rice flour with one-eighth each of corn flour and buckwheat flour.
- As pastry made with gluten-free flour tends to disintegrate easily, it helps if you roll it out between sheets of greaseproof paper.
- You can make bread without yeast using an ingredient called 'Arise'.*

The remainder of this chapter gives some meal ideas and recipes for people who want to avoid dairy produce and wheat or gluten. To help you find the recipes to suit you, each heading is marked **DF**

* 'Arise' is available from: Cirrus Associates (South West), Little Hintock, Kington Magna, Gillingham, Dorset SP8 5EW.

(dairy-free) or **GF** (gluten-free), or both, as appropriate. Weights and measures are given in both metric and imperial terms: stick to one system throughout each recipe.

Breakfasts

- Cereals with soya milk or fruit juice (**DF**)
- Toast with dairy-free margarine or nut butter (**DF**)
- Porridge made out of rice flakes, millet flakes, buckwheat flakes. Flavour with cinnamon, cloves and dates or fresh fruit, chopped nuts and seeds (**DF/GF**)
- Rice cakes with mashed bananas, almond or other nut butter and Whole Earth sugar-free fruit spread (**DF/GF**)
- Rice cakes with tahini and Marmite (**DF/GF**)
- Vitality Shake: mix equal measures of soya milk and orange juice; liquidize and add 1 tsp brewer's yeast and 1 tsp molasses; blend until smooth and serve chilled (**DF/GF**)
- Gluten-free muesli (see recipe below)

Gluten-free muesli (**DF/GF**)
(from *The Neal's Yard Bakery Wholefood Cookbook* by Rachel Haigh)

500 g (1 lb 2 oz) rice flakes
500 g (1 lb 2 oz) millet flakes
250 g (9 oz) sunflower seeds
250 g (9 oz) raisins
250 g (9 oz) sultanas
250 g (9 oz) hazelnuts
250 g (9 oz) dried apricots
90 ml (6 tbsp) desiccated coconut
250 g (9 oz) soya bran (optional, for added fibre)

Combine the ingredients and store in an airtight jar in a cool place. Serve with milk, yoghurt, soya milk or fruit juice; add a little fresh fruit if wished. Eat immediately or leave to soak overnight. Alternatively, cover with your choice of liquid, simmer gently for five minutes and eat warm. Makes 2.5 kg (4 lb 6 oz).

Starters and light lunches or suppers
Guacamole (**DF/GF**)
(from *The Neal's Yard Bakery Wholefood Cookbook* by Rachel Haigh)

This traditional Mexican dish needs really well-ripened avocados.

3 avocados
1 large tomato, finely chopped
juice and grated rind of 1 lemon
pinch of chilli powder or cayenne pepper
15 ml (1 tbsp) olive oil (optional)
salt and black pepper
black olives to garnish

1. Put the avocado flesh into a mixing bowl and mash with a fork or a potato masher.
2. Add the tomato and the lemon juice and rind.
3. Sprinkle over the chilli and olive oil, if using, and season to taste.
4. Garnish with black olives.
Serves 6.

Hummus (**DF/GF**)
(from *The Neal's Yard Bakery Wholefood Cookbook* by Rachel Haigh)

A blender is essential for this recipe. Make sure the chickpeas are thoroughly cooked before liquidizing. Chickpeas can be soaked for two to three days, which can help to eliminate the flatulence they otherwise might cause. Change the water night and morning if you do soak them for this longer period.

50 g (2 oz) chickpeas, soaked for at least 12 hours, overnight or longer (see above)
1 garlic clove, crushed
30 ml (2 tbsp) lemon juice
good pinch of salt

black pepper
50 ml (2 fl oz) olive oil
100 ml (4 fl oz) water or orange juice
15 ml (1 tbsp) tahini

1. Transfer the soaked chickpeas and their liquid to a saucepan. Top up with fresh water, if necessary, to cover the chickpeas. Cover the pan and bring to the boil. Lower the heat and simmer for about two hours or until they are cooked, i.e. no longer hard. Drain.
2. Place the garlic, lemon juice, seasoning, oil and water in a blender. Liquidize, then gradually add the chickpeas, blending until smooth.
3. Add the tahini and liquidize again, adding a little extra liquid if the mixture is too dry.
Serves 2–4.

Main meals

Caribbean stew (**DF/GF**)
(from *The Neal's Yard Bakery Wholefood Cookbook* by Rachel Haigh)
Quick and simple to make, this stew is given a truly Caribbean flavour by the creamed coconut and root ginger.

30 ml (2 tbsp) groundnut oil
1 large onion, finely chopped
1 red pepper, finely chopped
5 ml (1 tsp) grated root ginger
4 garlic cloves, crushed
1 small swede, cubed
1 small parsnip, cubed
1 large sweet potato, cubed
570 ml (1 pt) pineapple juice
30 ml (2 tbsp) tomato purée
60 ml (4 tbsp) creamed coconut
2.5–5 ml (1/2–1 tsp) chilli powder
salt and black pepper

1. Heat the oil in a medium-sized saucepan. Add the onion, red pepper, grated root ginger and crushed garlic. Sauté for five minutes, stirring occasionally, until the onion is soft.

2. Add the swede, parsnip and sweet potato to the saucepan and sauté for a further 3 minutes to seal in the flavours.

3. Add the pineapple juice, tomato purée, coconut, chilli powder and seasoning and simmer for 20 minutes or until the vegetables are cooked and tender.

4. Serve on a bed of brown rice.

Serves 6–8.

Aubergine pie (Melitzanpitta) (GF)
(from *Greek Vegetarian Cookery* by Jack Santa Maria)

olive oil
1 onion, chopped
4 tomatoes, chopped
2–4 cloves garlic, finely chopped
1 tsp salt
1/2 tsp freshly ground black pepper
1 tsp basil
225 ml (8 fl oz) yoghurt
225 ml (8 fl oz) cottage or curd cheese
2 tsp sesame seeds
1 large aubergine
225 ml (8 fl oz) crumbled feta cheese
1 tbsp chopped parsley or coriander leaf

1. Preheat the oven to 350°F/180°C/Gas Mark 4.

2. Heat 2 tbsp of oil in a pan and fry the onion for 2 minutes. Add the tomatoes, garlic, salt, pepper and basil and cook together for 5 minutes.

3. Mix the yoghurt and cheese together with the sesame seeds.

4. Wash the aubergine and trim. Cut into thin slices. Heat half a

cup of olive oil in a frying pan and fry the aubergine slices until golden. Remove and drain on absorbent paper.

5. Fill the bottom of a greased casserole or baking dish with some of the aubergine slices; cover with some of the tomato mixture and then with some of the yoghurt and cheese mixture. Put on another layer of aubergine, tomato and cheese as before. Cover with feta cheese. Bake in the oven until the top turns golden (30–40 minutes).

6. Serve garnished with the chopped herbs, with rice or baked potatoes and a green salad.

Serves 3.

Tofu burgers (**DF/GF**)
(from *The Foodwatch Alternative Cookbook* by Honor J. Campbell)

    5 ml (1 tsp) olive oil
    170 g (6 oz) leeks
    110 g (4 oz) carrots
    110 g (4 oz) mushrooms
    1 tsp oregano
    55g (2 oz) buckwheat or millet flakes
    225 g (8 oz) tofu, thoroughly mashed
    15 ml (2 tbsp) tahini
    15 ml (2 tbsp) tamari
    seasoning to taste
    45 g (1½ oz) sesame seeds

1. Chop the leeks finely, coarsely grate the carrot and slice the mushrooms. Put the oil into a heavy based pan and heat. Add the prepared vegetables and sauté for about 8 minutes.

2. Remove from heat, add oregano, flakes, tofu, tahini, tamari and season with salt and pepper. Stir the mixture well and then leave to cool for a few minutes.

3. Divide the mixture into 8 portions and mould each one into a ball. Roll each ball in sesame seeds until well covered, and then flatten each ball into a burger shape with a potato masher

or the palm of the hand. Grill or fry for about 5 minutes on each side.
Serves 4.

Swede and orange pie (**DF/GF**)
(from *The Neal's Yard Bakery Wholefood Cookbook* by Rachel Haigh)
Puréed swedes with a hint of orange and coconut make this an unusual dish.

30 ml (2 tbsp) soya oil
1 large onion, finely chopped
1 large red pepper, finely chopped
2 small turnips, finely chopped
1.5 tsp ground cinnamon
15 ml (1 tbsp) tomato purée
15 ml (1 tbsp) tamari
450 g (1 lb) courgettes, finely chopped
100 g (4 oz) mushrooms, finely chopped
salt and black pepper

For the topping:
1 kg (2 lb 3 oz) swedes, chopped
50 ml (2 fl oz) soya oil or 50 g (2 oz) butter
juice and grated rind of 1 orange
50 g (2 oz) desiccated coconut
salt and black pepper

1. Preheat the oven to 400°F/200°C/Gas Mark 6.
2. Boil the swedes for the topping for 10 minutes or steam them for 15 minutes, until tender.
3. Meanwhile, heat 30 ml (2 tbsp) oil in a medium-sized saucepan and add the onion, red pepper and turnips. Add the cinnamon, tomato purée and tamari and cook gently. Add the courgettes and mushrooms to the saucepan. Cook for a further 8–10 minutes or until the vegetables are tender. Season to taste.
4. By now the swedes should be ready. Drain well. Make the rest

of the topping: add the oil, orange juice and rind and coconut to the swedes and blend to a smooth purée in a blender or with a potato masher. Season to taste.

5. Put the vegetables into an ovenproof dish and spread the swedes over the top. Bake for 20 minutes until cooked through. Serve immediately with a crisp green salad.

Serves 6.

Puddings, cakes, sweets and biscuits

Strawberry mousse (**DF/GF**)

(from *The Neal's Yard Bakery Wholefood Cookbook* by Rachel Haigh)

This mousse is made without eggs or dairy products, but it is wonderfully rich and creamy. You will need a blender.

> 570 ml (1 pt) unsweetened soya milk
> 15 ml (1 tbsp) agar-agar flakes
> about 225 g (8 oz) strawberries, hulled
> 15 ml (1 tbsp) maple syrup

1. Pour the soya milk into a saucepan and add the agar-agar flakes. Bring to the boil and simmer for 5 minutes, stirring occasionally.

2. Pour the soya milk and agar-agar into a blender. Add the strawberries and the maple syrup and blend for 2–3 minutes until smooth.

3. Pour the mousse into a serving bowl or individual dishes and chill in the refrigerator for at least four hours.

4. Decorate with fresh strawberries before serving.

Serves 4.

Nerissa's chocolate (or carob) cake (**DF/GF**)

> 200 g (7 oz) rice flour
> gluten-free baking powder
> 30 ml (2 tbsp) cocoa or carob powder
> lashing of runny honey
> 125 ml (¼ pt) safflower oil

125 ml (¹/₄ pt) soya milk
2 eggs

1. Preheat oven to 375°F/190°C/Gas Mark 5.
2. Put all ingredients in a mixer and blend well. The mixture will be runny.
3. Pour into two sandwich tins and bake for 35 minutes.
4. When cool, spread with Whole Earth Lime Spread (or whipped cream if dairy-free not desired).

Chocolate cake (**DF/GF**)
(from Berrydales newsletter, June 1994 – see 'Suppliers' under Useful Addresses in Appendix)

75 g (3 oz) dairy-free margarine
250 g (9 oz) dark muscovado sugar
60 ml (4 tbsp) gluten-free cocoa powder
3 eggs
100 g (4 oz) ground rice or rice flour
75 g (3 oz) ground almonds
1 tsp gluten-free baking powder

1. Preheat oven to 350°F/180°C/Gas Mark 4. Line a 20 cm (8 in) tin with greaseproof paper.
2. Beat together the fat and the sugar till light and fluffy.
3. Bring 100 ml (3 oz) water to the boil, pour on to the cocoa, mix well, then beat into the creamed mixture.
4. Beat in the eggs, adding a spoonful of rice flour with each.
5. Mix the baking powder into the remaining rice flour and ground almonds and fold into the mixture.
6. Spoon the mixture into the tin and bake in the oven for approximately 35 minutes or till the cake is firm to the touch. Cool on a wire rack before cutting.

Millet and peanut cookies (**DF/GF**)
(from *The Cranks Recipe Book* by David Canter, Kay Canter and Daphne Swann)

60 ml (4 tbsp) oil
$^1/_4$ tsp salt
1 egg
75 g (3 oz) raw brown sugar
100 g (4 oz) ground peanuts
75 g (3 oz) raisins
100 g (4 oz) millet flakes

1. Preheat oven to 350°F/180°C/Gas Mark 4.
2. Lightly whisk together the oil, sugar, salt and eggs. Stir in the remaining ingredients until well blended. Roll the mixture into 10 balls. Place on a lightly greased baking sheet. Press each one down to flatten slightly.
3. Bake in the oven for about 15 minutes, until golden. Allow to cool on the baking sheet for a few minutes before transferring to a wire tray.

Brown rice digestive biscuits (**DF/GF**)
(from *The Foodwatch Alternative Cookbook* by Honor J. Campbell)

110 g (4 oz) brown rice flour
$^1/_4$ level tsp salt
$^1/_2$ level tsp gluten-free baking powder
45 g (1$^1/_2$ oz) dairy-free margarine
30 g (1 oz) sugar or 15 g ($^1/_2$ oz) fructose
45 ml (3 tbsp) goat's, sheep's or soya milk

1. Preheat oven to 375°F/190°C/Gas Mark 5.
2. Sieve together flour, salt and baking powder into a bowl. Rub in margarine and add sugar or fructose.
3. Mix to a stiff paste with milk. Turn on to a lightly floured surface and knead well. Roll out thinly.
4. Cut into rounds with 6 cm (2$^1/_2$ in) biscuit-cutter. Transfer on to a greased baking tray and prick well.
5. Bake for 12–15 minutes. Transfer to a wire rack to cool. Store in an airtight tin.

Potato shortbread (**DF/GF**)
(from *The Foodwatch Alternative Cookbook* by Honor J. Campbell)

170 g (6 oz) potato flour
110 g (4 oz) dairy-free margarine
55 g (2 oz) sugar
85 g (3 oz) ground almonds or cashews

1. Preheat oven to 350°F/180°C/Gas Mark 4.
2. Beat margarine until soft and creamy. Add other ingredients and work until a ball of dough is formed. Put into a greased 18–20 cm (7–8 in) round sandwich tin and press down evenly. Prick all over and bake for 35–40 minutes or until lightly golden brown. Cut into 8 wedges.

Fruit and nut chews (**DF/GF**)

100 g (4 oz) raisins
100 g (4 oz) stoned dates
100 g (4 oz) walnuts
50 g (2 oz) desiccated coconut

1. Using a mincer fitted with a coarse blade, or a blender, mince or blend the raisins, dates and walnuts together.
2. Add the coconut and work the mixture with the fingertips until it binds.
3. Form into thin rolls and cut into bite-size pieces.

Carob 'fudge' (**GF**)
(from *The Cranks Recipe Book* by David Canter, Kay Canter and Daphne Swann)

50 g (2 oz) butter or margarine
25 g (1 oz) carob powder
50 g (2 oz) clear honey
25 g (1 oz) soya flour

75 g (3 oz) ground almonds
5 ml (1 tsp) vanilla essence
25 g (1 oz) almonds, ground or chopped finely

1. Cream the butter and carob powder until well mixed. Add the honey, soya flour, ground almonds and vanilla and mix thoroughly.
2. Sprinkle the ground almonds on a clean, dry working surface and shape the 'fudge' into a roll, coating it with the almonds.
3. Cut into bite-sized pieces. Keep in the fridge until required.
Variation: For sesame 'fudge', replace 25 g (1 oz) ground almonds with 25 g toasted sesame seeds.

Useful miscellaneous recipes
Dairy-free mayonnaise (**DF/GF**)
(from *The Neal's Yard Bakery Wholefood Cookbook* by Rachel Haigh)

100 ml (4 fl oz) soya milk
60 ml (4 tbsp) lemon juice
10 ml (2 tsp) mustard powder
10 ml (2 tsp) finely chopped mixed herbs or
5 ml (1 tsp) dried herbs
salt and black pepper
200–300 ml (7–11 fl oz) soya oil

1. Put the soya milk, lemon juice, mustard powder, herbs and seasoning in a blender. Liquidize until smooth.
2. Gradually add the oil, with the blender still running, until you have a thick consistency.
Makes about 425 ml (¾ pint). Keep in fridge.

Cornmeal Yorkshire pudding (**DF/GF**)
(from *Good Food, Gluten Free* by Hilda Cherry Hills)

112 ml (8 fl oz) cornmeal
1 tsp salt

$^1/_2$ tsp marjoram (optional)
450 ml (¾ pint) milk or soya milk
4 eggs, beaten
1 tsp oil

1. Preheat oven to 350°F/180°C/Gas Mark 4.
2. Make paste from cornmeal, salt, marjoram and a quarter of the milk. Heat rest of milk in top of double boiler on direct heat. When it boils, add cornmeal paste. Stir until smooth. Place over hot water in double boiler. Cover. Cook gently until all liquid is absorbed. Remove.
3. When lukewarm, blend in eggs.
4. Oil large baking pan or individual ones, place in preheated oven.
5. Pour in mixture to half full. Bake for 10 minutes.
6. Remove. Dot with remainder of oil. Return to oven and bake for another 15 minutes.
The following two sauces are made without flour of any kind.

Foam white sauce (**DF/GF**)
(from *Good Food, Gluten Free* by Hilda Cherry Hills)
This sauce can be used for vegetables instead of standard white sauce.

2 egg whites, beaten to a peak
pinch of salt
onion juice to taste
45 ml (3 tbsp) soya milk
chopped chives or parsley

1. Sprinkle salt into beaten egg white and mix in onion juice.
2. Gradually pour on the hot soya milk while beating well until it thickens.
3. Add chives or parsley.

Golden cheese sauce (**GF**)
(from *Good Food, Gluten Free* by Hilda Cherry Hills)
Serve this sauce with vegetables, fish, hot hard-boiled eggs etc.

2 egg yolks
60 ml (4 tbsp) finely grated cheese
salt to taste
30 ml (2 tbsp) butter

1. Beat the egg yolks with grated cheese and salt.
2. Melt the butter in top of double boiler or bowl over pan containing boiling water; add egg and cheese mixture and stir until it has thickened enough. Thin with a little milk if necessary.

Mock cream (**DF/GF**)
(from *The Foodwatch Alternative Cookbook* by Honor J. Campbell)

1 level tbsp arrowroot flour
75 ml (5 tbsp) cold water
45 g (1½ oz) dairy-free margarine
sweetener to taste

1. Place arrowroot in a saucepan and add water, stirring all the time.
2. Heat and stir until the mixture thickens. Beat until smooth, then put in a basin and leave until completely cold.
3. Add margarine and beat well.
4. Sweeten to taste and continue to beat until fluffy. Use within 2 days.

Nut cream (**DF/GF**)

110 g (4 oz) cashews or blanched almonds
honey or maple syrup to taste
90 ml (6 tbsp) water

Blend or grind nuts to fine powder. Add rest of ingredients and blend until smooth and creamy. Chill in fridge.

Chapter 8

Psychological Treatment of IBS

Brenda Toner and Claire Rutter

Most people, if asked what they thought psychotherapeutic techniques involved, and how helpful they were, would probably answer that they are wholly focused on events which happened in childhood, and of use only in dealing with mental disorders. In fact, psychotherapy involves helping people with all sorts of problems, by 'talking treatments'. There are various different techniques, but they share the basic method of the therapist and the patient talking about events, thoughts and feelings that matter to that individual – for example, his or her problems, everyday lives, worries and fears. The therapist then pursues these discussions with the individual to gain a greater understanding of his or her problems and how they could be alleviated.

How can psychotherapy help people with physical symptoms, such as those in IBS?

Whatever your view is of why you have IBS, psychotherapy may be able to help you come to terms with your problem and, in some cases, may even help to reduce your symptoms, or provide you with some coping strategies to deal with them.

Researchers have found that what distinguishes IBS patients from people without the condition is the reactivity of the colon to environmental events. The changes in bowel activity associated with the disorder have been shown to be associated with heightened arousal of emotions such as anxiety and anger.

Since it seems that there is a link between IBS and stress, and since it is virtually impossible to avoid stressful situations, it makes sense to consider ways in which you might improve the way you cope with stress: this is where a psychotherapist can help.

Also, if your symptoms *are* associated with psychological factors, then a therapist will also be able to construct a programme of treatment that could help. Some of these factors are discussed later in this chapter.

The following stories demonstrate two very different responses to psychological treatment for IBS. Carol is a professional woman in her mid-thirties:

'I have been seeing Dr F on a six-weekly basis for about a year now. I was referred to Dr F by the gastroenterologist who had exhausted his treatment and that was the only thing we hadn't considered. I was reluctant at first, but on the other hand, I felt that I had to try everything. I was so frustrated at the doctors not having found anything tangible that a psychological link would have been better than nothing and would at least have given me something to work on.

'It was explained to me that the purpose of psychotherapy was to see if there was anything emotional that I had buried in the past which was not noticeable when I had a "well" gut but which is now manifesting itself in the form of pain, etc. now that I have an "unwell" gut. I can remember my first visit to see Dr F. I had been feeling dreadful all day at work – the pain was so bad that I had been pacing around the office (this is how I feel *every* day). I was worried about how I was going to get through my meeting with Dr F because I guessed it would mean my having to sit down for up to an hour, which I would find so uncomfortable. My office friends said that I should ask Dr F if I could talk to him while lying down, because if anyone should understand how I felt then he should. When I arrived I explained my need to lie down. Dr F's reply was to tell me to sit down and see if it got any better. I couldn't seem to get through to him that sitting made it worse and that the way I felt that day was how I feel every day and was not in any way connected with being nervous about our meeting.

'Dr F's attitude does not seem to have altered to this day. For example, on my last visit I stood up after about ten minutes and he asked me why I had stood up at that particular moment. In other words, were we talking about something which had touched a raw nerve, thus making my symptoms worse – I could have cheerfully swung for him! Dr F has discussed with me all areas of my life. One angle he explored was the possibility that my IBS was connected to the fact that I was in my thirties and unmarried! Why wasn't I married? Why wasn't I in a long-term relationship? Where are my children? I'm not normal! I have tried explaining to Dr F that I believe one shouldn't succumb to the pressure to be married, and one should marry when one feels it's the right thing to do. I believe that a person should not be made to feel abnormal if they choose to remain single. In my opinion, a person can lead a happy and fulfilled life without marriage. Dr F kept on implying that I had a "problem". I told him that surely it is only a problem if one is unhappy. I'm not unhappy with my life, apart from IBS. I see myself as "sitting on the fence" – i.e. a long-term relationship with children with the right person looks inviting but equally dating lots of different men and having lots of fun looks equally good too. It would take someone really special to make me take the leap. How on earth has this got anything to do with IBS?

'I don't think psychotherapy has helped me in any way whatsoever, nor do I think it ever will. The only benefit I could get from it would be to discuss the stresses and strains of having IBS and how I was coping with it. Sometimes I feel guilty about moaning to my friends about my IBS so I tend to keep quiet and let the frustration build up. After all, they heard all this three years ago and to continue moaning about it would just be going over the same old ground. There's nothing more to say, nothing more to add. I feel Dr F has been patronizing. He hasn't got a clue. This is nothing personal as I am sure he is a kind man and means well, but I don't know how much longer I shall continue trying to explain to Dr F that the only underlying emotional problem contributing to my IBS is the actual strain of having IBS.'

Anne has a totally different story, however. Although reluctant at first to be sent to a psychiatrist, she found that he was the only one who really understood and helped her. Anne's IBS symptoms were uncontrollable; she was in a lot of pain and suffered badly with diarrhoea and flatulence. She had lost a lot of weight, and was struggling to hold down a responsible job. She knew no one with IBS, and did not confide in others about her problems. She was becoming weaker and weaker, and more depressed by the day. Her GP did not seem to be helpful – she felt he dismissed her symptoms and believed she was neurotic. She did not feel she wanted to keep going back to her GP, who never seemed to offer any help. However, eventually he persuaded her to go to a psychiatrist, saying there must be a reason why she 'keeps getting all these symptoms'. Although Anne did not want to go to the psychiatrist, she now feels it's the best thing that happened to her. Anne sees Dr P regularly, and talks through all her problems and anxieties with him. She is lucky in that Dr P seems to understand:

'Until four years ago I was fine, went out to parties, travelled everywhere, etc. Then I began to get all these symptoms. I went to my GP, who thought I'd imagined it all; he thought IBS wasn't serious and I should just get on with it. He didn't understand, he didn't help. I felt weak, ill, my life was so miserable I just kept going back to him all the time, so in the end he thought I must have something psychologically wrong with me. He insisted I go to a psychiatrist but at first I wouldn't. However, over the course of a couple more visits he kept on about it, and because I didn't have any choice, I thought I had better go because I do need help. When I did go, I found him helpful. He was understanding, and really listened to me. He takes me seriously, he believes me when I say how bad I feel. I decided I would keep on going to see him because he promised me that, if he couldn't help me get better, he would send me to a consultant. He's helped me, because he actually believed that IBS is a problem. He believed that how I felt was genuine, and that it wasn't all in my mind. He could see that I was weak, and believed me whereas the GP wouldn't.

I could hardly get up the stairs to my GP, and I nearly collapsed one day. The GP acted as if I made it up. Dr P hasn't got rid of my symptoms, but could see that I couldn't go on, and he made me stop work. He thought I should because I was so ill, and travelling to town each day was making me far worse. Stopping work has helped me in a lot of ways. If I hadn't gone to him, I'm sure I would have had a nervous breakdown. He's been very good to me; if it wasn't for him, I don't know what I would have done.'

How successful is psychotherapy in treating IBS?

Assessing trials of psychotherapy for IBS patients is not straight-forward, given the varied nature of people's symptoms, and the lack of carefully controlled studies in this area. However, some research results do suggest that psychotherapeutic treatment may be beneficial.

In one experiment conducted in 1985, 33 IBS patients were given either medical or psychological treatments, after having six weeks with no treatment. It was found that the psychological treatments helped lower distress by reducing both anxiety and IBS symptoms. Another team of researchers gave 51 IBS patients medical care and 50 others short-term psychotherapy plus medical care: after treatment, those who had had psychotherapy had improved, feeling less pain and fewer physical symptoms. This improvement was still evident one year after treatment. In another trial, patients were given either medical treatment alone or medical treatment plus psychotherapy. Three months after treatment, the researchers found a significant improvement in the psychotherapy group on self-ratings of diarrhoea and pain, compared to their original condition, although no improvement in constipation. They stated that psychological treatment is feasible and effective in two thirds of patients who do not respond to standard medical treatment.

While these studies are promising in that they show that psychological interventions might be useful for people with IBS, much of the research in this area suffers from problems which limit interpretation of the findings: for example, in some studies the therapeutic techniques were not adequately described or monitored; and many people refused to take part in the experiments, which limits the generalizability of the results. However, the fact that the majority of studies were not carefully controlled and monitored does not make them worthless. Many people believe they have been helped by psychotherapy; and it has been claimed that psychotherapy can lead to a significant improvement, both in symptoms and in accompanying mood states, and that these improvements can be maintained for several months at least.

What to expect from psychotherapy

Therapists use different methods in their attempts to help individual patients overcome their symptoms. There are various basic types of approach, and each therapist will also have his or her preferred techniques and style. In the rest of this chapter, we will describe the different techniques you may encounter if you try psychotherapy, focusing in particular on the two main types of psychotherapy used in treating IBS: cognitive-behavioral therapy and exploratory psychotherapy. Whatever the particular approach used, most therapists will offer an initial assessment, at which you will be asked about your symptoms, relationships, family history, employment and so on. At this stage, you and the therapist can negotiate what treatment entails and what you hope to achieve – the 'treatment goals'. Also, you can discuss how long you are likely to be in therapy, and, if the treatment is private, the actual cost. At all times, therapists should ensure confidentiality. If you are having therapy under the NHS, you may be asked for details of your GP, and your therapist will usually notify him or her should you engage in treatment. If you are paying for private treatment, this may not happen; you should ask your therapist his or her policy on this point.

Group psychotherapy or individual psychotherapy?

Most of the techniques mentioned in this chapter can be conducted either in groups or individually. Which is chosen depends on the patient's preference, or sometimes on which is available in the patient's locality.

Group psychotherapy is typically conducted with a small number of individuals, usually between about 6 and 12, who all have the same problem(s). The advantage of the group approach is that the individual can derive comfort and support from observing that others have similar experiences. Also, in the case of IBS sufferers for whom the condition is a major hindrance to social life, it may provide the opportunity to make friends with people in a similar situation, without the embarrassment of either hiding or explaining the problem. The advantage of individual therapy on the other hand, is that the specific techniques are tailored more specifically to the patient's individual needs and goals.

Psychodrama

The earliest use of the group process in psychotherapy can be credited to the Austrian Jacob Moreno, who in 1910 combined dramatic and therapeutic techniques to create what he called 'psychodrama'. He conducted his therapy on stage, with people in the group playing key figures in the patient's life. He would also instruct patients to reverse roles to gain a greater awareness of how other people saw them. This may seem a strange method, but many have claimed that role-playing techniques offer patients valuable insights and feedback that help them to achieve a better understanding of themselves.

A Swedish study looked at the effectiveness of psychodrama and relaxation training in the treatment of IBS. Patients were invited to have conversations with their own stomach or gut, played by another group member. The aim here was to make the participants aware of the interplay between emotions and bodily symptoms. After the initial treatment, both symptom levels and anxiety levels dropped; however, symptom levels tended to rise again after three years.

Cognitive-behavioral group therapy

Cognitive behavioral therapists believe that what you think about the things that you do, and the reasons behind your actions, are as important as your behaviour. The aim of this particular therapy is to modify unhelpful or damaging beliefs as a means of overcoming problem behaviour. A team of researchers led by Brenda Toner in Toronto has recently completed a study investigating the use of cognitive-behavioral group therapy in treating IBS: this study will be used here as an illustration of the cognitive-behavioral method in practice.

The group consisted of one therapist and six IBS sufferers, who all started and finished treatment at the same time. Group sessions took place weekly for 12 weeks, each session lasting 90 minutes. One treatment session took place before the beginning of the first group session, in order to begin teaching people about cognitive-behavioral therapy, to establish initial rapport with each IBS sufferer and to identify treatment goals.

At each group session, there was a predetermined agenda set by the therapist as well as individual agenda items chosen by each group member for that session – for example, dealing with a stressful situation at work. The following items were always included in the group agenda:

- progressive relaxation exercises to begin the session (this involves tightening and relaxing each muscle group).
- individual members' agenda items (e.g. each member may report on something they want the group's help with).
- individual members' reactions to the previous session.
- members' own reports of their mental and physical state and any other significant events during the week.
- therapist's review of previous session's self-help assignments (e.g. the outcome of homework tasks).
- introduction of any new cognitive theory or technique for that session.
- discussion of selected individual agenda items (e.g. individuals

may agree to try out a new way of thinking about a problem or to carry out a particular task).

- new self-help assignments.
- summary of session.
- individuals' reactions to the current session.

The roles of therapist and patient

It is not surprising that people with IBS, who are suffering physical symptoms and pain, may interpret referrals to psychologists or psychiatrists as insulting and personally diminishing. The critical challenge to the therapist is to counter the implication that IBS symptoms are imaginary or caused by underlying mental problems. Only when this task is successfully addressed is a therapeutic alliance possible.

The therapist giving treatment does not consider him or herself an expert on your situation; on the contrary, they see you as the best person to evaluate your own experience and want to enable you to be a 'personal scientist'. Some IBS sufferers see themselves as victims of their disease or as devoid of control over their bodily reactions, and they may see stress as something which happens to them from the outside, over which they have little control. These beliefs need to be evaluated in the open.

An attempt to encourage you to be a personal scientist involves three steps. The first step is to encourage you to gather information about your thoughts and emotions in stressful situations. The second step involves asking you to examine whether there is any relationship between these pieces of information (therapists can be particularly helpful in this phase by pointing out possible connections between thoughts and feelings – e.g. the thought may be 'I am upset' and the feeling may be 'sad' or 'tearful'). Step three involves helping you to become aware of the beliefs which you have and to examine the extent to which the data you collect (your beliefs) are supported or not supported.

An example might be someone who believes that showing a need for emotional contact with others or giving overt displays of affection are signs of weakness. Gathering information may involve asking other people how they feel about the expression of emotion, examining the patterns of emotional expression in the family or recalling instances when you felt good about other people expressing emotion to you. In this way, feedback from others is used to challenge some of the beliefs you might have about expressing emotion as signs of weakness.

The value of the therapist taking this stance is that he or she avoids being in a position of telling you that he or she knows what is best for you. This may appear difficult at first: you may want the therapist to find the solution for you. At the same time, however, the therapist can reassure you that this process has been found to be helpful in the past, and that there is good reason to believe that it will continue to be helpful in your case. The questions asked by the therapist are phrased in a manner requiring judgement on the part of the IBS sufferer and evincing respect for his or her beliefs. The therapist does not generally assume the role of expert, but rather assumes that of facilitator.

This approach establishes the collaborative relationship that is central to cognitive-behavioral intervention. Goals (what you want to achieve) are mutually agreed upon and are developed in consideration of the individual's current status, his or her particular strengths, limitations or disabilities, and the more general goals for treatment. The result of this negotiation process must be the establishment of goals that the individual feels are obtainable as well as personally relevant to his or her particular needs.

Examples of common themes in cognitive-behavioral sessions
On the basis of previous research, we feel that there are several themes common to many individuals who come to us with IBS.

Thoughts, feelings and gastrointestinal symptoms In this type of therapy, interactions between thoughts (cognitions), emotions and gastrointestinal symptoms are explored. In particular, the cognitive-behavioral model is used to highlight how certain thoughts and underlying beliefs may lead to increased attention to bodily sensations and increased arousal and heightened sensitivity to pain and other gastrointestinal symptoms. The daily record of dysfunctional thoughts (i.e. thoughts which do not serve a useful purpose) is introduced and used during sessions to identify and alter these thoughts.

Coping with stress and anxiety Stressful situations are identified and coping strategies discussed; anxiety hierarchies are introduced. To construct an anxiety hierarchy, you are asked to identify situations that you find most stressful and then to rank them according to the degree of anxiety they produce on a scale of 1–100 points. When the ranking process is complete, specific anxiety-reducing methods of treatment are given. In addition, thoughts relating to these situations are identified, challenged and modified throughout the course of treatment.

Assertiveness Assertiveness is defined as the direct, honest and appropriate expression of opinions, beliefs, needs and feelings. Previous research and clinical experience have suggested that people with gastrointestinal disorders have particular difficulty in being assertive. Training and homework assignments are especially directed at challenging the underlying thoughts and beliefs that inhibit expressions of your opinions, needs and feelings.

Anger Techniques are introduced which help you to identify how reactive or easily irritated you are in various situations. The interplay among thoughts, anger, physiological arousal, non-assertive behaviour and symptoms is highlighted.

Social approval In cognitive-behavioral group work with IBS sufferers, assumptions frequently centre on three major issues: heightened need for social approval (wanting others to like you); perfectionism (the need for things to be perfect or 'right'); and the need for control (or certainty). Thoughts and underlying beliefs concerning a heightened need for approval from others are examined in the light of gastrointestinal symptoms. The relationships between the need to please others and difficulties with and fears of doing something publicly unacceptable are identified and challenged.

Perfectionism Thoughts about appearing less than perfect are identified and challenged. Cognitive and behaviour techniques are directed at working with group members to change extreme, all-or-nothing attitudes about being perfect.

Control Techniques and assignments are used to demonstrate the limitations of the control ideal. Some people with gastrointestinal disorders respond to their symptoms by trying to control aspects of their environment that may be associated with symptoms: this then paradoxically limits their freedom – that is, it has the opposite effect to that they intended. By trying to exercise control and achieve certainty in all situations, people lose opportunities to collect evidence that they can handle situations.

The final session

This session is spent primarily discussing progress to date towards treatment goals. Cognitive and behavioral strategies are reviewed in light of how you have been able to use them in daily living. Particular emphasis is placed on their continued use once treatment has ended.

How successful is this approach?

The results given here are only preliminary, as we have not yet obtained follow-up data, but nevertheless look promising. We found that IBS sufferers who had cognitive-behavioral group treatment experienced a lessening of depression, while sufferers who had conventional medical treatment actually had more depressive symptoms.

We asked IBS sufferers to fill out a daily diary on their IBS symptoms for two weeks before therapy, two weeks following therapy and again for two weeks six months after the therapy had ended. We found that IBS sufferers in the cognitive-behavioral group had less bloating following therapy compared to a group which only received information on IBS – e.g. the causes, symptoms and possible treatments. (This latter group was called the 'psychoeducational' group.) There was also a group who had medical treatment only. On a combined measure of diarrhoea and/or constipation symptoms, there was improvement in both the cognitive-behavioral and the psychoeducational groups compared with the group given only conventional medical therapy.

IBS sufferers in the cognitive-behavioral group found therapy to be more effective for them than sufferers in the other two groups (psychoeducational and medical). Specifically, members in the cognitive-behavioral group reported significantly stronger identification with the following statements:

- 'I am better able to cope with my symptoms as a result of participating in the group.'
- 'Participation in the group has helped me to cope better in other areas of my life that have turned out to be in crisis.'
- 'My IBS symptoms have improved as a result of participating in the group.'
- 'I look more on the positive side of things as a result of participating in the group.'
- 'My level of confidence has increased as a result of participating in the group.'
- 'I found the group to be more helpful than I had expected.'

In 1995, researchers Annette Payne and Edward Blanchard in the United States carried out a study comparing the results of patients receiving cognitive therapy with the results of both self-help groups and a waiting list control (people who are on a waiting list for treatment, but who are not receiving any treatment at the time of the study). The cognitive therapy patients kept a daily diary in which they recorded how bad their irritable bowel symptoms were, and the researchers also measured their anxiety and depression. Patients then underwent individual therapy for eight weeks, which consisted of increasing patients' awareness of the association between stressful and anxious thoughts and their symptoms. The therapist also trained patients in how to reinterpret negative thoughts, and how to combat depressing ones. The cognitive therapy proved to be extremely beneficial. The average reduction in irritable bowel symptoms was 67 per cent (compared with 31 per cent for the self-help groups and 10 per cent for the waiting list control). In addition, 9 of the 12 cognitive therapy patients were improved in terms of symptoms and health.

Exploratory psychotherapy

The principle underlying this method is that your physical and psychological problems arise from disturbances in significant personal relationships. Improvement in your interpersonal relationships should therefore result in a reduction of your symptoms. The creation of an interpersonal relationship with the therapist, who adopts a warm, friendly manner and expresses sympathy and understanding, allows your problems to be revealed, explored and understood.

The following outline of the different types of sessions used is based on the practice of a group in Manchester led by Drs Guthrie and Creed.

The initial session
The first session is quite long, lasting approximately three hours. The goals of this first session include establishing a firm working relationship between you and the therapist, and helping you to make a link between physical symptoms and psychological processes. The strategies used include: exploring irrational fears you may have about therapy; taking a detailed history of your symptoms; exploring in depth the personal meaning of your symptoms and their effect on you; assessing your early life experiences and contact with sickness. Specific techniques used include the use of statements rather than questions, and specific use by the therapist of bowel-related metaphors (e.g. 'full of shit', 'bunged up').

The intermediate sessions
The main goal of the intermediate sessions is to work on the problem areas identified in the initial session. Strategies include: exploring further the development of symptoms; identifying reasons for the continuance of symptoms; and linking interpersonal

difficulties outside therapy to interpersonal processes in the session. In addition to the techniques used in the opening session, the therapist will introduce the use of bowel charts to link bowel disturbance to interpersonal conflict.

The final session
The goals of the final session include the identification of positive changes that have occurred during therapy, and consideration of how these can be maintained after therapy has finished, and the exploration of any negative changes or feelings.

Using this model of exploratory psychotherapy, Drs Guthrie and Creed found that, compared to a control group, sufferers showed significant improvements on ratings of diarrhoea and abdominal pain, and this led to reduced health-care utilization for one year following therapy.

Stress management techniques

This section focuses on some specific techniques that psychotherapists may use in approaching the problems of IBS sufferers. Since more than half of patients with IBS report that their symptoms are made worse by stress, and more than half report an acute episode of stress preceding the first onset of symptoms, it is not surprising that psychotherapists have focused in particular on developing techniques for managing stress.

Arousal reduction training/relaxation training
The aim of this technique is to reduce and control emotional arousal and anxiety, using progressive muscle relaxation training, non-specific biofeedback training (discussed below), autogenic training or meditation. It is important to realize that all mental health professionals (psychologists, psychiatrists, nurses and social workers as well as therapists) may use these techniques.

Progressive muscle relaxation training is the most commonly used arousal reduction technique. The aim is to tense and then relax each major group of muscles in turn, while concentrating on the sensation within. This is an easy exercise that you can practise at home; cassette tapes with specific exercises recorded on them are available.

Some investigators have reported good results in IBS patients with these exercises alone. One psychologist used relaxation training together with brief psychotherapy in 20 IBS patients and reported significant reductions in psychiatric symptoms (depression and anxiety) as well as modest reductions in bowel symptoms.

Self-control

This technique works by the therapist getting the patient to recognize the onset of tension and then using arousal reduction techniques to guard off undue stress.

Biofeedback

This is a more technological method of stress management, and requires patients to be given information about their bodies which is not normally available to them. With the aid of electronic instruments they can either see or hear what is going on in their bodies; by observing how physical reactions are triggered, it is hoped that they can learn to control their bodies even when the amplifying instrument is removed.

Two types of biofeedback have been used in treating IBS patients, specific and non-specific. Non-specific biofeedback involves the use of the technique to teach relaxation, whereas specific biofeedback involves feedback on bowel motility itself to teach the patient to inhibit the response.

One psychologist applied biofeedback successfully on IBS patients: he used an electronic stethoscope to amplify bowel sounds and trained his patients alternately to increase and decrease the volume of sound. He reported that all five patients were able to learn this response, and that all five experienced symptomatic improvement.

Self-regulation

This is a method of self-control developed by Japanese researchers. The patient is instructed to get into a state of relaxed alertness, achieved by focusing attention on their breathing and body warmth (active thinking is discouraged). The patient sits upright, with a straight spine, palms placed flat on the thighs, legs comfortably apart with the feet touching the floor (ideally the patient should be barefoot). The patient is told to breathe gently, inhaling through the nose, and exhaling through the mouth. The patient is then instructed to say to him/herself: 'I am feeling relaxed.' Then the treatment begins. Each stage must be mastered before the next stage begins.

In stage 1, the therapist draws the patient's attention to the warmth of the palms on the thighs. This stage usually takes around five minutes to complete, but obviously it varies with individual experience. In stage 2, the warmth of the hands is suggested to spread to the forearms. In stage 3, the patient becomes aware of how their feet are touching the floor, and then focuses on the warmth in their feet. In stage 4, the warmth of the feet is suggested to spread to the legs. In stage 5, the patient focuses on the coolness of the forehead region (sometimes this is achieved by patients suggesting to themselves that the forehead region feels refreshed). In stage 6, the control of the internal organs is practised. This is usually achieved by moving one hand (either one) from the thighs to the abdomen, and then suggesting to oneself: 'My abdomen is warm.' In patients who have carried out a great deal of practice, stages 3–6 will take around five to ten minutes.

This particular technique was used to treat a teenager with IBS, and it was claimed that it improved his diarrhoea.

One research team evaluated this treatment and concluded that those IBS patients who were less anxious at the beginning of the treatment were more likely to show a significant clinical improvement. However, it was predicted that the more anxious patient simply needs longer, more intensive treatment.

Systematic desensitization

If you have symptoms of IBS that always seem to flare up in certain non-stressful situations, some psychologists would say that you have become 'conditioned' to respond thus. This means that you have learned to pair a certain situation (or behaviour) with the worsening of your symptoms. This would happen, for example, if your symptoms were bad during a particular non-stressful situation in the past, and you have tended to worry that they will worsen again if the situation is repeated: so, whenever you do encounter a similar situation (e.g. a car journey), you automatically feel worse. Once this connection is established, such sufferers tend to avoid these seemingly non-stressful situations, and so the connection becomes stronger.

In the treatment of this particular problem, therapists use a technique called systematic desensitization, which is designed to produce a decrease in anxiety associated with a feared situation (or object, or behaviour). This is achieved by using a gradual approach consisting of four basic steps. First, the patient learns to think of anxiety in terms of subjective units along a 100-point scale, where 100 is the situation that would create the most anxiety imaginable, and 0 is the calmest. For example, 100 might be being stuck in a traffic jam on a motorway with no services, and 0 would be thinking about going on a very short car journey with toilets at either end. Second, the patient would be given relaxation training (the exact technique used will vary between therapists). Third, the patient and the therapist work together to produce an anxiety hierarchy, ranking situations according to their anxiety-involving properties for that individual. Fourth, the patient progressively imagines being in each of the scenes of the hierarchy, starting from 0, while trying to remain relaxed. The patient will not move on to the next scene/situation until they are able to visualize the previous one without feeling any anxiety. This stage will vary in duration for different individuals, and will progress until the patient reaches the top of their own unique hierarchy. It is hoped that a previously feared situation will then be paired with an automatic relaxation response.

Combining medical and psychotherapeutic treatments

For a long time, IBS treatment was primarily medical, based on drugs and diet therapy, both of which provide only minimal relief from symptoms. More recently, published research has included multicomponent treatment packages or combined techniques, including various combinations of cognitive-behavioral, relaxation, psychodynamic and biofeedback approaches. For example, one team of researchers devised a combined treatment programme for IBS patients which included: education about normal bowel functioning; progressive relaxation; thermal biofeedback; and cognitive techniques for coping with stress. Those patients taking drugs for their condition, and following special diets, continued to do so. The subjects found significant reductions in abdominal pain and diarrhoea. It was reported that similar results were achieved when this combined technique was conducted in one-to-one therapy, but that some patients expressed particular satisfaction with the group format, through finding that they are not alone with IBS. (However, the cognitive treatment was found to be more successful in individual therapy, where each patient's needs and problems could be addressed in more depth.) Moreover, 57 per cent of the patients treated in this way were still experiencing clinical improvement in their condition two years later.

It is best to look upon psychotherapy as an addition to, or integrated with, medical treatment, not as an alternative to it. If you believe that you might benefit from psychotherapy, go ahead and give it a try. And remember, any treatment will be more effective if you believe in it, and are motivated to stick with it. The expectation that one will get better, the development of a trusting relationship with a therapist, and a strong desire that it will happen are essential ingredients of hope, and hope can have a powerful impact on our emotions and bodily responses.

Further aspects of psychological interventions

One important area that needs to be developed and incorporated into work with IBS is an appreciation of the distress that is caused by living with a debilitating chronic illness which arouses little understanding or empathy, and with which considerable stigma is associated, with trivialization of the condition widespread on the part of both society in general and the medical system in particular. Another area that needs to be considered is the influence of gender on IBS. Despite the repeated documentation of a significant gender imbalance in sufferers from the condition, with three women to every man, little attention has been devoted to gender issues in either the conceptualization or the clinical management of IBS.

The stigma associated with functional somatic syndromes

Nearly every medical specialty has identified a 'functional somatic syndrome' (FSS). These syndromes are usually defined by physical symptoms unexplained by organic disease. The term 'functional' implies a disturbance of physiological function rather than anatomical structure; because of the stigma associated with the term, various alternative labels have been used to describe FSS, including 'somatic disorders', 'health anxiety', 'physical symptoms unexplained by organic disease', 'unexplained medical symptoms' and 'psychophysiological disorders'. Three of the most common functional somatic syndromes on which increased research and clinical attention has been targeted during the last decade are irritable bowel syndrome (IBS), chronic fatigue syndrome (CFS, formerly known as myalgic encephalitis, or ME) and fibromyalgia syndrome (FS).

In Western societies in general, and in medicine in particular, illness is either attributed to impersonal causes and viewed as an accident that befalls the patient as a victim, or is viewed as psychologically caused, and potentially under the person's voluntary control. Pejorative moral connotations therefore become attached to a functional somatic disorder, often leaving patients believing that their problems are due to a psychological or moral defect or weakness in themselves, and are being treated as 'not real'. Women are especially alive to the possibility that their symptoms are not taken seriously, because research has found that disorders disproportionately prevalent in women are often trivialized or described as psychological in origin. Unfortunately, 'trivial' and 'psychological' are often equated, and therefore sufferers may not want to discuss psychological factors in their illness since to do so seems to provide further evidence that health professionals are not taking their symptoms seriously. When individuals with FSS are referred to a mental health professional, they may come into the consultation with the belief that the therapist does not think their symptoms are 'real' or serious, but 'all in their head'. The therapeutic alliance cannot be established unless the reality of the symptoms is validated. Our group finds that a psychoeducational session focusing on the interplay among psychological, social and biological factors in illness is helpful early on in the treatment of FSS.

In the persistent search for organic causes, both patient and doctor become frustrated and the doctor–patient relationship is compromised. This can lead to various outcomes that serve further to heighten the sufferer's distress and fuel the vicious circle of perpetuating factors. Because you are understandably hypervigilant to any hint that medical specialists, friends, family, employer or society are not taking your symptoms seriously, you may become even more determined to find the medical cause to very real pain and physical suffering. You may also experience added worry and self-doubt arising from the ambiguity of your illness. This lack of clarity in your experience may in turn heighten certain forms of behaviour, such as the rejection of any psychological influence in an effort to obtain medical and social validation for your suffering.

The gender issue in therapy

It is important to consider issues of gender in therapy because research suggests that gender plays a role in influencing individuals' reactions to various situations, as well as how they perceive themselves and are perceived by others. More discussion of this issue can be found in Chapter 11.

Several writers have suggested that, in certain fundamental ways, women experience a different social reality from that experienced by men. Accordingly, certain areas require added focus in therapy because of their relevance to women's social context. We have identified several salient areas in the lives of women who have received a diagnosis of IBS. These fall under two general themes: (1) a history of sexual and physical abuse; and (2) areas that have been influenced by gender role socialization, including physical functioning and relationship issues concerning nurturance, assertion and pleasing others.

Physical and sexual abuse One research team found that a history of sexual and physical abuse is a frequent, often undetected experience in women seen in gastroenterology clinics and is particularly common in patients with functional gastrointestinal disorders. Specifically, 44 per cent of a consecutive sample of 206 women seen in a referral-based gastroenterology practice had experienced sexual and/or physical abuse. Almost one third of the abused patients had never discussed their experiences with anyone, and only 17 per cent had informed their doctors. The same study also found that women with functional gastrointestinal disorders were significantly more likely than those with organic diseases to report forced intercourse, frequent physical abuse, incest, chronic or recurrent abdominal pain and more experience of surgery. Abused women were more likely than non-abused women to report pelvic pain, multiple somatic symptoms, more surgery and greater resort to health care. The frequency of abuse found in this study is similar to that reported in studies of women who suffer from chronic pelvic pain, but who, upon laparoscopy are not found to have anything gynaecologically wrong with them. Other researchers also found that approximately three quarters of female IBS patients had sexual disorders which may be related in part to findings of sexual abuse.

Hypervigilance and IBS Researchers have identified common thoughts concerning body functioning in women clients. These frequently involve concerns over losing control, doing something socially unacceptable, appearing less than perfect, having something physically wrong with one's body and not being able to control bodily functions through thoughts or behaviour. A common phenomenon is a hypervigilance or hyperawareness of any notable body sensation, with corresponding hyperconcern over the potential meaning of that sensation. Men as well as women may be subject to developing these thoughts and attitudes; however, girls undergo a socialization process that is more likely to emphasize appearance, self-control and restraint in physical activity. For example, in regard to gastrointestinal functions, while belching and passing gas are not usually socially desirable in public for either sex, girls and women are socialized into believing that these bodily functions are especially not 'ladylike' (e.g. 'belching and farting' contests are less frequent among female than among male adolescents). Moreover, bowel function is considered a taboo subject in 'polite' conversation, and talking about associated symptoms is viewed as lacking in good taste, embarrassing and even shameful, especially for women.

Monitoring exacerbates symptoms Many IBS patients report that their fear of experiencing bowel symptoms in public places often exacerbates the symptoms themselves, resulting in further avoidance of public situations. Such avoidance can lead to personal and social isolation, another factor in the stress and depressed mood experienced by clients with a diagnosis of IBS. The following example of a 37-year-old office worker highlights the anxiety associated with bowel functioning:

'Whenever I went to the office dinners, I lived in fear for weeks thinking of all the excuses that I could make for not attending. For two days before, I would try to eat as little as possible with the hope that my bowels would not act up. I always arrived early at the restaurant to scout out the toilets so I could try to choose a seat as close as possible to the washroom so that I could sneak away as unobtrusively as possible should I need to use the washroom. During the meal, I picked at the food but felt too anxious to eat anything. I was starving, but it was better than all the tumult that I could experience in my bowels when I ate in this situation. Every time my stomach rumbled, I felt like crawling under the table.'

Most individuals with IBS are sensitive to any changes in their gastrointestinal system. Individuals who have experienced embarrassment in social situations because of IBS enter such situations highly attuned to any signs that might signal pain or dysfunction of the gut. Once any such change is noted, the focus on this is amplified and the individual begins to worry and become stressed.

The following is a useful behavioral intervention to give clients a greater sense of power over their symptoms. Clients are instructed to monitor their symptoms every two or three minutes when they are experiencing them, rating them on a severity scale of one to ten. On another occasion when they are experiencing symptoms, they are instructed to try to focus on something that is not connected with their pain (looking out of the window, for example). After this, in the debriefing session, it is useful to ask how their symptoms were affected by the two different focus strategies.

Nurturance Clients with unexplained medical symptoms (including IBS) are often quite surprised to realize how poorly they nurture themselves. It has been suggested that these patients often go out of their way to help others, but do not take time to nurture themselves. Women with IBS often express pride in their ability to give practical and emotional support to their partners and children at home and to their colleagues at work. Neglecting herself can often mean that a woman in this situation is not attuned to her own psychological and emotional needs; however, a woman with severe IBS symptoms is forced by her gastrointestinal problems to be aware of her physical difficulties. Consequently, she is hindered in being aware of the connection between her own self-neglect, the resulting stress and its impact on her symptoms.

It can be seen that part of this cycle of denying one's need for self-nurturance and internalizing the belief that women gain pleasure from nurturing others is that a woman under stress may attempt to alleviate her stress by being even more nurturing of others. For women with IBS, this can be a potentially unhealthy coping strategy because these women often report that the more nurturing they are of others, the more nurturance is expected of them. This further self-neglect may result in greater personal stress as well as increased severity in associated bowel symptoms.

Non-assertion and need for approval Gender role socialization has encouraged girls and women to be non-assertive, putting others' needs before their own, not expressing anger and being attuned to other people's feelings. One consequence of this is that women have problems with anger and assertion more often than men. Common underlying beliefs that have been identified in women clients are central themes with women diagnosed with IBS. These include: 'I don't have a right to push my opinion on others,' 'It's better to please others, and selfish to please myself,' 'Others always come first,' and 'It's not ladylike to raise your voice or show anger.'

When individuals feel powerless or their needs are not being met, angry feelings will be evoked. In the absence of 'permission' to express these needs directly, women are likely to be more critical and self-blaming. Moreover, when women do behave in an assertive manner, it is often perceived by others as aggressive or inappropriate, again on the basis of gender role expectations. The relationships between the need to please others, the expression of anger, assertion difficulties and self-esteem need to be explored.

These empirical findings and clinical observations have implications for both the assessment and treatment of individuals with IBS. Health-care providers and researchers alike need to become more aware of factors such as the stigmatization, trivialization and shame that have been associated with IBS and the influence of gender role socialization, and to integrate this awareness into therapies.

We need to challenge society's negative view of bowel functioning. This is likely to be quite a struggle, since the stigma associated with 'the bowels' is very strong in our society. However, it is worth 'coming out of the closet' for, until this happens, many people with IBS will continue to suffer a debilitating and often misunderstood illness in silence.

Chapter 9

The Treatment of IBS by Hypnotherapy

Elizabeth E. Taylor

We have all heard of hypnosis – but how many of us have any accurate idea of its use? Old films and even modern cartoons leave us with images of swinging watches and domineering voices commanding the subject to 'Look into my eyes' and 'Go to sleep . . . sleep . . . sleep . . .' Equally worrying are the misconceptions created by the stage hypnotist who seems to be able, by the mere click of his fingers, to 'compel' his volunteers to caress a mop head, believing it to be a loved one's hair, or to cluck like a chicken or bark like a dog – all in the name of entertainment! These delusions give hypnosis a bad name. The stage hypnotist cleverly selects either exhibitionist or obedient 'volunteers' who enjoy playing the fool in public. The theatrical atmosphere and audience expectations do the rest. Further misconceptions arise from expressions such as 'putting someone under' and 'getting stuck in hypnosis', which encourage fears that the hypnotist will dominate the subject's mind.

All these notions are naturally off-putting, but none actually has anything to do with medical hypnosis, which for IBS sufferers is merely a tool to enable you to overcome the distressing symptoms that make your life a misery.

This chapter reviews information and research on the treatment

The author would like to thank her patients for allowing details of their cases to be published.

of IBS with hypnotherapy. It will discuss both physical and emotional considerations and will outline the different approaches available to suit different individuals. A detailed account of what to expect in both 'gut-directed' and analytical hypnotherapy will be given. Case reports are included, with the permission of the patients concerned, to provide examples: the individuals' names have been altered to protect their identity. Suggested mechanisms by which hypnotherapy may benefit IBS sufferers are outlined, together with details of the availability and cost of this kind of treatment.

What is hypnosis?

Hypnosis can be described as an altered state of conscious awareness. It is a natural state of relaxation, similar to daydreaming or the condition of complete absorption in an activity, such as reading, watching television, etc. You are aware and can hear people talking to you, but you remain entirely absorbed in what you are doing. In hypnosis, the imagination rather than the intellect is active. There is no loss of control: you and the therapist form a team, and if you are unwilling to cooperate, it is impossible for the therapist to effect a change. In the clinical setting, the hypnotherapist is unable to make you do or say anything you do not want to do or say. Nearly everyone can enter the hypnotic state. The depth of relaxation is irrelevant to a successful outcome, and it is usually the intelligent individual with a high motivation for change who achieves the best results.

What to expect
During an initial consultation, you and your therapist will get to know one another; hypnosis is explained, and any worries you may have about treatment will be discussed. At the second visit, hypnosis is induced. This involves listening to suggestions of deep relaxation – contrary to widespread belief, it does not involve unconsciousness and has nothing to do with sleep; you will be aware of what is said. Nevertheless you will allow yourself to enter an altered state of consciousness which is usually described

as a very pleasant relaxing sensation. The induction of hypnosis itself can be very beneficial and, when combined with further suggestions specific to you, can be used to eliminate or alleviate many common problems. Hypnotherapy is not a miracle cure; rather it is a state of awareness that can be used for self-help. A strong commitment on the part of both you and your therapist is essential for a successful outcome.

Some people worry about remaining in hypnosis indefinitely – that is, about getting 'stuck' in the hypnotic state. This is, in fact, impossible: as with sleep or daydreaming, people emerge naturally from hypnosis, particularly if there is a need to do so.

Can hypnosis help people with IBS?

This question was addressed by Dr Peter Whorwell, a consultant physician in Manchester, who with his colleagues carried out a controlled trial on hypnotherapy and IBS in 1984. He selected 30 patients with severe symptoms of IBS who had failed to respond to other forms of treatment. These patients were randomly divided into two groups. One group received individual half-hour sessions of hypnosis over a three-month period; the second group, acting as a 'control', was given the same amount of time and attention as the hypnosis group, but without the hypnosis sessions. All the patients discussed their symptoms and described any stressful incidents in their lives which they thought may have contributed to their bowel problem. They were also given a 'placebo' – i.e. tablets (sugar pills) which they believed would help their condition but, in fact, contained no medication. The idea behind this was to control for the 'placebo effect'. Very often, if a person expects a treatment to work, it does: the effect of the mind on the body is quite remarkable. If the hypnosis group improved beyond the level attributable to the placebo effect, this would constitute good evidence that the hypnotherapy itself was causing the beneficial effects rather than the placebo effect alone.

During treatment, both groups rated the severity of their symptoms (abdominal pain, bloating and bowel habit disturbance) on a daily basis and recorded their general feelings of well-being on a numerical scale. When these scores were compared for the two groups on completion of treatment, the differences between them were impressive: the hypnotherapy group showed a dramatic improvement on all measures, whereas the control group showed only a minor improvement. During a further study in 1987, Whorwell's original patients were followed up after a period of 18 months. All patients had remained well, although two had needed a top-up session of hypnotherapy.

The poor response of the control group was rather surprising; many other studies have reported the value of psychotherapy in the treatment of IBS, and it may be that the approach used in the control group was more of a general discussion rather than structured psychotherapy. Nevertheless, although a more structured approach might have reduced the differences between the two groups, this does not detract from the clinical effectiveness of hypnotherapy in IBS. Dr Whorwell's study was the birth of gut-directed hypnotherapy, a technique which is becoming more and more widely accepted. In 1996, Professor Houghton and colleagues at the University Hospital of South Manchester found that not only did hypnotherapy relieve the symptoms of IBS, but it also improved quality of life and reduced absenteeism from work.

It has been suggested that the improvement in Dr Whorwell's hypnotherapy patients might have been due to his personality and skill rather than the actual technique, but this has been disputed by other therapists who have produced similar if not identical results using the same technique. These studies leave no doubt that it is the technique which is successful rather than the personal attributes of the therapist.

This is Susan Backhouse's account of a visit to Dr Whorwell's clinic in Manchester, on behalf of the IBS Network:

'Dr Whorwell is well known for his treatment of IBS by using hypnotherapy. His success rate is high, especially with long-term sufferers. Nevertheless, in view of the time-consuming nature of the treatment – it is on a one-to-one basis and each session can last up to half an hour – and lack of sufficient funds, hypnotherapy is seen as a last resort treatment, to be tried when all else fails.

'We were able to sit in on two sessions of people being hypnotized. This was extremely interesting as neither of us had seen anything like it before. The hypnotist (Liz) started by talking to each patient about how they had felt since she had last seen them, and whether they were worried about any up-and-coming events.

'The hypnotherapy itself seemed to me to be like someone talking you through a relaxation exercise. Liz talked each patient into a state of deep relaxation and then concentrated on telling them about the positive ways in which they could control their bowels. She uses soothing imagery to relax and then tells the sufferers about their own strengths and capabilities. She tells them that they are in control of their bowels and their lives, that they will be able to cope with any difficulties during the coming week, that they feel confident and relaxed. Coping with IBS is inextricably linked to coping with life.

'We asked the patients what they thought of the hypnotherapy. They were both enthusiastic. It had helped them a great deal and made them feel more in control.

'The hypnotherapist assured us that hypnotherapy is more than just inducing a state of deep relaxation. From research it is apparent that it will slow down colonic activity, although how this happens is not known. We asked if anyone can be hypnotized and were told that eight out of ten people are able to "go under". We were also assured, as I'd heard before, that the hypnotist doesn't have control over the patient and cannot make her or him do anything that she or he would not normally do.'

What actually happens in gut-directed hypnotherapy?

Before making any attempt to find a therapist, it is essential that your condition has been medically investigated and a diagnosis of IBS has been made by a medical practitioner. Your next port of call is to contact a therapist trained in the gut-directed approach (*see* Appendix II).

The initial consultation

Having found a therapist, you will be asked to attend an initial consultation. This takes about an hour, during which the therapist will ask you questions about your condition and your general medical history. She or he will listen carefully to all you have to say; it is essential that a good rapport is established in this session. A caring and trusting relationship is a necessary component for successful therapy. She or he will ask detailed questions about your abdominal pain, bloating and bowel habits, and will also ascertain whether you have any problems with your 'upper gut' such as nausea, heartburn, reflux of liquid back into the oesophagus (gullet), etc. She or he will need to know if you have any gynaecological problems or back pain, and whether you feel tired for much of the time. Many of these symptoms are associated with IBS. The therapist may also ask if you have any emotional problems.

After completing the history, the therapist will explain the approach to you. She or he will show you pictures of the inside of your body and explain how the gut functions. Your bowel is a hollow tube surrounded by muscle. This muscle is controlled by the involuntary part of your nervous system: that is, the part which controls your breathing and heart rate – the part you don't usually think about. You will be informed that half of this system psyches you up and half slows you down, and that the system works in a very fine balance. The therapist will go on to explain that the nervous system moves the gut in waves of contraction and relaxation (peristalsis). When you have IBS, the muscles of the gut contract too hard and go into spasm. This causes abdominal pain, bloating and constipation or diarrhoea, or both. She or he will explain that you do have a medical condition (spasm of the bowel can be measured in the laboratory). We do not, however, know what causes the bowel to go into spasm.

Many theorists have suggested it may be caused by stress, and although we know that stress has a detrimental effect on the bowel, it seems likely that the anxiety and depression reported by many IBS sufferers is secondary to the disorder. Conventional medical treatment often fails, and you may have been told: 'There is nothing wrong with you,' 'Learn to live with it,' etc. This approach can only add to your burden. Your debilitating symptoms persist and are at variance with the assertion that nothing is wrong, leaving you in conflict. Because of the effect of emotion on the bowel, this can make your symptoms worse, and you become trapped in a vicious circle where physical symptoms and anxiety reinforce each other.

All this will be discussed in your initial consultation. The therapist will go on to explain that hypnosis itself can help to break this vicious circle and replace it with a healing circle of calmness, relaxation and confidence (CRC). If you are relaxed, it is impossible to be anxious. The therapist will then explain what hypnosis is and, with the help of a diagram, will explain the concept of the conscious and unconscious mind. We store information in the unconscious part of the mind, and while most of this is 'forgotten', these stored events affect the way we think, feel, behave and react. She or he will go on to explain what therapists call the 'critical factor', present in the conscious part of the mind (the part we think with). The critical factor protects us from unpleasant information, which we would prefer not to think about, leaking out of the unconscious part of the mind. We do not believe that there is a critical component in the unconscious mind, so if we can put positive suggestions in there, they will in turn change the way we think, feel, behave and react.

Hypnosis enables you to relax sufficiently to bypass the critical factor and make this possible.

How the therapy is conducted

The therapist then explains that two sessions of CRC therapy backed up by a daily relaxation tape are necessary to prepare your mind for symptom removal. You may have had IBS for many years, and your bowel will have formed a bad habit which will take time to break. After these two sessions, the therapist will commence gut-directed hypnotherapy. This uses a 'direct suggestion' approach: that is, suggestions related to symptom removal are directed into the unconscious mind. You will not be required to talk while in hypnosis or to release any uncomfortable emotions.

Following induction of hypnosis, ego-strengthening suggestions will be made. Ego-strengthening is a learning process consisting of repetitive suggestions designed to reprogramme your mind into positive thought. When these positive suggestions are repeated time and time again at each session you attend, they become firmly rooted in your unconscious mind and you will gradually notice yourself improving at a psychological level as your thoughts become more positive, confident and optimistic. This is a similar procedure to CRC therapy, but it is more directive and is designed to increase your determination to get well.

Following the ego-strengthener, you will be asked to place your hands on your abdomen and generate a sense of warmth and comfort in this area. This is a simple procedure in hypnosis. A sequence of suggestions relating to relaxation of the spasm in your bowel and personal control over gut function will then follow. (Some therapists prefer to use ego-strengthening suggestions *after* the gut-directed suggestions.) If you have the ability to visualize (make pictures in your mind), the therapist will ask you to visualize a river flowing evenly and comfortably, with no delays or hold-ups, no rushing or hurry. She or he will then ask you to picture the movement through your bowel in the same way. If you are unable to visualize, this option is merely left out of therapy.

How long does it take?
Gut-directed suggestions will be repeated for a further six weekly sessions and you will be expected to play a gut-directed hypnosis tape every day in between treatments. You should, by this time, be feeling a great deal better, and because of this, the next two sessions will be a fortnight apart. If you remain well, you will continue with your tape, but have no sessions for a further four weeks. You will then have a final session before discharge. Once you have this degree of control, you have the wherewithal to control your condition for the rest of your life. There will be times when you have the occasional flare-up (gut-directed hypnotherapy cannot cure IBS), but in most people, this is quickly overcome by playing the tape. Booster sessions are offered but are very rarely needed.

The full treatment package will be explained in the initial

consultation, and the therapist will tell you that this approach has a very high success rate (eight out of ten patients readily admit to feeling 80 per cent better after a course of treatment) but that the successful outcome depends on you. You need to be absolutely determined to learn to relax the spasm in your bowel and overcome your symptoms. Often during therapy you will begin to recover and then have a relapse. This is actually good news, because it gives the therapist the opportunity to help you to increase your personal control and determination to get well. Once you have overcome that 'blip', you usually improve steadily; and, more importantly, you will lose your fear of relapses which itself helps to prevent further ones. Once you have the ability to control any recurrence of abnormal spasm in the bowel, the condition is no longer a problem. All in all, you will need 12 sessions after the initial consultation for a successful outcome.

Brian: '*Hypnotherapy changed my life*'
Brian was a 55-year-old IBS sufferer. He had the classic triad of symptoms of pain, bloating and disordered bowel habit and felt tired for much of the time. He suffered from severe diarrhoea, passing up to 12 loose stools per day. His life had become dominated by his bowel movements. Venturing away from his daily routine was a misery. A day out required careful planning with regard to the whereabouts of public toilets and even a visit to his local town was problematic. Brian's professional background was in science, and he wondered how anything as 'airy-fairy' as hypnosis could possibly help him. However, he had a very open mind and was prepared to put his doubts to one side to make the effort needed for successful therapy. Gut-directed hypnotherapy was commenced and he began to improve after four sessions. This improvement was steady apart from a slight 'blip' on all three symptoms halfway through treatment. This was quickly overcome and improvement continued. Brian was discharged after 11 sessions, feeling a new man. His energy had returned with all symptoms of IBS eliminated. Follow-up at two years revealed that Brian had remained well. He leads a full life and his bowels are 'not even given a thought'. As he put it: 'Choosing

my words deliberately and carefully, gut-directed hypnotherapy literally changed my life.'

Brenda: '*When all else failed, hypnotherapy worked*'

Brenda was a 32-year-old professional woman. She had classic IBS with alternating constipation and diarrhoea. She had several emotional problems associated with the embarrassment of bloating in public and urgent need of the toilet. Thirteen sessions of gut-directed hypnotherapy coupled with counselling eliminated severe pain, bloating and bowel habit disturbance. On completion of treatment, she described herself as 100 per cent well. Follow-up at four years revealed that the benefits have persisted: she has had no flare-ups at all in that time. The latter is welcome but unusual news – most patients have the occasional flare-up from time to time, but they are quickly overcome by using the tape. Brenda has not used her tape since she weaned herself off it after completion of treatment. Brenda concludes by saying: 'When all else had failed, hypnotherapy worked, but I wish it had been suggested as an option sooner.'

Hypnotherapy and upper gut problems

If you have upper gut problems – nausea, heartburn, indigestion, reflux of stomach contents back into the gullet – the therapist will explain that your stomach is either secreting too much gastric acid (a clear fluid secreted by the glands of the stomach to assist digestion) or not emptying as it should. It is a relatively simple procedure to reduce gastric acid secretion or speed up the emptying of the stomach in hypnosis. Your therapist will ask you to place a hand on your stomach; she or he will then make a sequence of suggestions to reduce your gastric acid secretion and/or speed up your gastric motility (movement). Again, this procedure is enhanced by visual imagery if you have this ability. The therapist will include a post-hypnotic suggestion enabling you to control your gastric acid at any time simply by placing your hand in the same position and repeating a trigger word. As your gastric acid becomes normalized, your stomach can contract and empty properly, leaving you free from symptoms. Using this technique, control can be achieved in very few sessions. As with Dr Whorwell's experiments, scientific research has shown that relaxation under hypnosis can result in a significant reduction of gastric acid secretion and gastric motility as compared to a conventional form of relaxation.

Jenny: '*I wouldn't have believed it possible*'
Jenny is a 48-year-old manager. She has suffered from IBS, with constipation her predominant symptom, since a hysterectomy. She had the classic triad of symptoms, but described her abdominal discomfort as soreness rather than pain. She also suffered from severe heartburn. Gut-directed hypnotherapy was commenced, but Jenny initially proved to be a poor hypnotic subject and felt that there was 'nothing happening to her'. Nevertheless, despite her misgivings, she began to improve after the fourth session. Her heartburn was addressed at the fifth session with the gastric emptying technique described above. This was recorded on tape for her personal use and, as Jenny put it: 'I was astonished. My heartburn, which had been continual for two days, just went!' Both techniques were continued simultaneously for a further five sessions, after which Jenny was discharged, symptom-free. She has the odd 'blip' from time to time which she overcomes herself by using her tape. Jenny states: 'If I hadn't been there, I wouldn't have believed it possible.'

What alternatives are there to gut-directed hypnotherapy?
An experienced therapist can usually deduce from what you say during the initial consultation whether gut-directed hypnotherapy will be sufficient to control your symptoms. Some sufferers may need psychotherapy and/or analytical hypnotherapy before gut-directed hypnotherapy can be successful. Most of us have had traumatic experiences in our lives which can be deeply embedded within the mind. Therapists refer to this process as suppression or repression. These buried events can sometimes have a distorting effect on reality, resulting in unwanted psychological and/or physical symptoms. Working with an altered state of awareness, harmful repressed emotions can be accessed and eliminated. Clients can draw on their imaginative resources and be open to suggestions which encourage more helpful and

realistic attitudes. After 'spring cleaning' the mind, the client then has more room to accept gut-directed suggestions, and treatment is usually effective.

This process is known as a psychodynamic approach. If it is adopted, you will be encouraged to talk through any emotional problems. There is a wealth of psychotherapeutic techniques to draw on, and each therapist tends to specialize in one or more areas. The aim, however, is the same in all: to uncover buried traumatic events that are having an adverse effect on your health. When you have gained insight into and understanding of your problems, you can be taught how to deal with them in more constructive ways.

You may decide to undergo hypnotic regression. This is an analytical form of hypnotherapy designed to 'regress' you – take you back – to earlier upsetting events in your life which you have buried and forgotten about. Regression can be carried out in a number of ways. The therapist may establish a diagnostic scan. After fully explaining what is going to happen, she or he will then establish an 'ideo motor response' (IMR). This means that she or he will ask your unconscious mind to lift, say, one of your fingers; this happens without any conscious effort on your part. The therapist will then count from your present age down to the first year of your life, suggesting that your finger will lift at each year in which there has been an event or influence which is pertinent to your problem. Establishing the ages that need to be addressed usually takes up one session. In the next, the therapist will start at the top of the list, the age closest to your present one, and while you are in hypnosis, she or he will ask your unconscious mind to take you back to that age. You will relive, recall and re-feel those events or influences, and at the same time, your finger will lift to let the therapist know what is going on.

Most people talk through what is happening to them in regression, and this will be appropriately and sympathetically dealt with. This process is known as abreaction or catharsis. When the abreaction is worked through, the therapist will help you to return to the present, and will probably also give you some CRC therapy before bringing you out of hypnosis because you are likely to be very tired. You will then have the opportunity to discuss your experience and learn new ways to deal with whatever has come up. This process may sound daunting, but your unconscious mind will protect you and will only allow you to release what it is safe for you to release at that particular time. You will also have formed a trusting relationship with your therapist, who will have had personal experience of regression during training and, as a result, will be understanding and empathic. Most therapists feel privileged to be allowed to share their patients' emotional problems, and you can be assured that ethical therapists operate within strict confidentiality. The above procedure is repeated session by session until the IMR signals 'clear'. This process in effect clears out the mind, leaving you feeling a great deal better.

Other therapists may use a 'free float' regression. They, too, will establish an initial scan to get an overall picture, but then, rather than starting at the top and working down, they will use techniques to take you back to whatever event your unconscious mind is willing to deal with at that particular moment. Alternatively, some therapists may use regression to take you straight to the root of whatever is your particular problem. Each practitioner will use his or her discretion as to which is the best approach for you, and the end result is usually the same. Nevertheless, after regression some patients will still have symptoms of IBS, which will then need to be addressed using gut-directed hypnotherapy.

How can I be sure that a therapist is properly trained?

If you are going for a psychodynamic approach, it is essential that your therapist is qualified in psychotherapy as well as in hypnotherapy. Physicians practising gut-directed hypnotherapy in the National Health Service (NHS) are usually competent in managing the hypnotic state. If it becomes obvious that psychotherapy is necessary and they are not trained in this discipline, they have the facility to draw on hospital psychologists and psychiatrists. In the private sector, however, you need to be able to check that the therapist is properly trained. A competent psychotherapist/hypnotherapist is trained in a number of psychotherapeutic disciplines, which is a lengthy procedure. Thorough training in all aspects of hypnotherapy is also essential. Anyone can learn to induce hypnosis, but management of the hypnotic state is a different business altogether, and the study of applied psychology is just as important as thorough knowledge of hypnotherapy itself. Personal experience of therapy is also desirable and is an essential part of training. During training, students will have undertaken a comprehensive programme of study as well as taking practical and written examinations of a high standard.

An adequately trained therapist will hold a diploma in hypnosis and psychotherapy from a reputable college and will have documentary evidence to this effect. Therapists will belong to an approved association of psychotherapists, which will require them to keep up to date with new developments in the field and to follow a strict code of professional ethics. Such associations also have a disciplinary procedure to deal with any complaints.

The Register of Approved Gastrointestinal Psychotherapists and Hypnotherapists (*see* Appendix II) was formed in 1993 to provide hypnotherapy and psychotherapy to sufferers from gut disorders, both in the private sector and within the NHS. The Register is a properly constituted body with a strict ethical code. You can be sure that all members are professionally trained by a reputable college in both psychotherapy and hypnotherapy before being trained in the gut-directed approach. The Register's constitution requires members to have formal continuing supervision after completing their diploma, and Register members are also required to have additional supervision in the gut-directed approach.

What happens if I have gut-directed hypnotherapy and fail to improve?

This will become apparent after the first few sessions, and both you and your therapist will need to make a choice either to change the approach or to stop the treatment. If there is no change at all in your condition after six to eight sessions, you may conclude that gut-directed hypnotherapy is not going to help you. If this is the case, your therapist will probably already have suggested that you might want to look at yourself in more detail and go for the psychodynamic approach. Most people are happy to do this, but if you are not then do not be persuaded into doing anything against your will. It is your life and your condition, and your views are important. On the other hand, there is little point in continuing gut-directed hypnotherapy, and you may want to think about visiting your general practitioner or trying another form of complementary medicine (*see* Chapter 10 for discussion of these types of treatment).

Mary: '*Therapy taught me not to hold back*'
Mary is a 45-year-old IBS sufferer who came to us for gut-directed hypnotherapy. She suffered the major triad of symptoms plus upper gut problems. Constipation was her most severe symptom: Mary had not had a bowel movement without the use of suppositories for the past 18 years. She works part-time as a secretary and needed to get up early every morning to use the two or three glycerine suppositories necessary to open her bowels. This performance was causing social, domestic and emotional as well as physical problems. Gut-directed hypnotherapy was having little or no effect on her severe abdominal pain, bloating and constipation, although gastric emptying therapy had reduced her nausea and reflux of gastric acid.

Mary was convinced that her constipation was caused by unresolved problems in her childhood. She requested hypnotic regression, and this, coupled with psychotherapy, proved to be an extremely beneficial but also a lengthy procedure, lasting 18 months. Hypnoanalysis revealed a number of incidents in childhood that she was 'holding on to'. She thus interpreted her constipation as holding on to the past. She had grown up in a restricted environment with little freedom to do what she wanted to do. Many traumas were overcome, but a major incident involved her wanting to continue her education after school. This she was denied by her father, and as a result, she had become dependent on other people's approval for her own happiness. 'I wanted to please my father at the expense of myself.'

Resolution of this incident was the beginning of natural bowel movements. Gut-directed hypnotherapy was recommenced and her constipation continued to improve for a period of two months, after which she relapsed. By this time her suppository use had been reduced to half a suppository as necessary. On more and more occasions she was able to open her bowels naturally.

It was expected that this relapse would be overcome with direct suggestion, but this was not the case. Counselling revealed that Mary was not particularly happy in her job; deep down she wanted to start her own business, but was afraid to take the plunge because of her past trauma. Having resolved to go ahead, this time for herself rather than to please others, her bowel began to function once more. Mary reports: 'Therapy taught me not to hold back; I can now make my own important decisions.'

Mary still uses the occasional half suppository. She has many natural bowel movements, but these tend to be irregular. She still has occasional abdominal discomfort, but nevertheless she is choosing to live her life the way she wants to live it and as a result her constipation continues to improve. Mary is slowly being weaned off treatment. She is no longer concerned about her condition and describes herself as 99 per cent well.

Personality and limitations
Without determination to overcome the symptoms of IBS, gut-directed hypnotherapy will almost certainly fail. Your motivation is the key to a successful outcome. If you are unduly depressed, your motivation will be poor, and a short course of anti-depressants from your GP may be helpful to lift your mood sufficiently for treatment to be successful.

Almost everyone can be hypnotized if they want to be. Some people are unable to relax sufficiently because they have a psychological block: that is, they resist deep relaxation for fear of uncomfortable feelings leaking out of the unconscious mind into the conscious. This type of problem would almost certainly need a more psychodynamic approach. Others do not want to be hypnotized for various reasons, including fear of 'mind domination', usually derived from the misconceptions of the stage hypnotist. This can usually be overcome by a sensitive explanation in a trusting, therapeutic relationship. Some patients are afraid that they will not be able to enter the hypnotic state; this also can usually be overcome. Hypnosis is a learned ability, and if you want, expect and allow it to happen, you will gradually, session by session, drift deeper and deeper into relaxation.

Some patients feel they have not been hypnotized; these are usually in what we call a light trance. Depth is unimportant to a successful outcome (see the case study of Jenny above), but the difficulty is convincing you of this. If you feel nothing has happened, you are unlikely to believe that gut-directed hypnotherapy can help you. However, as your symptoms reduce, you will become more confident. Light-trance patients sometimes need one or two extra sessions simply to alter their belief that nothing is happening.

The effects of the direct suggestion approach can be influenced by age: we expect less striking improvement in the elderly than in younger or middle-aged sufferers. Nevertheless, I have successfully treated an 88-year-old gentleman. Again, if the elderly are motivated to change, direct suggestion is beneficial. Older people can also benefit from gut-directed hypnotherapy combined with general counselling.

A further limitation is a long history of psychological problems; however, this only limits the gut-directed approach. If you belong to this category and are willing to address your emotional problems, a psychodynamic approach followed by gut-directed hypnotherapy can bring about enormous improvements in both your psychological and physical health. The response rate from gut-directed hypnotherapy in patients with chronic constipation coupled with eating disorders tends to be poor. If this is your case, and you are motivated to change, your first step should be to seek a therapist who specializes in eating disorders. When this particular problem has been overcome, gut-directed hypnotherapy may be beneficial.

Attitude is always important. It is necessary to accept that you have IBS, and that this is unlikely to go away. However, if you have no symptoms (or very mild symptoms) then the condition is no longer a problem. If you are expecting a miracle cure from hypnotherapy, you will almost certainly be disappointed. As previously mentioned, the major triad of symptoms in classic IBS consists of abdominal pain, abdominal distension (bloating) and disordered bowel habit. If you have the major triad of symptoms, are not overly psychologically disturbed, are determined to overcome your symptoms and have an open mind, you will almost certainly benefit from straightforward gut-directed hypnotherapy. If you have only one or two of the classic symptoms, success from this approach is less certain; however, if you are not a classic case but are prepared to look closely at yourself, a psychodynamic approach is usually successful.

There is still stigma attached to psychotherapy; please don't let this put you off. Everyone has problems and everyone stores incidents in their unconscious mind. It takes courage and commitment to address the problem, but if they can be released and dealt with in a warm and confidential environment, you may feel completely different.

Ellen: '*Love changes everything, but hypnotherapy does it better*'
Ellen is a 58-year-old professional woman. She had been diagnosed as having IBS six years previously. Her only symptom was severe diarrhoea: up to 17 loose or liquid stools per day. During the initial consultation, it became obvious that she had a multitude of emotional problems. It was these that she wished to address.

A diagnostic scan confirmed a host of traumatic incidents in her past. Regression was commenced and, one by one, these painful memories were brought to the surface. Through this process, she gained insight into and understanding of her problems, and supportive psychotherapy helped her to resolve many conflicts. She came to the conclusion that her diarrhoea was an expression of running away from these painful memories, and with that understanding, the frequency and urgency of bowel action began to reduce.

Ellen is a very strongly motivated lady and put a great deal of effort into her treatment. Regression was completed in 16 weeks, during which time her diarrhoea had reduced to half without addressing the gut. She needed only six sessions of gut-directed hypnotherapy to complete her treatment. At discharge she had only occasional diarrhoea. On completion of treatment, Ellen commented: 'It has been said that love changes everything, but hypnotherapy does it better!' Follow-up after one year revealed that she had continued to improve both psychologically and physically. She gives no thought to her bowels at all and is enjoying life.

In general, diarrhoea-predominant IBS sufferers or those with alternating diarrhoea and constipation tend to respond to gut-directed hypnotherapy better than constipation-predominant sufferers. Nevertheless, the direct suggestion approach has helped a great many constipation sufferers, particularly if they have the classic triad of symptoms.

In my experience sufferers from IBS tend to be intelligent, caring people who are motivated to help themselves. It is this type of individual who will respond best to complementary therapies.

Why is hypnotherapy beneficial?

Apart from the obvious explanation that hypnosis is a useful tool with which to access repressed material in the psychodynamic approach, how it is effective in straightforward gut-directed therapy remains a mystery. Various ideas have been put forward. It has been suggested that, as hypnosis has a beneficial psychological effect, reduction of stress with increased relaxation and coping skills explains the successful outcome. On the other hand, therapists have found that general CRC therapy, although it reduces anxiety, has little effect on the symptoms of IBS. This explanation also implies that stress is the cause of the condition.

An alternative explanation is that hypnosis affects the actual functions of the gut. Dr Whorwell pointed out that the gut and brain share the same nerves and hormones. If emotional and gastrointestinal symptoms are related, physiological changes may be induced by a 'central mechanism' operating at brain level. A study by Whorwell and his colleagues in 1992 looked at the effects of hypnotically induced emotion on the bowel; their results suggested that certain emotions have a striking effect on the bowels of IBS sufferers, and their observation that the induction of hypnosis reduced colonic activity goes some way towards explaining the beneficial effects of gut-directed hypnotherapy in IBS. A further study suggests that improvement in IBS patients after hypnotherapy may be partly due to changes in visceral sensitivity (sensitivity of the abdominal organs). It may also interest readers to know that gut-directed hypnotherapy is clinically effective in cases of inflammatory bowel disease, gastric ulcers and oesophageal problems.

In the absence of more specific facts we can only assume that gut-directed hypnotherapy operates by a variety of mechanisms in IBS patients at both a physiological and a psychological level. Undoubtedly, however, for the vast majority of IBS sufferers, hypnotherapy works either by direct suggestion or as a tool to 'spring clean' the mind.

Availability and cost

Gut-directed hypnotherapy is available in several NHS hospitals. However, lengthy waiting lists are a problem. It is certainly worth asking your GP if this treatment is available in your local hospital, and asking him or her to refer you. An increasing number of GPs are subscribing to this treatment within their NHS budget, although they tend to treat only their own patients. (*See* Appendix II for physicians practising within the NHS.) The practicalities of obtaining treatment in the NHS are not always straightforward. Once a diagnosis of IBS has been made, you are unlikely to be offered hypnotherapy. Medical treatment together with a sympathetic explanation of your problems will be effective for some people; however, many more are left with a distressing condition that affects them not only physically but socially and emotionally as well. If these people were offered hypnotherapy sooner rather than later, they would probably be spared unnecessary suffering. Apart from this, in the long term there should be a substantial saving to the NHS. It has been argued that it is costly to fund hypnotherapists, which is why gut-directed hypnosis is used only as a last resort. On the other hand, one patient cited above (Ellen) cost £598.44 a year in drugs alone, and had been treated thus for over five years. After hypnotherapy plus a follow-up period of 12 months, she was costing the NHS £55.12 per annum, a cost which reflects medication for an additional medical problem: all IBS medication has been discontinued.

We must also consider cost to the state. A number of patients are so debilitated by this condition that they are receiving incapacity benefit. After treatment the majority of patients are able to relinquish their need of benefit and return to work.

Gut-directed hypnotherapy and psychodynamic therapy are available nationally in the private sector through the Register of Approved Gastrointestinal Psychotherapists and Hypnotherapists (*see* Appendix II). Practitioners charge according to their overheads and it is worth shopping around for the right therapist to meet your needs and your pocket.

In the discussion of hypnotherapy in this chapter, I hope to have dispelled some of the misconceptions created by stage hypnotists and the media. I have described medical hypnosis as an altered state of consciousness, a pleasant state of relaxation which allows positive suggestions to enter the unconscious part of the mind. I have outlined relevant research and given a detailed account of what to expect in both gut-directed hypnotherapy and analytical hypnotherapy, using illustrative case studies. I have described the limitations of treatment and discussed speculative suggestions as to how gut-directed hypnotherapy may operate. The short answer to this question is that we do not know: nevertheless, gut-directed hypnotherapy is extremely effective for the majority of IBS sufferers, and the alternative psychodynamic approach is available for those who need it.

To close, here are two IBS Network members' experiences of hypnotherapy:

'I decided to try hypnosis for my IBS with great trepidation. I think to most of us the word "hypnosis" brings to mind the typical stage act with people being made to do silly or strange things without knowing they are doing them. Believe me, this is not possible. I found a qualified GP who also practised hypnosis as I felt that he would know about IBS and what the range of symptoms includes. I was lucky in that, when I first met the doctor, he was very pleasant, understanding and "normal". He did not charge me for the first appointment, during which he explained about hypnosis, how it works, how you should feel, etc. He also explained that different people can be hypnotized to different levels – for example, if you are a relaxed person, you are likely to respond more easily than someone who is tense. He then hypnotized me for a short while to let me decide if I wanted to go ahead with treatment. By this time, I had got myself into quite a state worrying about what was going to happen to me, so I was very surprised that, once I was lying down and he had started to count, I could gradually feel myself relaxing and feeling more and more comfortable. I left the surgery wondering what on earth I had been worrying about as I had been pleasantly surprised by how simple it all was and how relaxed I felt.

'I had six appointments, and although I did not actually have any improvement in my IBS symptoms during that time, I was gradually feeling more relaxed generally. I felt I would have liked more appointments, but the doctor said I had progressed as I should and that, if I used the cassette he had recorded for me two to three times a week, I should see further improvement. He also said that if in the future I felt I wanted to take things further, he could attempt to hypnotize me to a deeper state where he could look into my past to see if there was anything there that could have triggered IBS, but this could be a very upsetting experience and it needed careful consideration as to whether some things are best left in the past.

'Within a couple of weeks of finishing the hypnotherapy, I did have three months when my IBS was a lot better and I do think it was because I had a time of being more relaxed. The problem I found with being left to use the cassette was finding the right time to listen to it because you need complete privacy and the peace of mind to know you are not going to be disturbed so that you can relax completely. I have not been able to use the cassette regularly as at present I have a four-year-old and very little privacy. When she goes to school I do intend using the cassette regularly and will see if I get any improvement again. The only question mark left for me about hypnosis is whether one hynotherapist's treatment would be different from another's. My hypnotherapist only used relaxation suggestions, and I wonder if another one would refer to the IBS and make suggestions to you about ways of controlling the symptoms?'

A man in his twenties gives the second account:

'The first thing I do when I go for my hypnotherapy sessions is to answer questionnaires about my symptoms: pain, bloating, diarrhoea and so on. I have to mark on a scale how bad my symptoms have been. Then I talk to her about my week, what I've been doing, whether it was a good or bad week. It's like a mini-counselling session. The last was my sixth session (out of ten) and the doctor compares my notes now with my notes from the last session. This is all before the session begins. Then I sit down and close my eyes and relax for the session. She tells me to relax, to think of my abdomen, to hold my hands over my abdomen . . . she keeps telling me to relax, saying this warm feeling over my stomach is taking the pain away. She builds it up over the 20 or so minutes . . . saying the feeling is getting hotter and all the time telling me to relax. Then towards the end of the session she'll say things like, "You will be confident . . . you can take on anything", and so on.

'I feel very relaxed after the sessions. I'm fully aware of everything that's going on around me. I'm quite clear that the reason my symptoms have improved so much is the hypnotherapy. I had all sorts of drugs before, they didn't help me in the slightest, but this is really good. I also have tapes given to me by the doctor which I try to use every day. I'm very lucky, because all this is on the NHS.'

Chapter 10

Treating IBS by Complementary Medicine

Susan Backhouse

Since the 1980s there has been a surge of interest in 'alternative' or 'complementary' medicine. These terms suggest almost a sideline to traditional Western medicine, but in fact, many of the various therapies have been successfully healing people for thousands of years. Certain sectors of the medical establishment have often failed to take these disciplines seriously because, it is claimed, there have been few scientific studies to test their efficacy (although more are being undertaken as mainstream interest increases). The practitioners of complementary medicine, however, respond that their results and methods of working are not testable within the framework of conventional medical research. In addition, many will say that they have stood the test of time. An important factor to take into account is that, unlike a trial of a new drug, research into complementary medicine will not profit big business concerns; and certain medical training establishments, in the United States particularly, have been significantly influenced by the financial support of the pharmaceutical industry. This has meant that, since the beginning of the century, mainstream Western medicine has become more and more synthetic drug-based. Medical training centres which emphasized a more holistic idea

The author would like to thank Barry Alexander, Kate Burford, Kris Burroughs, Peter Conway-Grim, Dr I. P. Drysdale, Christine Evans, Victor Foster, Nerissa Kisdon, Penny Nunn and Dr Christine Page for their help in preparing this chapter.

of healing were not financed to the same extent and so were more likely to flounder.

Although often thought of as the father of Western medicine, the Greek Hippocrates had ideas about health that were very much in tune with those of complementary practitioners. He firmly believed that treatment of a specific complaint should be carried out only as part of the treatment of the whole person; and he stressed the importance of diet to people's health as well as their habits and the environment in which they live.

What is complementary medicine?

Complementary, or holistic, medicine is based on the idea that the physical, emotional and spiritual aspects of a person make up an integrated whole. Each individual is also connected to their family, their environment and the world around them. Thus a practitioner will look at, and attempt to treat, the whole person, rather than particular symptoms or a specific disease. This means that one person with certain symptoms may be given different treatment from another person showing the same symptoms.

A holistic approach is one that sees ill-health as a sign that the body, mind, spirit and emotions are out of balance with each other. It acknowledges the body's great power to heal itself, although therapies may be used to stimulate this power. Holistic medicine does not try to attack a diseased part but aims to support the entire person and guide him or her towards health.

Complementary medicine is different from orthodox Western medicine in that the emphasis is on you taking responsibility for your own health and well-being. It is inadvisable to look upon your practitioner, as some people look upon their doctors, as someone to whom you can hand over responsibility for your health. The complementary practitioner should be seen as a facilitator, someone who can support and encourage you, as well as stimulate your body's own unique ability to heal itself.

Choosing a therapist

Because of the recent increase in interest, there are now many different therapies available to choose from, especially if you live in a city. However, the vast majority of them are costly (usually from £25 upwards for an initial session and £20 upwards for treatments thereafter). A few therapies are available on the NHS, and maybe, in time, that will become more common; also, you may be able to attend a training college for a reduced fee. For more information on these colleges, and on NHS availability, contact the umbrella group for the therapy in which you are interested (*see* Appendix II). Occasionally, in some areas of the country, complementary practitioners will be part of a local LETS barter scheme (Local Economic Trading Schemes – ask in your library or Citizen's Advice Bureau if there is one near you). But for most people, at the present time, going to a complementary practitioner means parting with a significant sum of money if you want to give it enough of a chance to work. Therefore it is important that you choose your therapist carefully. The following guidelines will help you.

- As the law stands at present, anyone can use the title 'acupuncturist', for instance, whether or not they are adequately trained. To safeguard yourself, contact the umbrella group for the therapy in which you are interested. You will then be able to find out what training those on their register will have had to undertake. You will also be able to enquire about their code of ethics and complaints procedure. They will let you have a list of practitioners in your area.
- Find out about the therapy you are interested in before approaching a particular therapist. Take responsibility for knowing about your own treatment.
- When you make contact with therapists, ask them how long they have been qualified and whether they are a member of a recognized representative organization.
- Ask them if the therapy is available on the NHS. If not, ask

them how much they charge and whether they operate a sliding scale, if this is relevant to you.

- Ask them if they have had many patients with IBS, and what their success rate with this condition is.
- Ask them for how long they expect you will need treatment. Although this will only be a guide, and they may be reluctant to pin themselves down, it could give you some idea as to how much the whole course is going to cost you. Treatments for conditions such as IBS often go on for a year or more.
- You may wish to ask them for the name of one of their clients whom you could contact for a reference.
- Ask them if patient records are confidential.
- Ask what insurance cover they have.

In the following sections, the most popular complementary therapies available in this country, and some of the more unusual ones, are discussed in more detail, with particular reference to their use in treating IBS.

Chinese medicine

Chinese medicine has very ancient beginnings. Between 479 and 300 BC, a book was compiled that has much similarity with modern thought on preventative medicine. It states that ailments must be cured before they arise, by proper diet, rest and work, and by keeping the mind and heart calm. This book, the *Nei Ching*, described the circulation of the blood through the body, which was not discovered by the Western world until the 17th century. Anaesthesia was administered by Chinese surgeons as far back as the third century BC, and the catheter, which was 'invented' by Western medicine in 1885, was described in a Chinese medical book in the 7th century BC. The concept of stress-induced illnesses, thought by some to be a relatively modern idea, was also known to Chinese healers thousands of years ago.

Central to Chinese medicine is the idea that our health depends on the balance of the body's motivating energy, or *chi* (pronounced 'chee'). *Chi* flows throughout the body but is concentrated in meridians, or channels, underneath the skin. The meridians are connected to the body's organs and functions. *Chi* has two opposite qualities – *yin* and *yang* – and the purpose of treatment is to restore the balance between the two. *Yang* energy represents maleness, light, heat, dryness, contraction, strength, activity, sun, spring, summer; *yin* is characterized by femaleness, receptivity, tranquillity, darkness, coldness, moisture, swelling, weakness, passivity, earth, autumn and winter. Although *yin* and *yang* are opposites, they are not hostile to one another. Each needs the other; without one, the other could not exist. *Yang* is not superior to *yin*, nor is *yin* superior to *yang*. Contrast this concept with traditional Western thinking where masculinity is superior to femininity, objective is better than subjective, quantity is better than quality, activity better than passivity. Chinese medicine teaches that the whole order of the universe results from the perfect balance between the two forces of *yin* and *yang*, and that similarly our health depends on this crucial balance within our bodies.

Yin and *yang* are represented, for example, by the dilation and contraction of the heart; the exhalation and inhalation of the lungs; and the functions of the parasympathetic and sympathetic nervous systems. According to the Chinese, all diseases are the result of an imbalance between *yin* and *yang*. In the body, too much *yang* manifests itself as acute pain, inflammation, spasms, headache, high blood pressure, irritability and excitation. Too much *yin* might appear as dull aches, chilliness, fluid retention and discharges and is characterized by weakness, exhaustion and debility. By restoring the balance of the energy system, Chinese medicine aims to stimulate the body's own healing powers.

Modern Western medicine is coming to the same conclusions in some respects. For instance, many Western physicians believe that if the sympathetic and parasympathetic nervous systems are not in harmony with each other, illness will surely follow. Science tells us that a harmonious functioning of the nervous systems and a well-balanced disposition is essential in order to avoid some of the stress-induced diseases which are so rampant today

– high blood pressure, heart trouble, stomach ulcers, headaches, insomnia, etc.

Chinese medicine teaches that the stomach and spleen are the 'mothers' of the bowel. The idea is that, if the 'mother' is tired and therefore deficient, she cannot properly nourish the 'child' – in this case, the colon. A practitioner of Chinese medicine would aim to strengthen these organs together with the bowel for anyone suffering from a bowel disorder.

Chinese medicine also sees the emotions of grief, melancholy and sadness as inherent to colon *chi*. Not only is the colon affected adversely by these emotions from without, but it can itself give rise to these emotions, which are believed to exacerbate IBS. It might be interpreted that an IBS sufferer is holding on to some sort of grief, or harbouring a sense of loss. There may be deep disappointment about oneself, one's own life, the hopes and dreams one had, and this will affect the bowel quite profoundly. Chinese lore teaches that it is essential to give up these emotions that one might be holding to give the bowel a good chance of recovery.

Acupuncture

Acupuncture is an ancient medical system, dating back over more than 2,000 years. The word itself is a Western one meaning 'needle piercing', but the Chinese term is *chen chiu*, which means 'needle moxa'. Moxa – the powdered leaves of the mugwort plant – is sometimes burned on the skin or on the end of the needles to create a gentle heat which facilitates the treatment.

The idea of having needles stuck in your body has been alien to many Westerners until recently. It sounds as if it would be very painful. However, the needles used in acupuncture are so fine that, when they are inserted, it is usual to feel nothing more than a slight tingle or a dull ache.

For those people who are afraid of needles, or for children, the acupuncture points of the body can be massaged or pressure can be applied with a probe. Modern technology has seen the arrival of electro-acupuncture and laser treatments in which the acupuncture points are stimulated by a low-frequency electrical current, applied with a probe or with finely tuned laser beams.

It has been discovered that the stimulation of acupuncture points induces the release by the brain of morphine-like substances called 'endorphins', which have pain-relieving properties; acupuncture is used extensively for pain relief, and has been used as an alternative to more conventional anaesthesia in many surgical operations.

The theory behind acupuncture has been developed through the ages and is based on the idea that the meridians, along which flows the life energy *chi* are connected to the body's organs and functions, and along these meridians are found the points that the acupuncturist manipulates to regulate the flow of energy and restore health. Although there doesn't seem to be a definite anatomical structure to the points, they can be detected electronically.

An acupuncturist will attempt diagnosis by careful and thorough questioning and observation. You will be asked about past illnesses, details of the current problem, your general energy level, and family traits and tendencies. Your practitioner will attempt to assess the functioning of all your body's systems, and your face and body features will be carefully observed. You will be asked about your response to changes in the weather, your taste preferences, your feelings and phobias. On each visit, six different pulses will be felt and your tongue will be inspected. The acupuncturist will aim to build up a full picture of you so that your current problem can be seen in perspective.

With the rise of AIDS, there has been some concern about the safety and hygiene aspects of acupuncture treatment. The British Acupuncture Association and Register say their members have to use needle sterilization techniques approved by the Department of Health, which are considered to be completely effective against hepatitis and AIDS. Many practitioners use disposable needles.

Acupuncturists will say that they treat the person, not the disease, so a question such as 'Can acupuncture cure IBS?' can only be asked as 'Can this person be cured of their IBS using acupuncture?' and can only be answered after the practitioner has examined the patient. However, it is said that acupuncture can have an effect on almost any illness as long as the degenerative process in the tissues of the body is not too extensive, which, of course, does not apply to IBS. Many practitioners will work in cooperation with other therapists if it is deemed to be useful in particular cases.

One practitioner believes that acupuncture is very effective in IBS cases where the link with stress is strong. He says that, in his experience, those patients whose stress is relieved by the treatment get much better, while those whose stress stays much the same don't improve. As it is believed that acupuncture can be particularly helpful in alleviating stress, if you feel this is a major factor in your IBS it may be worth a try. The same practitioner says that he would normally expect some change after three or four treatments, with significant improvement after ten. If there is no result after ten sessions, he advises trying something else.

It is worth noting that, as some acupuncture points are not suitable for use on pregnant women, it is important to tell your practitioner if you are pregnant or trying to conceive. This advice would apply for any therapy.

Lizzie has been receiving acupuncture for a year. She's 40 years old and has had IBS for five years. She has been happy with the way her acupuncturist has treated her and has found him to be very sympathetic. He has attempted to get a picture of her as a whole person and to try and understand what the reasons might be behind her symptoms. However, she says:

'I feel that the sessions don't really help as much as I might have hoped. I usually feel better for a day or two after each session but the symptoms get worse again. Sometimes I feel that the symptoms increase again when I am nervous or tense. Occasionally I get panic attacks when I am alone and my insides go crazy. I feel a bit silly admitting this as outwardly I appear to be confident. I have scarcely mentioned this to the practitioner. I pay £22 per acupuncture session and wonder whether I am wasting money but continue to go.'

As well as the acupuncture treatment, Lizzie was given dietary advice – a balanced wholefood diet avoiding coffee, too much wheat and alcohol.

Gillian, who suffers from chronic constipation, first tried acupuncture 20 years ago. She attended the sessions weekly for some months. She found it very beneficial and achieved a better bowel function. However, when she stopped the treatment the constipation returned. She later saw another acupuncturist but this time experienced no benefit and the practitioner advised her not to continue the treatment, which Gillian felt was honest of her. A third time, Gillian found the needles very painful and was unable to continue the acupuncture because the discomfort was causing a lot of tension. Interestingly, a non-IBS-related stomach problem cleared up soon after.

Caroline is aged 43 and had had IBS for over ten years. She originally went to her acupuncturist for neck and arm pain; this disappeared after five treatments and her IBS also greatly improved.

Others have also found acupuncture very helpful, as illustrated by one of our IBS Network respondents:

'I have two very accurate indicators of the degree of stress in my life. Both I could do without! One is eczema on my hands and the other is IBS. My IBS began even as a toddler. As a child I sat for hours at the bottom of the stairs, hugging my tummy before heading off for school. As my life went on, I learnt to accept that I would have to rush to the toilet five, six or even seven times before an appointment, and that exams would be accompanied by severe gut ache. No one seemed to question it, so I thought that I'd go on like that for ever.

'In my first job after university, I found myself under a great deal of pressure and, at the same time, my personal life was going badly wrong. My IBS took over with a vengeance and became the centre of my life for some months. I was being sick, spending large chunks of time rushing to the toilet and generally feeling wretched. Doctors and hospital appointments left me feeling more hopeless. I was given anti-spasmodic tablets and left with the assumption that this would be it for the rest of my life – not a very attractive prospect.

'At that time acupuncture was pretty new on the British health scene, and a friend and I wondered if it could help us over hay fever. Never thinking that it could help my problems with my gut, I went off to my first appointment. When the acupuncturist put the first needle in my hand to show me that it didn't hurt, my hand became red and throbbed. Puzzled, I told him that, although it wasn't hurting, it certainly was doing something.

'The acupuncturist asked if I had something wrong with my large intestine. When I told him my history, he said that he could probably cure that but not to hold out great hope for my hay fever. I could have kissed him!

'Six treatments later, I felt well enough to take some decision about my life which started to relieve some of the stress I was under. Up until that time, I felt so terrible that I couldn't see a way forward at all. After eight treatments I was able to stop going to the acupuncturist with the knowledge that I could go back if I needed to.

'That was 16 years ago. I am still someone whom stress first strikes in the gut; the difference is that I feel that I can do something about it. When my gut gets bad, I make an appointment to see the acupuncturist, have a few treatments and I'm back to normal. In fact, there haven't been so many times since that first lot of treatments that I have got that bad. I feel that knowing that there is something that will relieve the symptoms is part of the battle and helps me to keep my guts under control.'

However, two other IBS Network members, both women in their thirties, found the experience unpleasant:

'After trying acupuncture, the practitioner said she didn't know what else to do. I found acupuncture extremely uncomfortable and sometimes painful and was relieved to give it up.'

'I only went four times. The woman put needles in my stomach, but mostly in my legs. They tingled but were not particularly painful. Then she left the room for 20 minutes. During this time, the needles became more and more painful. I wanted to pull them out but was scared in case I pulled them out wrongly or something. I didn't like to call out – I didn't know whereabouts in the building she was. So I waited. When she came back, I told her to get the needles out quickly, it was so painful. She said I should have called out. It didn't improve my symptoms at all – if anything, it made them worse. The woman said the pains were due to my negativity. I never went back.'

Chinese herbalism

Richard Lucas, in his book *The Secrets of the Chinese Herbalists*, says that these healers do not claim to cure anything: rather, they simply work to support and assist nature in its endeavour to heal the ailing organism. The herbalists of China believe that non-poisonous plant medicines supply to the body the appropriate constituents it lacks, in a way similar to natural foods.

Chinese herbalists use many herbs for bowel disorders, including yellow dock (normalizer and regulator of bowel function), blackberry root (astringent, with a strengthening effect when used as a remedy for diarrhoea), slippery elm (soothing, mucilaginous, aids easy passage during bowel movements, absorbs foul gases in the body) and garlic (used as a remedy for diarrhoea and other intestinal disturbances, anti-bacterial).

Shiatsu

Japanese shiatsu is based on the meridian energy system as applied in traditional Chinese medicine. Instead of needles, the shiatsu therapist uses touch to rebalance the energy – *chi* – at relevant points along the meridians, or anywhere on the person which is felt either to have an excess of, or to be deficient in, energy. The aim is to tone and strengthen the particular functions of the organs within the body, as well as give a feeling of well-being and deep relaxation. The practitioner applies pressure to the body using thumbs, hands, elbows, knees or feet. Stretching and structural adjustments may also be used. The recipient is clothed and lies or sits on a futon mattress on the floor.

Kris Burroughs, a shiatsu therapist, explains her view of IBS:

'The large intestine is closely associated with the lung and also the skin in Chinese medicine. These form an immediate interface with the external environment and a means of cleansing the body from waste and toxins. IBS can be associated with retaining the breath in the chest and an inability to let go, to exhale the carbon dioxide-loaded breath. This can be likened to a state of constipation and retention of the faeces in the colon.

'I would work with the breath, as a means both of cleansing and of releasing physical and emotional holding patterns. Often IBS sufferers feel a need to control themselves and memories of trauma over childhood toilet training (control or lack of control of their anal sphincter) may surface, perhaps that their shit, or how or where they shit, wasn't OK. This may have led to over-control or a disownership of that part of themselves. There may be alternating patterns of withdrawing into themselves for security (constipation) and moving out into the world in a more assertive or retaliating way (diarrhoea).

'Problems with the colon are often related to the spleen, the "mother" of the colon in Chinese medicine. This is associated with nourishment, security and a sense of inner trust of the self. If there has been insufficient mothering and mixed messages about both physical and emotional feeding, this will necessarily affect the kind of digestion, absorption and retention of food and how we feel about our products of digestion.'

She goes on to describe how she treats a client:

'A session usually begins with palpation of the *hara* [belly] – the central reservoir of our *chi* – and this enables the practitioner to decide which meridians to focus on during the session and is itself a treatment. In fact, the entire shiatsu session can be viewed as both diagnosis and treatment – not only where and how the practitioner touches but what form of verbal communication takes place with the client. This may range from emotional counselling to advice about physical exercise, spiritual practice or diet.'

Many therapists believe that a healthy way of eating is essential for people with IBS. Shiatsu practitioner Barry Alexander says that slow and thorough chewing of the food is of supreme importance because, he says,

'If animal or vegetable protein hits the bowel incompletely digested in the previous stages of gut absorption, then the caecum section of the colon will be forced to flood that whole area of the colon with white blood cells to neutralize this rotting protein. Because the colon is not designed to deal with undigested protein particles it protects itself in this way, but inefficiently, and the detrimental effect to the colon gives rise to the multitude of pathologies associated with IBS and other related colon problems.'

Shiatsu practitioners may accompany their treatment on the large intestine meridian with special techniques incorporated in what is called *hara* (belly) massage. They may also recommend the Japanese way of self-massage of the abdomen or *ampuku*, which can be very effective. It is believed to prevent stagnation of blood, fluids and *chi*, which can cause various problems including bowel disorders. An additional technique which the patient may practise for him or herself is to stimulate the acupuncture point Colon 4, which is between the index finger and thumb, above the web, on the fleshy part. This is something that can be done yourself by massaging the point, using your other thumb in an upward direction towards the wrist and towards the index finger. The point can be massaged on both hands.

Barry Alexander says that treatment for IBS must be consistent if absolute improvement is to be obtained. He believes that, in the early days, treatment should be at least weekly for, say, the first eight sessions. After improvement, sessions can be less frequent. Successful shiatsu treatment will stimulate *chi* so that the bowel can be regenerated and healed; full recovery of the bowel may take up to a year, depending on the severity of the problem. He goes on to say:

'It is important to choose a shiatsu practitioner who possesses strong *chi* in him/herself and can project it to where he/she wants it to go. In this way, spectacular results can be achieved. It also matters how the practitioner thinks. If there is no conviction in his/her treatments, the results will not be good.'

And on *chi*:

'*Chi* is that force which accompanies all of life, without which there is none. *Chi* is the very energy and meaning in the message you are reading right now. It is the desire to help. It is the power behind vitality. It is grace in all its meanings, and is the power behind action.'

Denise tried shiatsu for a number of conditions including IBS. She has had IBS for over ten years and had frequent acute abdominal pains which were very difficult to deal with and which were not relieved by anti-spasmodic drugs. She speaks well of her therapist, whom she enjoys going to see and whom she finds very supportive and sympathetic towards her health problems. She reports feeling very relaxed once the treatment is over. Since her first visit some months ago, she has had no pains from IBS.

Homoeopathy

The principles of modern homoeopathy were established in the 18th century by a physician, Dr Samuel Hahnemann. He was disillusioned by the medical practices of the time, which so often did more harm than good. He believed that we humans have the ability to heal ourselves and that the physician's task is to discover and, if possible, remove the cause of the trouble, and to stimulate the body's own vital healing force. By experimenting on himself and his supporters, he discovered that many substances which caused symptoms in a healthy person would ease the same symptoms in someone who was ill; amazingly, he also discovered that the smaller the dose he used, the more effective it was. The homoeopathic remedy is produced by a special method of dilution until virtually nothing of the original substance is left. It is then given in tablet, liquid, granule or powder form.

The remedies are given with the intention of removing symptoms by rebalancing energies in the body. In contrast to the approach in conventional Western medicine, the patient is treated rather than the disease. This means that one person with IBS might be given different remedies from another person suffering from the same condition, even the same symptoms.

The remedies come from many different sources: plants; substances such as sand, charcoal, salt and pencil lead; drugs such as morphine, cocaine and arsenic. However, all are diluted in the special manner so that poisons are no longer poisonous, innocuous substances become effective and all have great power for healing – for the right person. For anyone else, they would have no effect. Because of the minute doses involved, there are no side-effects, although as the healing starts, symptoms may get worse before getting better. Homoeopathic remedies are safe for babies and children, and for pregnant women.

During the first consultation, the practitioner will take a detailed case history of the patient. Homoeopaths have a particular interest in what makes the symptoms worse or better – for example, certain foods, stress, warmth or cold, etc. They will look at the general health of the individual, the aspects of his or her personality which make him or her unique as well as the particular symptoms being experienced. As the patient's personality is often discussed in some depth, it will inevitably lead to some counselling. Dr Christine Page, a medical doctor and practising homoeopath, believes that all homoeopaths should have some counselling skills or be ready to refer the patient to a specialist.

Dr Page describes what she looks for at the first consultation:

'Having taken a full homoeopathic history, I, personally, also take a history of a daily diet and check that there are no excesses (or deficiencies). Foods which are known to make IBS worse include wheat products, tea, citrus fruits and tomatoes. The problem of candida overgrowth would also be assessed, especially if there is a history of recurrent antibiotics. Dietary advice may well be given or referral to a nutritionist.

'In the first consultation I aim to record a set of parameters which relate to the specific illness, general health and the mind. From these, I select one remedy from thousands which hopefully matches these parameters as closely as possible. This remedy may be given as a single dose or regular doses, depending on the individual. With homoeopathy, once the symptoms clear you stop the treatment. Even with one powder it is possible to see the cessation of all symptoms for life.'

She goes on to describe the part she believes personality has to play in IBS:

'My own feeling is that IBS is associated with relationship issues when the patient is often uncomplaining and lets things go, rather than speaking out. [He or she] looks for peace rather than conflict. There is often a love/hate relationship especially with family and a need for both closeness and space and yet an inability to ask for either. There is also a strong conscientious energy, trying to do a good job and yet often resenting the neediness of others.'

Dr Julie Allen has been a practising homoeopath for over 20 years and has a high success rate with IBS sufferers. She uses hypnotherapy and psychotherapy with homoeopathy and believes that a large part of the problem with IBS is of a psychological nature. She says that, in the majority of patients that she has treated over the years, stress, anxiety and deep-rooted psychological problems have predominated. If the patient is unwilling to change their lifestyle and attitude, she says, they may only obtain temporary relief from either homoeopathic or conventional medicine.

Maria is in her seventies and has suffered from IBS for about 35 years. When she was diagnosed as having 'spastic colon' in 1963, her consultant told her she would be on drugs for the rest of her life. She wasn't helped in any way and became dependent on the Libraxin she was prescribed. After a year, she was determined to wean herself off the drug, and did so over the next six months.

What Maria found hardest to deal with was the many days when she felt completely unwell – feverish, constipated, with a feeling of general malaise. The only way of getting over it was to go to bed for two days and to eat just stewed cooking apples and milky rice pudding.

Her practitioner treats her with both acupuncture and homoeopathy. When she first went, she was very ill with her symptoms. She was relieved to find that, in the practitioner, she experienced for the first time someone who knew what she was talking about and who did not treat her symptoms as of no account, a waste of time.

> 'She said she had treated other people with this trouble, she could improve the quality of my life, renew my energy, and make me feel much better – she did *not* say she could "cure" me. I began to feel better very soon, and this was lasting, although it was several months before I was feeling really well.'

Maria found that tension in her lower back disappeared, as did a swelling of fluid under her skin that had been there for a year, which was proof to her that the treatment was working. After going every three weeks, she now attends three-monthly sessions for a general booster. She also has a Bach Flower formula to suit her (*see* pp. 264–5) and the practitioner also recommended a slippery elm drink and Quiet Life tablets. At £25 for the first consultation and £15 for each visit thereafter, Maria feels it is expensive but worth every penny:

> 'I still have some of the symptoms at times, but never so severe, and only very infrequently, after great stress, for instance. I am now much stronger and fitter than I have been for many years. It is such a pleasure to be well after nearly half my life drifting from one ill patch to the next.'

Angie, a 40-year-old nurse, was diagnosed with irritable bowel syndrome some 20 years ago. Her symptoms were relatively mild up until the last three years, when she has suffered with more diarrhoea, abdominal pain, severe nausea, bloating and wind. A year ago she began to see a homoeopath who is also a medical doctor:

'She has helped me to recognize certain patterns and issues in my life with which I wasn't dealing effectively and how this was affecting my physical health. Her treatments helped me feel stronger and more confident – people commented I seemed like a different person – with a resultant decrease in IBS symptoms, but, more importantly, [it gave me] the ability to cope more effectively with them and not go to pieces when they did occur.'

Not everybody speaks of homoeopathy so highly. Gwynneth is a 75-year-old housewife and retired teacher. She has suffered from diarrhoea and nausea for the last two years. She saw a homoeopath for six months, and spent £80, but felt it did not relieve her symptoms. The practitioner suggested she tried the Hay diet for the diarrhoea, and this was of some help.* However, she stopped the treatment when she began to feel that the remedies he was giving her (primarily for sinusitis) were contributing to her bowel problems.

Treatment may last years, as Maureen found out. She has been seeing a homoeopath for four-and-a-half years:

'This may seem like a long time, but one of the first things she told me was that there was no quick cure, just a long-standing improvement. During my course of treatment the pills have been changed many times and I still take two pills every other day, or every day if needed.

For the past year, I have been 90–95 per cent free from IBS – I won't say cured as I still have little setbacks.'

---

* The theory behind the Hay system is that starches and sugars shouldn't be consumed at the same meal as protein and acid fruits; *see* pp. 107–8.

Herbalism

The use of plants for healing goes back, no doubt, as far as we humans do! Archaeological evidence has shown that Neanderthal people of 60,000 years ago may have had knowledge of medicinal plants. In the beginning, prehistoric men and women probably put most plants into their mouths. Many were innocuous, some were nourishing, some made them ill and a few killed them. Some, they found, relieved symptoms of sickness or pain and a few caused hallucinations. The plants in these last two categories became their medicines.

Much of our knowledge of herbalism has probably been acquired over the ages by trial and error and handed down from one generation to another. It is only really in this century that herbal or 'natural' remedies have *not* been at the forefront of medicine. On more than one occasion in recent years, scientists have developed a drug that is less effective and more toxic than the original herbal remedy. Of course, there are areas in which herbal medicine has remained important, especially in the pockets of surviving aboriginal cultures where modern Western medicine has remained relatively unknown and where plants still provide the only medicines.

Medical herbalists disagree profoundly with the orthodox or 'allopathic' approach of finding, isolating and synthesizing an active ingredient from a plant – for example, aspirin from willow bark, quinine from cinchona bark, digoxin from foxglove. They believe that the active ingredient, when taken out of the context of the whole plant, is incompatible with good health: there are many other elements in the whole plants which have an important part to play in the natural balance. For example, dandelion leaves are a strong diuretic, but it is not necessary to give a potassium supplement with them, as is usually required with a diuretic drug, as they are a rich source of potassium themselves.

Like many other complementary therapies, herbalism aims to stimulate the body's own powers of healing. It does not suppress the symptoms; rather, it assists in the restoration of balance and harmonious functioning of the body. The discharge of toxins is encouraged, which can often make the patient feel quite unwell for a short time while the cleansing process is taking place. This is important, as an underlying toxicity would, herbalists believe, prevent a lasting equilibrium from being established.

Although you can buy herbs and herbal remedies for specific complaints over the counter, qualified herbalists would say that they will treat you as a whole person, rather than a collection of symptoms. A herbal preparation made specifically for you by an experienced practitioner will address the underlying imbalance, rather than simply aim to alleviate the surface symptoms. Herbalist Peter Conway-Grim points out:

'The interest in peppermint oil is a good example. Peppermint can be useful in the treatment of IBS, but only in certain circumstances and within certain limits. When treated as mere pills to be popped, herbs will be only occasionally effective. Likewise, the quality of herbs is also important. The chamomile [which has anti-inflammatory, sedative and tissue-healing effects on the gut] used in commercial teabags is not of medicinal standard and will be unlikely to offer much help.'

Another herbalist, Christine Evans, looks at diet and dietary habits in great detail, often with the use of questionnaires, so that she can make recommendations as to how they might be altered to help the healing process. The first consultation includes a detailed investigation of the whole patient. It may take an hour or more and includes an in-depth medical history, abdominal palpation, examination of the irises, skin, tongue, nails and other physical diagnostic features. Christine looks for general signs of the patient's overall condition such as signs of debility, and physical, mental and emotional exhaustion. Blood pressure and pulse are assessed.

She describes how she prescribes with the IBS patient in mind:

'The herbal formulae chosen would be quite individual, being composed of a number of complementary herbs which would not only address the root cause, but [also] strengthen weakened organs and systems within the body. For instance, anti-inflammatory, antispasmodic, demulcent, soothing and cleansing herbs may be given to heal the intestinal wall, along with herbs to tonify or calm the nervous system, provide nourishment and balance specific related organs such as the liver, pancreas, spleen or kidneys. In addition, any nutritional deficiencies, which are frequently present, are assessed and corrected. This is very important as many patients are severely debilitated, which impairs the body's ability to heal. The herbs themselves supply vital nutrients in an easily assimilable form, thus strength and vitality is restored and many other seemingly unrelated symptoms are frequently improved.'

After years of suffering and misery, when she seemed to be getting worse and worse, Patsy decided to get rid of all her drugs and, as a last resort, to try a local clinic of herbal medicine run by a former nurse and midwife. The herbalist told her she was run down because of the continuous diarrhoea she suffered, and she was put on 13 different minerals and nutrients straight away. She was advised to go on the Hay diet (*see* pp. 107–8) and to avoid all processed foods, tea and coffee. Patsy was also put on a three-day fast which, she was told, was a cleansing process to rid her body of all the toxins she had accumulated. She felt quite ill for a day or so, with severe headaches, but was told this was to be expected, like going through 'cold turkey' after giving up drugs. Two years ago, she wrote:

'I stuck it out as I thought anything was worth it to get rid of my IBS. I have slowly got better. For the past three months I have not had diarrhoea at all. My nails and skin have improved and many people tell me I look so much better. Also, my blood pressure has reduced so I have also been able to cut down on the tablets I have been taking for 15 years for that.

'The downside of this is that it has so far cost me £200 which, as a pensioner, has been difficult to find, but it has been worth it.'

One of the clinics run by this herbalist is now able to take, at reduced fees, patients who have been referred by their GP.

Gillian visited a different herbalist many years ago. After a very thorough medical history was taken, she was prescribed a medicine which was to help a number of problems she had apart from constipation. She consulted the practitioner every four to six weeks, but, although the medicines she was prescribed were generally helpful, she didn't sustain any long-term improvement to any of her health problems, including her IBS.

Aloe vera

Recently a lot of attention has centred on the healing properties of aloe vera, and descriptions such as 'wonder plant' and 'miracle cure' have been used in media articles. Supporters believe aloe vera to have all-round qualities, and it has been said to cure IBS. Is there any substance to these claims?

Aloe vera is a member of the lily family and looks like a cactus. It is known to have anti-inflammatory and antibiotic properties, and the history of its use in herbal medicine goes back thousands of years. It is claimed that sufferers of both constipation and diarrhoea can be helped by aloe vera because of the way in which it regulates the bowel.

Paul Hornsey-Pennel, in his book *Aloe Vera: The natural healer* (Wordsworth, 1995), says that aloe vera is especially beneficial to those with bowel disorders. He cites how the plant bathes the intestinal tissue, softens and cleans out impacted toxic layers and helps the body assimilate and process food. It is also claimed that it can ease the pain associated with IBS.

To date, there appears to have been little research to assess the value of aloe vera. According to the *Daily Mail* (14 February 1995), however, an American study concluded that aloe vera juice is able to break down and loosen impacted material in the bowel. It is also believed to help in detoxifying the colon, and to have no harmful or irritant effects on the bowel, although the Aloe Vera Information Service (PO Box 52, Bordon, Hants GU35 0UP) suggest you contact them if you are epileptic, prone to hyperactivity or pregnant.

Medical herbalists and other practitioners are cautious about the 'cure-all' claims that aloe vera has received in the media and from commercial interests. Alison Tyas, a medical herbalist, says,

> 'Although it wouldn't be my first choice, considering it is a great healer and its anti-inflammatory properties, I can see how aloe vera could be useful. However, if something is claimed to be a 100 per cent cure-all, it is simply not true. I have used aloe vera occasionally but not for IBS.'

Sufferers of IBS were asked whether they'd tried aloe vera for their condition and what the results had been. Judith wanted to stop taking drugs for her IBS and was recommended aloe vera juice by her regular pharmacist. She experienced a strong reaction,

> 'I was told it would "cleanse my system" and, boy, did it do that! The two weeks during which I forced this vile liquid down were the worst two weeks since my IBS began. My IBS tends to come in bouts, but it became a constant nightmare of day-and-night vigils in the bathroom while taking this "miracle cure".'

And Mary took the product for about a month after hearing a talk about it at a health fair. She says,

> 'I found that it did not help to relieve my symptoms at all, and now regard it as a waste of money, although perhaps I should have persevered longer.'

All accounts weren't negative, however, as Pauline shows:

> 'I used the concentrated juice for about three months. After about a month, the griping pains seemed to diminish and the "looseness" of motions seemed to be less frequent and intense. After three months, I decided to give the aloe vera a rest (about a month ago). I am lately finding that I am having griping pains

and loose bowels more frequently again. I shall take aloe vera again for a while to see if things improve.'

Evening primrose oil

Workers at Addenbrookes Hospital, Cambridge, conducted a study in which they found that women whose IBS symptoms were severe during their menstrual period were helped by taking evening primrose oil. One group of women took eight Efamol capsules containing 500 mg of evening primrose oil daily, and another group took placebo capsules (containing olive oil). They found that just over half the patients taking the Efamol reported an improvement in symptoms, while none of those taking the olive oil capsules improved. This seems a strong effect. However, improvement did not take place straight away – it usually began in the second month of administration, but in some cases was not apparent for over three months. The researchers suggest that their IBS patients may be deficient in some essential fatty acids that are contained in evening primrose oil. It is not suggested that evening primrose oil will help all IBS patients – just women whose symptoms seem to vary with the menstrual cycle. Women with IBS should keep a diary of symptoms, and see whether this is the case. If so, they should see their doctor and discuss the possibility of taking evening primrose oil. However, evening primrose oil is very expensive and its benefits are not proven.

Bach flower remedies

Edward Bach, a renowned Harley street physician and bacteri-ologist, developed his method of flower healing in the 1930s.

The remedies are presecribed not for the physical complaint, but for the patient's state of mind and mood. The principle behind the Bach flower remedies is that negative and inharmonious states of mind will not only hinder healing and recovery, but are the primary cause of sickness and disease. For instance, someone who is extremely fearful or anxious will have their vitality depleted. The body loses its natural resistance to disease and the person becomes vulnerable to infection and illness. Edward

Bach said: 'There is no true healing unless there is a change in outlook, peace of mind and inner happiness.'

All the remedies are derived from the blossoms of wild flowers, bushes or trees. None of them is harmful or habit-forming or has any side-effects. A few drops of the remedy are taken in a little water.

According to your moods and emotions, you might be prescribed rock rose for terror or extreme fear; aspen for vague fears of an unknown origin; gorse for feelings of hopelessness and despair; pine for feelings of guilt; or vervain for tension and over-enthusiasm. The composite remedy, Rescue Remedy, was formulated for use in emergencies. It is composed of five remedies for shock, terror and panic, mental stress, desperation and for the faraway feeling which often precedes loss of consciousness.

Bach flower remedies are often used in conjunction with other therapies.

Naturopathy

Naturopathy is both a philosophy and a therapy, which aims, like many other complementary therapies, to stimulate the body to use its own power to heal itself. The philosophy, and some of the methods used in naturopathy, date back to at least 400 BC (although 'modern' naturopathy is about a hundred years old), when Hippocrates stated that only nature heals, providing it is given the opportunity to do so. He also believed in the importance of food as medicine and that disease is an expression of purification.

Naturopathy is based on three principles: (1) that the body has the power to heal itself through its own vital force; (2) that disease is the body's way of trying to get rid of anything that is preventing its organs and tissues from functioning properly, whether this is chemical (e.g. an imbalance in the body's chemistry due to dietary deficiency or excess), mechanical (e.g. physcial damage due to poor posture or injury) or psychological (e.g. illness caused by stress and anxiety); and (3) that the whole person – body, mind and spirit – must be considered and the patient seen as a unique individual who might respond and react quite differently to the next person.

According to the General Council of Naturopaths:

> The task of naturopathic practitioners is twofold. First, to educate their patients to take more responsibility for their health and to assist them to understand the fundamental laws of health relating to rest, exercise, nutrition and life-style. Second, using natural therapies, to increase the vitality of the individual and to remove any obstructions, chemical, physical or psychological, which may be interfering with the normal functioning and internal harmony of the organs and tissues.

A practitioner might use various therapies to stimulate the healing process, including: the prescription of a natural diet, which may or may not be specific and controlled, depending on the practitioner and the patient; fasting; structural adjustment such as osteopathy, chiropractic and remedial exercises to rebalance the body; hydrotherapy, which is the use of water in various ways, both internally and externally; advice on a healthy lifestyle – relaxation, exercise, the cultivation of a positive attitude, etc; and education, so that patients are able to take responsibility for their own health. It isn't unusual for patients to experience an initial worsening of their symptoms as part of what is called the 'healing crisis'.

Naturopaths aim to help restore their patients to a point where they no longer have a use for treatment and can maintain good health themselves through whole food, fresh air, exercise and positive thinking.

Dr I. P. Drysdale of the British College of Naturopathy and Osteopathy has this to say about treating patients with IBS:

> 'Practitioners such as ourselves treat individual patients uniquely. However, there are certain basic elements of treatment which are common to most sufferers of IBS. For example, the types of treatment that a naturopathic osteopath would use are manipulation of viscera [organs of the abdomen], together with

dietetic advice and a certain amount of counselling advice, stress being an important input to the IBS syndrome.

'What I think is unique about our particular philosophy is that we combine rational dietetics with counselling and a physical hands-on treatment, and this approaches the patient's situation on at least three levels. As these three are integrated from the practitioner point of view, we feel this is most beneficial to the patient.

'Generally when treating irritable bowel syndrome, it ultimately depends on patient cooperation and willingness to follow the particular lifestyle outline that is given.'

Katie was recommended to a college of naturopathy and osteopathy by her reflexologist. The following is her account of her treatment there.

'The first visit cost £15 for an hour's consultation and treatment. Further visits cost £10 for half an hour. They work on the basis of treating the whole person and look at body structure, mental make-up and biochemistry (nutrition).

'On the first visit I discussed my symptoms with a trainee osteopath who was due to qualify at the end of the month. She took details of my medical history, including any previous operations, and asked whether I was taking any medications. I explained the symptoms of IBS and she asked whether I had had any previous treatment.

'She asked me to undress to my underwear and stand in front of her. She checked my posture and felt along my spine, and also felt around my stomach/colon area. She then left the room to discuss her notes and diagnosis with a qualified osteopath. (A fully qualified osteopath will see you if the student is not sure about anything.)

'When she came back into the room, she explained that my colon on the left side was very "tight" and constricted and this is why the muscle went into spasm. She then explained how she would manipulate various muscles in my stomach and belly area.

'She pressed quite hard along the line of my colon and it was quite sore on the left-hand side. She also worked on an area to the left of my lower back which she told me corresponds with the digestive system. This was very painful. She worked on these areas for about ten minutes.

'At the end of the session, she asked me to complete a diet sheet and to post it back to her. This recorded everything I ate for one week. She also showed me how to massage the colon area myself and said I should do this for a few minutes every day if possible. She said that, by doing this, I would help to push the contents along and disperse any gas.

'Since I saw her I have had no morning upsets at all. [Previously, Katie had regularly passed frequent loose motions in the morning.] My colon area was quite sore for a few days, as was the area in my lower back where she had been treating me. I have had just one movement most days, although some days I have gone once more after lunch or later on. On these days I feel unwell until I go to the toilet for a second time. I have only had one day when I went three times in total. I have not used Imodium at all since the first visit.

'On the second visit, my diet was discussed. I was advised to try to cut down, or preferably cut out, sugary drinks and have plain water or fruit juices diluted with water instead. I should have a bowl of salad each day to include two green leafy vegetables. I was also asked to try to eat protein foods separately from carbohydrates. It was suggested that I should change what I have for breakfast as I usually have a cereal such as Rice Krispies which contain a lot of sugar. Unfortunately this discussion took up the whole half-hour appointment and I was disappointed that there was no time for any treatment.

'I have booked a third appointment as the osteopath said that I would probably benefit from three or four more treatments, although this was for [another problem] rather than the IBS. She said that, by continuing to massage my colon myself, I could keep the problem under control and altering my diet would help to "clean up" my system.

'I really do feel that this is the answer to my problems. I

just wish that my own doctor had advised me of the benefits of massage to the colon when I first had IBS.'

Reflexology

The principle of reflexology is that there are areas in the feet and hands which correspond to all of the glands, organs and parts of the body and that these can be manipulated by using the thumb and fingers on these areas.

Reflexology has been used for 5,000 years in China, but at the beginning of the 20th century, an American called Dr William Fitzgerald claimed to have discovered that there are ten electrical currents running through the body from the top of the head to the toes. All the organs, glands and nervous systems of the body fall within the areas covered by these currents. The theory is that crystalline deposits form around the nerve endings, preventing the electrical currents from 'earthing' through the hands and feet. Pressure on the hands and feet will break up the deposits and allow the currents to 'earth', restoring balance and enabling a smooth flow of energy throughout the body.

It was in the 1930s that Eunice Ingham developed a map of the feet which related to the entire body, all parts being connected to specific areas, or reflexes, on the hands and feet. Sensitivity in a particular area on the foot is believed to be a sign that there is congestion or tension in the corresponding part of the body. Pressure and manipulation on that part of the foot sets in motion therapeutic benefits within the body.

Reflexology aims, like many other therapies, to create a balance within the body in order that good health may be achieved or maintained. A consultation will start with the practitioner feeling the feet and noting where the sensitive areas are. A case history may then be taken. The feet will then be massaged and pressure applied, paying particular attention to those areas which indicate crystalline deposits and blocked energy. Most people find the treatment extremely relaxing and soothing, even though some areas of the feet may be quite sensitive. Results may be seen after two or three sessions, but in cases of long-standing disorders, progress may take a lot longer.

Nadia is 43 and has had IBS for a year. She was told that it was probably caused by a hysterectomy she had had some months before the onset of her IBS symptoms. These include passing stools about five times in the morning, which is exhausting for her and causes her to feel very low and anxious first thing. She says she finds it difficult not knowing what each day will be like. Some days she can be 100 per cent, but not know why, and on other days, she feels so bad that she just wants to stay indoors.

Nadia has been receiving reflexology treatment weekly for seven weeks. She pays £14 for an hour. She has found the practitioner very sympathetic, questioning her thoroughly about her general health as well as IBS, listening well and remembering every detail. After six treatments Nadia noticed a great improvement and felt elated, but sadly it only lasted for a week.

She would recommend that other sufferers try reflexology, mainly because she believes anything is worth a shot. She herself found it a worrying treatment, however, because:

'She kept picking up other points of the body that indicated trouble. In my case, it was neck, shoulder, adrenal gland, spleen, urethra and womb – which I haven't got!'

Stephanie saw a practitioner who treated her with aroma-therapy and homoeopathy as well as reflexology. Her symptoms consisted of wind, severe constipation, urgent visits to the toilet in the morning and cramping pains, as well as panic, lack of energy and a general feeling of unwellness. She received the treatment weekly for a year. Stephanie was pleased with the practitioner's sympathetic and caring attitude. She wasn't cured by the treatment but, as she says, it was helpful:

'The treatment helped to a certain extent by relaxing me, as by that time I was extremely tense and probably at my lowest level. However, the relief was not really beneficial in the long term. I must stress, though, that mentally it helped greatly as, having been told by the medical profession that this was just the way I was and I would have to live with it, I felt so alone and uptight, and I was becoming afraid to leave the house. Now, I no longer felt alone and was extremely thankful that someone felt I wasn't a stupid woman who was probably imagining all these symptoms anyway.'

Katie tried five sessions of reflexology for her IBS. She was very happy with the practitioner, who treated her for two-hour sessions at the one-hour rate of £15, made various dietary suggestions and discussed her case with other therapists, looking for ideas, but although stiffness in her neck benefited, her IBS did not improve at all.

Rena was sceptical about trying reflexology at first, but her story is a positive one. As she says:

'I am the type of person that shuns various herbs and home remedies, but when my IBS was at its peak, I was persuaded to try it. I had a treatment and was violently ill the next day. I had another the following week and can honestly say I felt better. I had two more treatments in five weeks and I now have a treatment every five weeks. My reflexologist has put together a small potion of herbs and liquidized it, and if I feel unwell, I rub a little on my stomach at night and by next morning I feel fine. I am pleased to say that, apart from the odd bout, I have been virtually IBS-free.'

Colonic irrigation

The technique of colonic irrigation, or colonic hydrotherapy, was apparently first recorded in 1500 BC and has been used by various traditional and complementary practitioners since then. Using sterilized equipment, warm, filtered water is gently introduced through the rectum and into the colon. Special massage techniques are used so that the water progressively softens and expels faecal matter and compacted deposits, which are then piped away with the waste water. The idea is that it rids the body of the build-up of toxins in the gut which can otherwise be reabsorbed into the blood, causing, or contributing to, a variety of illnesses.

A session takes about 30 minutes. Herbal preparations may be used, and regular colon implants of lactobacillus acidophilus are given to assure normalization of bowel flora. Afterwards you may experience improved mental clarity and a greater feeling of well-being.

The Colonic International Association recommends that this treatment is used in conjunction with other therapies. They say that, by improving elimination, the response to dietary, homoeopathic, herbal, manipulative and other therapies is also markedly improved. Treatments need to be regular over a period of one or two months, and they recommend six-monthly treatment to 'maintain inner cleanliness and good elimination'.

Gillian suffers from chronic constipation and flatulence. She found that colonic irrigation gave her more of an instant relief from being very constipated than any long-lasting benefit. She says:

'Treatment is not uncomfortable for the most part and lasts about 30 to 40 minutes. However, it is expensive – I paid £46 for the first session and £35 subsequently – and practitioners seem to be few and far between, perhaps because inserting tubes in the anal canal and pumping water wouldn't be a job that would appeal to a lot of people!'

Gillian was told that, immediately after treatment, it is common to empty the bowel thoroughly and sometimes to be constipated again immediately afterwards, which is what happened to her. However, the system then, apparently, readjusts itself. She decided she wouldn't continue with the treatments as, for her, it provided no long-term benefit.

Another patient who suffered from severe constipation – going for as long as two weeks without having a bowel movement – was simply advised by his specialist to take laxatives if he didn't have a bowel movement after more than five days. The laxatives, however, didn't work. He had heard about colonic irrigation and made some enquiries. He takes up the tale:

'I took my courage in my hands and made an appointment! It was one of the wisest things I had done – the relief! He gave me about eight treatments – two a week for two weeks and weekly afterwards, put me on a course of herbs and psyllium husks, lots of water and it has made such a difference.'

Aromatherapy

Aromatherapy uses essential oils, extracted from the roots, stalks, flowers, leaves or fruit of a plant, to heal the body. For thousands of years, people have used aromatic oils to soothe, relax, create spiritual atmospheres and protect from infection. The modern form of aromatherapy is about 30 years old.

The odour of essential oils can influence the state of mind. They can also help to reinforce the immune system and have antibacterial, antiseptic and disinfectant properties.

The essential oils are combined with vegetable oils and used in massage, put in the bath or heated in special burners, to create a regenerative and healing effect on the body. Aromatherapy can be especially beneficial in easing stress and anxiety.

As with most practitioners of complementary medicine, a qualified aromatherapist will start by taking a detailed history of your health and lifestyle. Useful oils for treating IBS might include lavender, clary sage, neroli, jasmine, marigold, vetivert (all good for anxiety); eucalyptus, juniper, black pepper, lavender, rosemary (may help to ease pain); rosemary, juniper, black pepper, fennel (may help constipation); lavender, neroli (massage with these can ease diarrhoea and stomach cramps); and peppermint (good for digestive problems).

Essential oils contain potent substances and should only be blended by a qualified aromatherapist. Certain oils should not be used in pregnancy (these include hyssop, marjoram and myrrh), or for babies and very young children. Oils for use on elderly people should be diluted to half strength.

Florence felt uncertain on her first visit to an aromatherapist but found it to be a very enjoyable experience:

'I had been suffering from pain for some time. Someone I met just by chance told me she had been going to an aromatherapist for chronic headaches, and she said she was much improved afterwards. She also said the aromatherapist was qualified and belonged to the International Federation of Aromatherapists and also the British School of Reflexology. Amazingly, she said she paid £30 for three hours. I made an appointment with the aromatherapist – she said to allow three hours for the first session. She spent half an hour taking my medical history, asking about illnesses, feelings, family members, etc. Then she explained that she was going to make up the oils for the massage based on the information I had given her. She spent a few minutes doing this, and then asked me to smell the oils to see if they were acceptable to me – I didn't like the smell of the first oil, and so she adjusted it with other oils, to one which I did like. I then undressed down to my underwear, she covered me with towels and I lay on the special couch. The room was fairly dark, and it was all very discreet. She massaged my back and neck, then covered these parts with a towel, and then started on another part of my body. So for those people who are a bit nervous of a massage, they have nothing to worry about. Your body is covered up, and only exposed bit by bit! Although I was anxious at first, I soon relaxed, and when she had finished I realized another two-and-a-half hours had elapsed! I was so relaxed it was hard to get up and drive home. I went again the next week; it was only £25 this time, but it still lasted two-and-a-half hours. This time I enjoyed it more because I wasn't anxious as I knew what was going to happen and she was no longer a stranger to me. I think it did help with the pain. I have only been three times so far, but each time I have felt good afterwards and I feel positive it has benefits for me. I wondered how I could spare three hours for this, but on the other hand, it makes me relax for this time, whereas otherwise I would probably be rushing around. I don't know that it would help people whose IBS had been caused by medical problems, but I'm sure it helps people who are stressed out. I also don't know what part the oils play – I think it might be the actual massage which helps most. I know £25 is a lot of money, and I certainly couldn't afford to go every week, but I am going to try to go every month – I am lucky to have a good job to be able to afford this.'

Meditation

Meditation for health and harmony has been used for thousands of years, and there are now many forms. Basically, though, meditation involves sitting comfortably in a quiet place, and focusing your mind – either through looking at a selected object, such as a candle, or repeating one word for the duration of the meditation. The word is called a 'mantra'. Concentrating on the one word or object, or on your breathing, can help focus attention and calm the mind. When somebody meditates, his or her breathing slows down, as does the heart rate. Meditation relaxes the muscles, and reduces oxygen consumption. When you practise meditation regularly, you may find that you can respond much more calmly to stressful situations.

Although you can meditate without learning the technique from others, or from books, you may find it easier if you do. You can obtain some simple books on meditation from your local library. There are courses at which meditation is taught – for instance, a popular one is transcendental meditation (TM), associated with the sixties and the Beatles. This involves sitting with your eyes closed for 20 minutes twice a day, repeating a mantra. The mantra is chosen for you by a teacher of TM to suit your particular personality. The word is meant to be as relaxing and tranquillizing as possible.

Meditation is said to relieve tiredness, dissolve deep-rooted stress and leave the system feeling calmer and more alert. Some IBS sufferers have found meditation very helpful.

Relaxation

Most of the books written for the IBS sufferer recommend

relaxation as a way of coping with IBS. This is not surprising, as any pain or medical complaint is aggravated by worrying, tension and stress. It is well known that people with the same complaint will experience pain differently; people who try to maintain a positive outlook, however hard this is, fare better than those who become depressed and believe that they will never recover. Consequently, any technique that decreases your stress levels and helps you to take life at a more even pace must be beneficial.

One of the best ways to relax is to learn to breathe properly. Many of us breathe too shallowly at the best of times and, in times of tension or pain, almost forget to breathe at all! Your body needs a good supply of oxygen at such times and deep breathing will help you to calm down.

Try this simple exercise for about ten minutes:

- Sit on a straight-backed chair with your feet flat on the floor (if your legs are too short, put a cushion under your feet). Keep your spine straight – imagine a thread attached to the crown of your head pulling it up towards the ceiling. Rest your hands loosely in your lap.
- Breathe slowly and deeply through your nose. Concentrate on the rise and fall of your navel. As you breathe in, say to yourself 'Peace in,' and as you breathe out, say Tension out.' Imagine the good, peaceful feelings that you are breathing in and all the worry, stress and bad feeling that you are breathing out.

You may also like to try this calming exercise:

- Stand with your feet hip-distance apart with your arms loosely by your sides.
- As you breathe in, slowly raise your arms out to the sides and up above your head.
- Hold the breath and stretch as far as you can with your arms. Then slowly exhale and lower your arms.
- Repeat, to the rhythm of your breathing, six times at first, increasing as you practise more. If the arm movements are done slowly it will encourage you to breathe in and out more deeply.

The following exercise is often used by teachers of yoga and other relaxation methods to relax the whole body:

- In a warm, quiet room where you won't be disturbed, lie on your back on the floor or sit in a straight-backed chair. Rest your arms by your sides if you are lying down, or loosely in your lap if you are sitting, with the palms uppermost.
- Concentrate on breathing deeply and slowly, feeling the gentle rise and fall movement of your navel.
- Imagine your feet and tense each one by pointing it downwards and curling your toes, and then relaxing.
- Tense your lower leg by pointing your foot towards your head, feeling the stretch, then relax and repeat on the other side.
- Tense and relax your knees and your thighs.
- Move up to your buttocks and then your stomach and tense, then relax the muscles there.
- Think of the small of your back, tense and then relax it.
- Move up your back and tense then relax your shoulders and your chest.
- Clench one fist tightly and then relax and let go. Repeat with the other hand.
- Tense and then relax your upper and lower arms.
- Move up to your neck, tense and relax the muscles there.
- Tense your jaw and chin, then relax them.
- Clench your teeth together and pull your mouth into a big, false smile, then relax.
- Close your eyes tightly and wrinkle up your nose, then release the tension. Raise your eyebrows as high as you can and relax them.
- Go through all the parts of your body, thinking about tensing then relaxing them. Be aware of how the muscles feel when they are tense and how they feel after you relax them.
- Continuing to breathe slowly and deeply, let your body give up to the pull of gravity. Rest like this for at least ten minutes. Concentrate on your breathing. If any unwanted thoughts come to mind, let them come up and through you and out of you.
- As you complete the relaxation, begin to move your feet and

legs, then your hands and arms. Move your neck and head and slowly open your eyes.

Faith healing

Healing by the laying-on of hands is generally performed free or at little cost as such healing is often part of the healer's service to the community, inspired by religious beliefs. You usually can give a donation, as large or small as you want. Spiritual healers tend to believe that there is a flow of energy from a higher force, or God, which can heal through the medium of the healer. It is often said that disbelievers can 'block' the healing energy by setting up a 'barrier'.

'In 1984 I had ten sessions with a lady healer which I'm convinced did a lot of good. Since then the pains have been very infrequent and of much less severity.'

'I went to a spiritualist place. I sat in a warm room and the woman put relaxing music on – it was very nice. Then she put her hands on my shoulders and asked me if I felt the warmth. She said it was energy flowing through her to me, as a vessel of God. I did feel a warmth, but I believed it was just the pressure of her hands. She then moved her hands around various parts of my body. I didn't like it, I felt uncomfortable, and what's more, I couldn't believe in it. I wanted to, but I couldn't. I went about six times, but I never felt any different. She said it was because I was resisting belief.'

An Overview

How does complementary medicine differ from traditional Western medicine?

There are significant differences in the way holistic and allopathic (orthodox Western) medicine look at health and disease. Holistic medicine aims to maintain health; illness is seen as a deviation from health. Allopathic medicine, on the other hand, is preoccupied with disease, and health is taken to be a deviance from disease. In orthodox medicine, diagnosis is of primary importance. Within complementary medicine, diagnosis is of lesser importance; instead, signs and symptoms are noted (including pulse-taking, observing body language, dietary habits, etc.) so that a whole picture can be built up.

In Western medical research, there is often talk of the 'placebo effect'. A placebo is a supposedly inactive substance or procedure that unaccountably produces benefits for the patient. It is often looked upon as a nuisance factor which researchers have to account for when assessing their results. Sometimes, when people's health is improved by complementary medicine, it is dismissed as 'just the result of a placebo effect', and therefore somehow unreal or inferior. However, for many complementary therapists the aim is, as A. V. Conway put it in his article 'Assessment of Complementary Medicine: Revolution or evolution?' in the *Journal of Complementary Medicine*:

> to bring patients into a position where they have more choice in the beliefs that they have about themselves, and as a result of exercising that choice, and changing their beliefs about themselves, they get better. It is unclear why this subtle, natural and cooperative process should be considered somehow inferior to treatment where a patient has something 'done' (medication, surgery, etc.) to him, to 'make' him better. The placebo effect can be extremely powerful . . . Placebos do not just help people feel better, they can dramatically affect physiology.

Within complementary medicine, there is often more of a desire to see the patient as the 'expert' when it comes to their own health. The practitioners are interested in the patients' explanations of their problems and, to some extent, their reasoning behind it, as well as their ideas and reasoning about what should be done. Often practitioners will have to take up and discuss 'hints' from their patients, especially if the latter are not used to discussing their health in this cooperative way. Learning how the patients see their own problems may also be helpful to practitioners when deciding on treatment. Having said this, practitioners will not usually see the patients as having the same expertise as themselves. After all, it is the practitioners who have been consulted for help and advice.

Probably the major difference between the two ways of thinking is that, while orthodox medicine attempts to destroy or suppress what is believed to be causing the illness, through drugs, surgery or radiation, complementary medicine seeks to defeat disease by strengthening the whole person's defences.

Here's how C. W. Aakster, in a Dutch study on complementary medicine, contrasted the two approaches (in his article 'Concepts in Alternative Medicine' in the *Journal of Complementary Medicine*):

> If a disease is something with a non-understandable Latin name, which can only be measured by experts and which can only be cured by doctors, who know the solutions, the doctor is by definition someone who should have had at least seven years of university training, a man (rather than a woman) with great authority (expertise), who takes the lead in the patient's problem-solving. If, however, diagnosis is of the functional type, and the therapeutic measures are of a rather simple nature and require the full and active cooperation of the patient (a profound change of dietary habits, regular exercise, etc.) then medicine becomes more manageable. It reverts to the patient and may lead to deprofessionalization, by merely emphasizing basic rules for healthy living, the responsibility of the patient . . . seeing the person as an integrated whole, as the patient sees himself.

In addition, most complementary practitioners and their patients choose such disciplines because they want to avoid the harm done by drugs which aren't compatible with the body and cause side-effects, as well as painful diagnostic tests and mutilating operations.

Others, however, may choose alternative medicine because they see it as having almost mystical qualities. If these patients are helped, all well and good; but they may also be particularly vulnerable to ineffective practitioners or even charlatans.

A criticism sometimes made is that some people seek out

complementary treatments as a last-ditch attempt, a clutching at straws, after orthodox medicine has failed them. Again, the sceptics say, these people may be easily taken advantage of. The answer to these criticisms, of course, is better regulation of complementary practitioners and the availability of their treatments on the NHS, or at low rates, so that patients are protected.

The wind of change?

Much of 20th-century medical science in the West has based its thinking on the idea that a disease is a distinct entity (a 'thing'), separate from the person who has the disease. Research methods have also emerged from this perspective, which is one of the reasons why it is difficult to evaluate complementary medicine using such methods. There is some indication, however, that this may be changing and that a more holistic way of conducting research may be developing. Dr David St George, senior lecturer in clinical epidemiology at the Royal Free Hospital School of Medicine in London, has this to say: 'Research is being undertaken to explore the new holistic paradigm. If this shift is really taking place – and I personally believe it is – we are right in the middle of it, and no one has a full picture of how it will emerge.' Explaining what this would mean, he goes on to say:

> The body would no longer be seen as an impersonal bi-molecular machine, but as a multi-layered hierarchical system with consciousness at its core. Disease would be seen to arise from different levels within the hierarchy and treatment would focus on self-correction, using the therapist as an external catalyst, stimulus or mirror, rather than focusing exclusively on external bio-engineering.

Dr St George also believes that complementary medical research should equally focus on basic scientific research into the theories and mechanisms which underpin the various methods.

It is clear that there is a growing interest in complementary therapies among some sections of the allopathic medical profession. In this country, there are already more than 300 GPs who practise acupuncture and 250 who use homoeopathy, and many are osteopaths. Nurses, in particular, are taking courses in massage, nutrition (it is ironic that this should be needed in addition to the basic training), aromatherapy, reflexology and counselling. The British Medical Association has called for a 'familiarization course' on complementary medicine to be included within the medical undergraduate curriculum.

During the research I did for this chapter, it was clear that many sufferers were satisfied with the way they were dealt with by complementary therapists, sometimes in favourable comparison with the approach of doctors and specialists. They often cited the thorough case histories that were taken, the caring and sympathetic attitudes – and, of particular importance to IBS sufferers, the feeling that they were being taken seriously, sometimes for the first time.

It was also clear, however, that complementary medicine, as a whole, cannot guarantee to help IBS sufferers. There are some positive cases, where the sufferer's IBS has been virtually eliminated; but more often relief is only temporary, and symptoms return after treatment stops, or the relief experienced is minor, vague or elusive. Some sufferers in this position may find it hard to break away from receiving the treatment, hoping that they will get better but at the same time wondering how much they are being helped. This dilemma can be particularly acute in view of the large amounts of money that are sometimes being spent.

Philippa, who suffers from abdominal pain with bloating and vomiting, says:

'In desperation I tried some alternative remedies, to no avail. I went to a homoeopath, who thought it was a gynaecological problem, and an osteopath, who said it might be the appendix. Confused? So am I!'

And Moira, who is 50 and has had IBS for over 20 years, was not helped by the treatments she tried:

'I have not found orthodox or alternative therapies very helpful. I have read widely on the subject and tried everything suggested without much success. I was managing a health food shop when my problem began and had been involved with alternative therapies for some time. I felt very guilty when natural methods I would advocate for others had no effect on me!'

On a more positive note, complementary medicine has a well-deserved reputation for increasing a person's sense of well-being and overall health. Many therapies are pleasant and extremely relaxing. IBS sufferers often say, even if their symptoms remain, that they feel better able to cope with their condition.

It is clear that no one therapy stands out as being particularly beneficial to IBS sufferers. Potentially, all may have something to offer; but you need to be able to make an informed choice. A great deal depends on the individual practitioner, and, of course, on you as the patient. As Dr Christine Page, who is both a medical doctor and a homoeopath, says:

'I don't think that homoeopathy is unique. Many therapies look at the whole person and most work towards restoring balance and not just suppressing symptoms, as with orthodox treatment. The patient eventually makes the decision and will be attracted to one form of therapy more than another. Sometimes personal recommendation will sway them in one direction. There is no therapy better than another and it depends very much on the therapist and the patient rather than the therapy. Orthodox medicine also has its place and can be used if necessary in harmony with complementary care.'

And the last word goes to Gillian, who has tried various different forms of complementary medicine:

'It is apparent from my own and [others'] experiences that different treatments work differently for different people and that there is no one effective treatment to suit everyone. I imagine that one's personal belief system about a particular treatment may well have a positive part to play in the outcome as well. At the very least, it must surely help to suspend judgement and keep an open mind – however, merely believing in a particular form of treatment (a kind of placebo effect) doesn't seem to be enough in itself to guarantee an effective outcome! But, I think, the opposite – not believing in a treatment at all – would probably be sufficient to ensure it has little chance or potential to help!'

Chapter 11

Women and IBS: Misdiagnosing the problem

Christine P. Dancey and Margo Steeden

Many people who receive a diagnosis of irritable bowel syndrome wonder at some point whether they are really suffering from another disease. Often the symptoms are so severe that you may think, 'It can't be IBS.' First, it should be emphasised that most people who are given a diagnosis of IBS are correctly diagnosed. However, if the symptoms get progressively worse over time, or are accompanied by bleeding, a thorough investigation should always be made; if you are in any doubt, you should return to your GP.

Unfortunately, however, misdiagnosis can sometimes occur. In this chapter, we are going to give you some accounts of women to whom this has happened. All of the women were initially told that they had IBS but were later found to have either endometriosis or inflammatory bowel disease. While they all had symptoms consistent with a diagnosis of IBS, they also had some that were *not* typical of IBS. These stories are not included to scare you or to undermine your confidence in your doctor; rather, they will provide useful information. In particular they will show you how difficult it was for these women to be rediagnosed, once they had had an initial diagnosis of IBS.

The core symptoms of irritable bowel – abdominal pain, diarrhoea and/or constipation – can often occur in other gastrointestinal diseases. The doctor has to decide, on the basis of your symptoms, whether to diagnose IBS or to refer you for hospital investigations to rule out a more serious disorder. Some doctors, however, are reluctant to refer patients for diagnostic testing as the tests are expensive and, in most cases, the results are negative (i.e. no evidence of organic disease is found). Also, people who undergo these tests often find them stressful. Therefore, some who have been diagnosed with IBS have not had thorough diagnostic tests for gastrointestinal disease.

Further, these core symptoms can also occur in the gynaecological disease endometriosis. Many women who have been diagnosed with IBS and are referred for hospital investigations are tested for gastrointestinal disorders *only*. These tests – barium enema, barium meal, sigmoidoscopy – are designed to rule out *bowel* disease; they give no information on whether you have endometriosis. Many women who have experienced symptoms such as abdominal pain, diarrhoea and/or constipation have been diagnosed with IBS when, in fact, they have got endometriosis.

Conversely, some women who have been finally given a diagnosis of IBS have undergone many hospital tests and operations because the medical practitioners thought that their symptoms must be gynaecological. Women have been known to have hysterectomies to cure their symptoms, only to find that the symptoms remain afterwards. However, most diseases with which IBS is confused have specific disease processes that show up on investigation (e.g. tumours in the case of bowel cancer, adhesions and cysts in the case of endometriosis), and so the likelihood of misdiagnosing IBS instead of one of these is likely to be far less than the likelihood of a woman receiving a diagnosis of IBS when she really has endometriosis. IBS fluctuates in severity and frequency, but people tend to improve or stay the same over a long period of time; other diseases are progressive, and get worse over time.

Misdiagnosis is a problem that can occur in every area of medical diagnosis. However, medical practitioners feel that, in the case of IBS, the chance of this happening is small. For instance, according to Professor Sidney Phillips of the Mayo Clinic in Rochester, Minnesota, studies have shown that only a few people with IBS are later rediagnosed. For example, one study followed 77 patients over six years; in only four cases (just over 7 per cent) was the diagnosis of IBS changed. Another found that 5 per cent of their patients had been incorrectly classified. However, because so many people have IBS, these relatively small percentages translate into a substantial number of misdiagnosed people!

Misdiagnosis of endometriosis as IBS

Endometriosis is a condition in which the lining of the womb – the endometrium – is found in unusual sites outside the womb cavity. Symptoms can include painful periods, deep pain during sexual intercourse, bleeding between periods, muddy discharge, pelvic pain (continuous or cyclical) and infertility, with the most common symptom being pain. It is currently believed that around 10 per cent of women are affected by endometriosis, but this figure is considered an underestimate as many women escape diagnosis. The Endometriosis Association in the United States found in 1988 that 3 per cent of women with endometriosis had previously been given a diagnosis of IBS. In 1996, the National Endometriosis Society (NES) in Britain reported that 7 per cent of a large survey of sufferers – more than 2000 women – had been incorrectly diagnosed as having IBS or Crohn's disease.

Many recent studies have highlighted the need to consider endometriosis during the evaluation of unexplained digestive complaints such as IBS. They note that, because endometrial tissue can sometimes attach itself to the bowel, certain symptoms that are usually present in IBS – such as abdominal pain, distension and bloating, constipation and diarrhoea – can also be present in endometriosis. Therefore, they argue, the reason for the misdiagnosis is 'symptom similarity'. However, symptoms such as painful intercourse, bleeding between periods and muddy discharge are not typical of IBS, and yet women experiencing these symptoms have been misdiagnosed.

Further, some doctors have persisted in a diagnosis of IBS even though women have noted a direct connection between their abdominal pain/bowel symptoms and their menstrual periods, and have not referred these patients for a gynaecological check-up. Thus, although symptom similarity can cause confusion initially, there could be other reasons for a misdiagnosis. First, research has indicated that medical practitioners' stereotypic beliefs about their patients can have an effect on the diagnosis and treatment prescribed; the gender of the patient is one example. A woman experiencing abdominal pain, for instance, may be told by her doctor, 'It's your monthly period . . . it's normal . . . it will settle down once you have a baby,' or they can be told that the pain is 'all in your mind' because the doctor can find nothing physically wrong. These sorts of remarks can often trivialize a woman's experiences and make her feel that she is wasting the doctor's time. It can also mean that a thorough investigation (by both a gastroenterologist and a gynaecologist) does not take place, and the reason for the abdominal pain is not discovered.

Second, certain disorders such as endometriosis and IBS are not considered sufficiently serious by some doctors and are therefore not always fully investigated. Researchers have reported that 'failure to appreciate the existence of this condition [endometriosis] often delays prompt therapeutic intervention'. This is borne out by a survey carried out by the National Endometriosis Society in 1996, which found that the time from respondents first perceiving symptoms to finally being diagnosed with endometriosis is, on average, just over seven years. Of the sample, 10 per cent had been referred to a urologist, 6 per cent to a psychotherapist or psychiatrist and 18 per cent to a gastroenterologist. IBS is often thought to be a trivial disorder. When medical practitioners can find no evidence of organic disease (as is the case with IBS), they often pronounce the verdict: 'There's nothing wrong with you.' This is also the case with many women suffering from endometriosis – in the NES survey, 11 per cent of doctors said that the women's symptoms were 'nothing'; 5 per cent that they were 'normal', and 2 per cent that patients would 'grow out of it'. A stereotypic view of a patient or a disorder can therefore also lead to misdiagnosis and mistreatment.

We decided to carry out research at the University of East London into the misdiagnosis of endometriosis as IBS. The focus of the research was the experiences of the women as articulated by the women themselves. Our intention was not to 'objectively measure' a list of data and then produce our 'findings', but by giving women the opportunity to articulate their own experiences, in their own terms, to better understand and improve the health care of women and any future research.

The 20 women who took part in the study, all of whom had been initially diagnosed as having IBS but were later found to be suffering from endometriosis, were asked to write about their experiences during their illness and the events that took place during its course. When the letters written by the women were examined, two main themes were identified: 'women's experiences of the medical consultation' and 'women making sense of their experiences'. The extracts that follow are a sample of the full research.

Women's experiences of the medical consultation
During consultation, many women reported that their doctors could find nothing wrong. However, there were differences in how doctors approached this. For example, some chose to give the absence of a 'problem' a name – that is, IBS – while others prescribed treatment for this 'non-problem' by saying that the women should 'have a baby', – and still others said that the 'problem' was 'all in the mind':

'At the age of 38, I noticed bright red blood in my stools at the time I was menstruating. A male locum GP told me that my symptoms were impossible! The following month I told my regular male GP. He thought it was nervous in origin, maybe IBS or colitis. He said I was a "sensitive flower". I had told him at least two years previously of experiencing pain low down in my left abdominal area. No physical examination took place.'
'During my period, I had such severe stabbing pain I had to go home from work. The flooding was terrible . . . I felt insecure if I wasn't a few steps from a toilet. I was also opening my bowels half a dozen times a day in the first two or three days of a period, and I had an odd stabbing pain in my left side, at hip level. The

doctor put this pain down to IBS and had no suggestions for the menstrual problems except the usual one of "Have a baby".'

In both of these accounts, the women's accounts of their symptoms were ignored or their experiences were trivialised and invalidated. One woman was told that she was a 'sensitive flower' by her GP, thus trivializing her pain and symptoms, and by a locum GP, she was told that her symptoms were impossible – thus she was not believed. The woman in the second account is told to 'have a baby' to help with her menstrual problems; this presumes that the woman will *want* to have a baby and indeed that it will 'cure' her problem. (In fact, women should *never* become pregnant simply because it may relieve symptoms of a certain condition.) In this second account, even though there were physical symptoms indicating a specific problem, the doctor implies that they were all in the woman's mind.

Women's experiences can also be ignored by their doctors if they do not match the doctor's idea of what is wrong – the doctor's medical knowledge. Even when women noted a direct connection between their abdominal pain/bowel symptoms and their menstrual periods, the doctors still insisted that the diagnosis should be one of IBS:

'I explained to the GP the difficulty I had in understanding a diagnosis of IBS when there appeared to be a direct connection to my menstrual cycle ... I explained that I could understand such a coincidence happening once or twice a year, as it well might if I really did have IBS, but the fact that it was happening without fail every month in time with my period cycle surely suggested a possible connection between the pain and menstruation. My GP said nothing except that the symptoms were typical of IBS. I explained that I had neither diarrhoea nor constipation ... I tactfully explained that I could not see how my symptoms bore any relation to IBS. He repeated that they were typical of people with IBS.'

Women making sense of their experiences

In light of the misdiagnosis and mistreatment of their illness, the women in our study reflected on the ways in which they had made sense of their experiences. Many of them began to question their own perceptions of the pain and symptoms because they had been told so many times that's 'Nothing is wrong.'

The accepted view in our society is that 'the doctor knows best'; doctors have the 'knowledge' and patients are dependent on the diagnosis and treatment given to them. In one particular study on doctor–patient consultations, a patient expressed dissatisfaction with the diagnosis given by the doctor. The doctor responded: 'I will tell you what is wrong with you, I will tell you what your symptoms are, and I will tell you what to do. I am the doctor and you will kindly not forget that fact.'

The women in our study often felt let down by their doctors; they had turned to them for help and had placed their trust in them and yet they did not receive what they needed. In most cases, it had taken several years to get a correct diagnosis, even though some of the women had sought opinions from different doctors and had visited hospitals many times:

'After all these years, I am now free from pain. At the time I was diagnosed as having IBS, I felt only anger towards the specialist who had been telling me to "just keep taking the tablets" – but I was not convinced I had IBS. We place our trust in doctors and believe what they tell us, and after a while you wonder if it's all in the mind.'

'. . . towards the final diagnosis [of endometriosis] I realised it was definitely worse at the time of my period. During this time, I felt very put down by the medical profession. I began to believe I really was neurotic and making a fuss about nothing . . . I believe that it has had a long-term effect on my self-confidence. I was very relieved when I was diagnosed with endo, to know that I was not imagining the pain and discomfort I was feeling.'

Throughout the course of their illness, these women experienced much unnecessary pain and suffering. They knew what they were experiencing, they knew it wasn't IBS, they questioned the diagnosis. However, the diagnosis did not change.

Their knowledge and experiences were ignored. The doctors had asserted their position of power within the consultation; so the women stopped questioning the doctors and started questioning themselves.

These assertions and 'knowledge claims' made by some medical practitioners resulted in serious consequences for these women; diagnostic errors were made and their illness was mistreated. Throughout these accounts, women's experiences were invalidated and trivialized by their doctors. Because the women's experiences of their pain and symptoms did not match 'medical knowledge', the symptoms were often assumed to be psychosomatic – 'all in the mind' or 'not possible'. As a result, many of them underwent years of suffering, their health was compromised and their confidence undermined.

Misdiagnosis of inflammatory bowel disease as IBS

Inflammatory bowel disease (IBD) is an umbrella term for two related diseases of the bowel: ulcerative colitis (UC) and Crohn's disease (CD). Although UC and CD are two distinct diseases, they are both chronic and potentially life-threatening. They share many of the same symptoms and the specific causes of both are unknown.

Ulcerative colitis is a chronic inflammation and ulceration of the lining (the mucous membrane) of the colon and rectum. The principal symptom of UC is diarrhoea, which can be violent and may also contain blood, pus and mucous. Accompanying symptoms can include abdominal pain and loss of appetite leading to a loss of energy and weight – it is not uncommon to find weight loss of between 20–30 kilograms (44–66 lb). People with UC may experience periods of remission, but the disease very rarely goes away completely. Consequently, once someone has an attack they remain at risk from further attacks. UC can occur at any age; however, it mostly affects people in their thirties and forties, and slightly more women than men.

UC is a lot less common than IBS, affecting only 5–10 people per 100,000 of population.

In Crohn's disease, an inflammatory process penetrates all layers of the bowel, which leads to thickening of the bowel wall and scarring, and can cause bowel obstruction. It also differs from UC in that it can involve any part of the intestinal tract, from mouth to anus, but most frequently affects the small bowel, the large bowel or both. As with UC, common symptoms are diarrhoea (sometimes bloody) and abdominal pain. There may also be weight loss, and sometimes fever. As in IBS, sufferers experience periods of remission and exacerbation. Over half of the people diagnosed with CD are young – under the age of 22 – and more men than women contract it. CD affects around half as many people as UC.

Certain symptoms that are present in UC and CD can be present in IBS – abdominal pain and diarrhoea, for example. Therefore, initially, it is possible for doctors to diagnose mistakenly IBS instead of inflammatory bowel disease (although this is rare). However, *extreme* weight loss and blood in stools are *not* symptoms of IBS and they should always be fully investigated. Unfortunately, once a diagnosis of IBS has been made, it can be difficult to obtain a referral for investigation – a vicious circle! Unlike IBS, both UC and CD are potentially life-threatening disorders, and they are also extremely debilitating.

We wanted to explore women's experiences of the misdiagnosis of inflammatory bowel disease. All of the following accounts come from those who were initially diagnosed as having IBS, but were later found to have either UC or CD. It is important to realise that this is a rare occurrence. However, knowing this is not much consolation to the women who wrote to us!

Women's experiences of the medical consultation

Like the women who had been diagnosed with IBS when they really had endometriosis, the women with CD or UC who wrote to us frequently gave accounts that focused on the way that they had been treated during the medical consultation. It appears that IBS is sometimes diagnosed, not only on the basis of the symptoms, but because the woman fits the GP's profile of an 'IBS sufferer'.

'I believe my GP stereotyped me when diagnosing IBS – I was a young student and was therefore under a lot of stress. She made up her mind and then dismissed me.'

'Whenever I went to my GP, he would look at my notes and say things like "Why are you so nervous?" Even the family thought it was all in my mind.'

'I was sent to the hospital to see the gastroenterologist. After various X-rays and an endoscopy, I was told that it was only IBS and that most of it was "in the mind".'

These quotes are very similar to the ones related by women with IBS, as well as those with endometriosis, when being given a diagnosis of IBS. Women felt that they were not listened to. Even when some of the symptoms did not match typical IBS, the GPs in these women's vignettes discounted them as unimportant. Women felt that, because their doctors thought they were 'stressed', they were not taken seriously:

'My GP in Oxford thought that I suffered from stress and would tell me to calm down as it worsened my IBS. I did not feel stressed at all! . . . It is disappointing that three different GPs did not take a teenage girl seriously.'

'My doctor didn't take me seriously and told me to eat a high-fibre diet, gave me laxatives and fibre drinks. He told me I had IBS and I was constipated, even though I was going to the toilet at least 15 times a day, up to 30 times or more. I was losing weight and being sick and I was in a lot of pain. He didn't do any tests and told me I was too tense.'

'I was treated very unsympathetically by the doctor who said I had irritable bowel syndrome. Even though I was suffering from diarrhoea, I was put on a high-fibre diet and given a pamphlet! . . . Doctors seem very ready to diagnose any stomach/bowel complaints as IBS . . . People *know* when they are seriously ill (I did) and this should be taken as important.'

Labelling the patient – the effects

As in the cases of endometriosis misdiagnosed as IBS, once these women had the label of 'IBS', it was difficult for them to challenge the diagnosis when symptoms became worse or changed in some way. Some were so upset by the attitudes of their GPs that they were reluctant to go back to the doctors when they needed to. This is no doubt very rare, too, but that it happens at all is worrying.

> '. . . I decided to see my GP. The pain and diarrhoea were constant by this time, but his first reaction was to tell me to "go and find something to occupy myself – idle hands and all that!" . . . I explained that . . . I was the sole "breadwinner" for my three children . . . I was very distressed at the GP's attitude . . .'

> 'I visited my doctor (very worried) and he decided I had IBS and he quite literally told me to go away and stop being so neurotic – he had decided that my "sensitive", "highly strung" personality was the cause of the problem! . . . I was terrified to return to my doctor because of my "neurotic" label.'

As in the cases given at the beginning of this chapter, the women's experiences of medical consultations sometimes led them to doubt themselves. Were they imagining it? Were they really neurotic? Perhaps there was nothing wrong with them!

> '. . . I had become conditioned to thinking of my illness as untreatable and myself as an inadequate and thoroughly neurotic person who was worrying myself into an imaginary illness . . .'

> '. . . he [the GP] referred me to a bowel specialist . . . he checked me over and decided to send me for a sigmoidoscopy . . . that was when I was diagnosed as having irritable bowel syndrome. I was sent home after being told there was no cure for it and to eat a high-fibre diet. I was so mad because I knew there was something wrong with me.'

Although this is only a preliminary exploration of these women's accounts of their experiences, it has identified some areas of concern. Like the endometriosis sufferers, medical practitioners' stereotypic beliefs about their patients can have an effect on the diagnosis and treatment prescribed. If doctors believe that the typical IBS sufferer is a neurotic woman, then women who seemingly fit this profile (and who of us wouldn't be stressed by having to cope with difficult and embarrassing symptoms that seem to have no explanation?) are likely to be diagnosed as having IBS. Like the endometriosis sufferers, sometimes these women with inflammatory bowel disease were told that their problems were due to being 'nervous' or 'stressed'. Again, like the endometriosis sufferers, many of these women began to question their own perceptions of their symptoms, because they had been repeatedly told that it was 'only IBS'.

These accounts are interesting, and not only because they show how these particular women were treated when it was believed they were suffering from IBS. They show how IBS itself is trivialized – 'It's nothing. Stop worrying and it will go away.' IBS is not taken seriously. The medical practitioners in these women's accounts did not give the impression that they believed IBS was a valid illness that needed to be taken seriously and properly treated.

The research presented here does not attempt to make generalised statements that will apply to all women, nor indeed to all doctors. It relates to a number of individual women who have been diagnosed and treated inappropriately by some doctors. However, it is hoped that it will help women to articulate their own experiences – experiences which should never be trivialized, ignored or reduced to being 'all in the mind'.

Professor Talley, a gastroenterologist at the Mayo Clinic with a special interest in IBS, says that IBS patients have real symptoms that originate *in the gut* (not the mind). He also points out that, although IBS patients frequently have psychological problems, such problems have often been linked in the past to other diseases that were once thought to be psychosomatic but are now known to be organic. It is not surprising that people who live with chronic symptoms on a more or less daily basis find they are affected psychologically. However Professor Talley says:

. . . there is no evidence that the symptoms of IBS are imagined or that these patients are just chronic complainers with a low threshold for bodily discomfort.

Consequently, women going to a doctor's surgery because of symptoms that the GP believes are due to IBS should be listened to, taken seriously, and be treated in the same manner as women who have any other disorder.

What you can do to avoid misdiagnosis

Gain information
People with IBS often suffer more than other people with backache, headache, tiredness, etc. This is not surprising, since they have to live with a chronic condition. Some IBS sufferers find they have less usual symptoms – nausea and indigestion, for instance – but these are all within the normal range of symptoms. If you have had a diagnosis of IBS, read up on the condition and make sure that you do not have symptoms inconsistent with the diagnosis – bleeding in between periods, for instance.

Go back to your GP if your symptoms change
It may be that, over time, your symptoms change in quality, or symptoms may appear that were not there before, and which seem to you inconsistent with the diagnosis of IBS. *In this case, go back to your GP*. Sometimes people can suffer from IBS and *other* diseases. Just because you have IBS, it doesn't mean you can't later suffer from endometriosis, for instance. Your doctor should take you seriously, especially if you suddenly begin to suffer from new symptoms after a long time with the old ones!

Change your doctor if you are unhappy with him or her
If you find your GP is unsympathetic, then *change your doctor*. Although this may be a bother for you, it is better to find a doctor with whom you can have a supportive relationship than stay with one you are not happy with. You do not have to tell your doctor you want to change.

You simply find a new one and then ask to be registered with him or her.

How do you find a new doctor? The best way is to ask friends and neighbours, or to sit in the surgery and start talking to the patients waiting there! You can also ask for a pre-registration appointment with a GP. This doesn't mean you will be given one, of course, but there is nothing to stop you asking. If you are given an appointment, you can have a general chat with the doctor to find out if you want to register.

Sometimes doctors are unable to take new patients. If you can't find a doctor you want to register with and who is taking new patients, you can write to your local Family Practitioners Committee, asking them to find you one. You can get the address of the FPC at your local library or a doctor's surgery.

Chapter 12

IBS among Children and Teenagers

Christine P. Dancey, Rachel Fox and Claire Rutter

It has been said that IBS is the most common gastrointestinal problem in children, yet although there is much research on childhood asthma, diabetes and other conditions, there is hardly any awareness of IBS in childhood. There is, however, quite a lot known about abdominal pain in children, who may be given a diagnosis of 'recurrent abdominal pain' (RAP). At least one in ten children suffer from RAP. However, RAP is not the same as IBS. Children with IBS suffer from abdominal pain *plus* some of the other adult symptoms of IBS – bowel problems and incomplete evacuation, for instance.

We first became aware that there were many child sufferers of IBS when nearly half of a sample of IBS Network members said that they had experienced bowel symptoms as children. We knew that adult sufferers find living with IBS quite problematical, and we wondered whether children were affected in similar ways. We thought that children might find IBS particularly difficult as they can have less control over when they can go to the toilet – at school, for instance, they are often not allowed to go when they need to. And then, perhaps, children do not talk to their friends about their bowel problems, increasing their feelings of isolation and embarrassment.

How common is irritable bowel syndrome among teenagers?

In 1996, Sue Thomson and Christine Dancey (of the University of East London) studied nearly 1,000 children at a comprehensive school just outside London. Each of the pupils was given a questionnaire asking about various symptoms, including the symptoms of IBS. They were asked to indicate whether they had suffered from various symptoms in the previous week only; if they had been asked about the previous year or the previous few years, no doubt most of them could have said 'Yes' to all the symptoms.

Only 2 in 100 children suffered from what we call 'diagnosable IBS' – that is, three or more symptoms. This was good news – there were a lot fewer child sufferers than adult ones. However, 16 per cent had experienced one or more symptoms, the most usual being incomplete evacuation of the bowel, and abdominal pain. The least reported symptoms were the usual adult ones – diarrhoea and constipation. Pupils with bowel symptoms were found to have more headaches and to feel different from their friends. They said that they were embarrassed to talk to their friends and teachers about their health, and that their health problems stopped them going out with their friends as much as they would have liked.

How do adults remember IBS affecting their teenage years?

Once we had found out that children *do* suffer from IBS, we decided to carry out further studies to give us some insight into how children feel about living with IBS. Since no study has really focused on IBS in adolescence, we couldn't be certain that teenagers suffer in the same way as adults, if indeed they suffer at all. To discover this, we first had to find the youngsters. Since they don't tend to join the IBS Network, it was necessary to have them referred by gastroenterologists. This would obviously take some time, so in the meantime, we spoke to IBS Network members who had suffered from bowel symptoms when teenagers, to get some idea of how IBS had affected them.

These people remembered that the most vivid and earliest symptom of irritable bowel syndrome was abdominal pain, which varied from severe rhythmic cramps to a dull ache. They said that, even though the pain was bad, they were still able to attend school regularly and participate in school life, although it was suggested that a lot of the enjoyment was removed because of worry about the pain or other symptoms.

'The pain was just horrendous. I used to get diarrhoea a lot. I was always having accidents and I always carried a spare pair of knickers with me when I was at school.'

Respondents focused not only on the pain itself, but on the fear and anxiety that the experience engendered. The fear was generally linked to confusion as to what could be causing such pain.

'This was when I was 13. The pain could be either side, and I would be at school. It would perhaps come on in the afternoon and I'd be curled up on the bed for two or three hours and then it would gradually subside – the doctors could never find any reason for it. I felt washed out, exhausted and quite depressed.'

Some of the women mentioned the embarrassment they felt as teenagers:

'I wanted to tell my friends but I was too embarrassed. Even now I find it embarrassing because you know that people don't like to talk about toilet things.'

Toilet availability

The availability of toilets is a frequent issue with adult IBS sufferers, and the people we talked to said that they remembered this being the case when they were young, particularly at school. Toilet availability evoked quite an emotional response in the women interviewed, who felt that problems with access to toilets had contributed to either the start or the maintenance of their IBS. For instance, issues about the locking of toilets were raised

by most women, as well as not being let out of class to go to
the toilet.

> 'We had a toilet at each end of the school, and I remember
> going to one and it was locked, and thinking, "Oh, I'll be able
> to make it to the next one," and I got to the next one and that
> would be locked ... On a few occasions, I actually ran home
> from school to go to the toilet. I remember it being a constant
> problem.'

However, the women felt that they had coped well with school
life, given the difficulties they faced.

School trips and other outings

School trips were remembered as having been difficult, due to
the pupils not knowing whether they would be able to find a
toilet when they wanted one. They remembered that sometimes
their IBS stopped them going out – for instance, with their
friends.

> 'It made a difference to my life, because basically when I was in
> pain I couldn't talk about it to anyone, because they wouldn't
> understand. I felt my whole life had to stop. Obviously, when
> I was in pain, I just came home and coped with it but they were
> really painful times.'

'Am I exaggerating?'

Some of the IBS Network members remembered doubting
themselves. They had had no way of knowing whether such
symptoms were 'normal', or whether they were exaggerating
symptoms from which other people also suffered.

> 'I knew I had really bad stomach ache. It was like "Is there anyone
> else who is sitting around me who is in this much pain? . . ." You
> can't really say, it's still like a taboo. You can't discuss it. It makes
> you an outsider, and I think, even as a child, you want to belong
> to part of a group.'

Some felt that other people, including doctors, didn't take them seriously:

'I just felt that the doctor didn't believe me, and was giving me something just to get me off his hands ... It just made me give up ... I just remember that they didn't think it was anything at all.'

Since some years had passed between their teenage experiences and now, it might be that the memories of these IBS Network members have become distorted over the years. Therefore, although this small study suggested to us that IBS in the teenage years could affect adolescents' social and school lives, it was important for us to talk to teenagers directly.

How do teenagers view their IBS?

We talked to young people, aged 11 to 16, who had been diagnosed as having IBS by a qualified medical practitioner. Our aim was to understand what it was like for the children and their parents to live with IBS and how they had coped with the problems that the illness brings. We also interviewed one parent of each of the young IBS sufferers; in all cases, this was the teenager's mother. The questions that we asked had been decided on beforehand, so that everyone was asked about the same things, but rather than asking the children and mothers to give yes or no answers, we aimed to make the interviews more like normal conversations. The areas covered in the interviews included the history of the illness, family communication and the effect of IBS on school life, social life and future plans. Each interview usually took about three quarters of an hour. All of them were taped and later transcribed, and from these transcriptions, we looked for common experiences, problems and ways of coping.

Symptoms
All the children we spoke to had experienced severe abdominal pain and altered bowel habits, particularly diarrhoea; some had

also had bloating, nausea, and blood and/or mucus in their stools. These symptoms can obviously be very distressing, both for the children and for their families. Sarah, a 15-year-old, described how she felt when she first started to get the symptoms:

> 'Well, it was mainly really, really bad stomach pain. When you're little, you don't understand what it was. I mean, I can't really remember before it . . . All I can remember is the pain, really, really bad, and I can remember saying to my Mum and Dad, "I'm dying, I'm dying – get the doctor . . ."'

One of the parents described her child's symptoms:

> 'Well, it was the screaming pain, because she wasn't a child to make a noise and she would sit on the toilet and scream.'

All the children had times when they didn't have any symptoms or when the symptoms were not so bad. The symptom-free periods varied from a few days to a few months, but symptoms usually reappeared for no obvious reason. The length of time that the children had suffered with IBS ranged from 3 to 14 years (one teenage boy had suffered the symptoms since birth).

Getting a diagnosis
There was also quite a difference in the length of time it took for a diagnosis to be made. For some, it took only two or three visits to the doctor, but others had spent a year or more constantly returning to their GPs and having to press them for a referral to a specialist, who finally told them what was wrong. Some of the teenagers and parents felt that, at first, they had not been taken seriously enough by their doctors. It's important to find a GP who is understanding and sympathetic and who you feel is taking you and your child seriously. If you are not happy with your doctor, you can always ask to see another in the same practice (if there is more than one). If not, or if the second GP proves equally unsympathetic, you could consider changing to a different practice (*see* pp. 297–8).

Is your child imagining it or making it up?

The time leading up to a diagnosis of IBS can be terrible for both teenagers and their parents, particularly if the symptoms have gone on for months or even years. The youngsters to whom we talked often said that, before they had been told that they had IBS, they sometimes felt that no one believed that their symptoms were real. One 16-year-old boy explained:

> 'It's annoying, really annoying because people say, "Oh, you're not really ill, you can go to school" when they don't actually know how bad it is. You're sitting there going, "Well, I wish you could feel the pain then."'

When repeated tests seem to show nothing, some of the children even started to doubt themselves. A 14-year-old boy said:

> '. . . First of all, I thought it was just me making it up, just doing it to myself. Then I told Mum and Dad and they said, "Oh, you're just making it hard for yourself, you ain't got nothing." Then when we went to the doctors, and then when they done this thing in the hospital [a test] and nothing come up, I thought, yeah, it's all my fault, 'cause there was nothing.'

Most of the parents had worried at one time or other that the symptoms might have been invented to provide an excuse to stay off school. Some had worried that their children might be being bullied and were pretending to be ill in order to stay at home. Although it is natural to have these worries, it is important to try and reassure children that they are being believed – the symptoms can be very frightening and it is important that they feel that they have someone to talk to about it. It is possible that fear about school could be triggering symptoms, but that doesn't mean that the children and their fears shouldn't be taken seriously.

IBS can be frightening

The time before a diagnosis is often very frightening and confusing for both adolescents and parents. Not knowing what is causing these symptoms can lead, naturally, to fears of a serious or even life-threatening illness. For many of the parents in this study, the time leading up to the diagnosis was the most worrying. One parent describes how she felt:

> 'Well, oh my God, I was so scared, you know, because my mind was going, that it could be cancer of the stomach or something. I didn't know what it was so I was worried, and you know, while he was having the tests, it was terrible . . .'

Again, teenagers need to be reassured by parents, and it is best if parents do not transfer their own fears to their child.

All of the youngsters we spoke to had visited the doctor frequently with their symptoms, and most had had various tests done, including scans, X-rays and blood tests as well as some more intrusive tests, before a diagnosis of IBS was made. Of course, these tests may be useful in ruling out any more serious illnesses, but it can be very worrying waiting for the results and then wondering what can be wrong when test after test seems to show nothing is actually causing the symptoms. It can be particularly difficult for parents, and many of those who took part in our research talked about feeling helpless and confused during this time. It can be very upsetting to see your child having all these tests, but one important finding that we made was that all the children we spoke to seemed to take the tests in their stride and did not seem overly worried about them. It can help for both child and parent to ask the doctor who is doing the tests to explain what the tests are for and what the results might mean, and to discuss *fully* with the child what the tests will involve before any are agreed to. Finding a helpful and sympathetic doctor can make all the difference at this time.

Living with IBS

Once a diagnosis has been made and after the initial relief that the illness is not life-threatening, other problems can arise. There may be the fear that the diagnosis might be wrong and something more serious has been missed, and also the concern that little can be done to relieve symptoms. Again, finding a doctor that you and your child trust and feel comfortable with can help to reassure you, as can talking to others who have had similar experiences. Life then has to be worked around the illness which is, by its very nature, unpredictable. Most of the children in this study had learned to live with their IBS, and they tried not to let it get in the way of the things they wanted to do. However, the feeling that they were unable to help their child overcome the illness often left the parents feeling frustrated, confused and helpless. One mother explained:

'. . . Total helplessness. I mean, I'm OK with things I feel I can help with or do more, but as a mother, when you're watching your child in pain and you want to take that pain away from them, it's awful. I've said to her, "If I could put my hand inside your stomach and tear the pain out and put it into mine, I would do." I would take that pain, double, treble, it's a dreadful thing . . .'

The same mother later described the frustration she feels when the pain returns after a symptom-free time:

'. . . you just go through it. I'm sick of it, you know, and I'll say "Let's do something, let's sort it out once and for all." The number of times I've said, "I'm not going through this again, we've got to do something about it." I said, "I'm your parent. I'm supposed to do something about it."'

However, despite the frustration, doubts and general upset that can occur when a loved one has IBS, it is important for parents not to pass on any feelings of blame or act as if the child is being a nuisance.

Worrying about IBS
One of the things that makes IBS such a frustrating and confusing illness for both sufferers and their families is not knowing what is the cause of the symptoms. Many of the children we interviewed described themselves as worriers and believed that they became

more stressed about things such as exams and school work than perhaps their friends or other people might. Some parents described their children as highly strung and thought this might play a part in the symptoms. Other children and parents were sure that stress was *not* the cause or a trigger. Some had found that particular foods or drinks seemed to set off a bout of pain or diarrhoea. In some cases, there was another family member with IBS and this led some of the youngsters and their parents to believe that it might somehow be a hereditary illness which is triggered by something, either stress or diet. Some of the parents, however, were at a complete loss as to what might be the cause of the symptoms. Two we spoke to had tried making lists of all the foods and drinks consumed by their children as well as possibly relevant events that they had experienced, in an attempt to find out what might be triggering the symptoms. Although this can sometimes be useful, these parents could find no clue as to the cause. Several of the children also spoke of the illness as coming out of the blue with no obvious cause or trigger.

Treatments for IBS

Just as there seems to be no one cause or trigger for IBS, neither, unfortunately, is there one treatment or medicine that will help everyone. Various treatments had been offered to the children in our study, both before and after diagnosis, including prescribed medicines – anti-spasmodics, anti-diarrhoeals, bulk fillers and peppermint oil. Some had tried more alternative therapies, such as aloe vera juice, boiled barley water and brewers' yeast. One girl we spoke to was symptom-free for two years following a course of hypnotherapy, which can have particular advantages for children, involving no drugs but with some degree of counselling. However, again, while this may be effective for one person, it may do nothing for the next.

How does IBS affect school?

Anyone who has suffered with IBS (or knows someone who has) knows how disruptive the illness can be to many aspects of everyday life, and not surprisingly, this is also the case for children. School life is one area which can be badly affected by the illness. In our study, all the children had had days off from school because they either felt ill or were worried that they might become ill, although happily none of them found that their school work had suffered as a result. This is very similar to the accounts given by the adult sufferers earlier in this chapter.

Toilet availability Before a diagnosis is made, children may find that their problems stem from unsympathetic teachers. Some of the difficulties that the children in this study talked about included being made to wait until break-time to use the toilet. Not only is this quite impossible sometimes as well as very painful, but by the time break-time arrives, the toilets are full of other students – and having to rush to the toilet with a bout of diarrhoea can be a bit embarrassing, to say the least.

School activities Other problems can include being made to take part in games that can make the symptoms worse or even bring them on, and taking part in school trips. Some of the children in our study had missed out on school trips because they were worried about the symptoms starting while they were away from home.

Problems with your child's school

Parents, too, may find that they have problems with their child's school. Many of the parents we talked to had been continually asked by the school why their child was ill and absent so often. This can be very frustrating, particularly before IBS is diagnosed and you don't know yourself what is causing the illness or even the *name* of the illness. Some parents said that, because of the pressure put on them by the school, they sometimes felt torn between sending their child to school ill, which parents are obviously very reluctant to do, or keeping them away from valuable lessons. For working parents, being frequently asked to pick up their child from school because he or she is ill and difficulties with arranging for someone to look after their child when he or she is at home ill can cause problems with employers.

Sometimes a parent may even have to take time off from work, and again this can be particularly difficult when there is no apparent reason for the child's illness. Unfortunately some of these pressures may be passed on to the child.

In most cases, these problems seem to lessen once a diagnosis is made. Parents are able to let the school know that their child has IBS and explain his or her needs. Teachers are usually sympathetic once they know what the problem is, and in some cases, they might make special allowances for the child. For example, one child was given a 'hall pass' so that he wouldn't be stopped if he was seen walking in the corridors during class time; this meant that he could make his way quietly to the toilet whenever he needed to. This sort of innovation should be encouraged as it is important for a child suffering from IBS to feel safe and cared for at school.

In a large number of cases, the parents in our study were able to make things a little easier for their children at school, keeping teachers informed about what was wrong with their child and making sure that there was a member of staff to whom their child could go when the symptoms were bad. Having regular contact with the school can also help parents to feel less worried about their child in terms of their school work and with the knowledge that their child would be treated sympathetically if he or she became ill while at school.

How does it affect their social lives?
For the children we talked to, the worst part of living with IBS, apart from the actual symptoms, was the restrictions it put on their social lives. Some of them said that they didn't take part in social activities such as playing football or going to a friend's house for tea because they were worried that their symptoms might suddenly become bad. Others talked about how they sometimes felt angry and frustrated that they were unable to socialise in the same way as their friends. As one young sufferer told us:

'Well, I just feel annoyed that it should be me, 'cause none of my friends have got it and they can go out and do things and I can't.'

One of the aspects of IBS that the children felt made socialising hard is its unpredictability. Often it is the *fear* of symptoms coming on as much as the actual symptoms which stopped them from taking part in social activities. Again, this is similar to the experience of adult sufferers. One of the young sufferers explained how the unpredictable nature of IBS restricted her life:

'. . . the way you don't know when it's going to come on, the unpredictability of it and not knowing when it's going to be there and not knowing how bad. Sometimes, you know, the pain isn't that bad and I can bear it, then sometimes it's like absolutely really, really bad. Not knowing the level of the pain and not knowing when it's going to be and the actual pain itself is the worst thing.'

As well as the restrictions on more everyday activities, important events may also cause some problems. Both parents and children talked about the fear that, when a big event was coming up, such as a family wedding or bar mitzvah, symptoms would be bad.

Teenagers think positively

Despite the restrictions that the symptoms put on them, all of the youngsters we talked to remained very positive, determined not to let the illness stop them from doing the things they wanted to. They all seemed to have found ways in which they were able to cope, mainly by just getting on with life, trying not to think about their IBS and carrying on as normally as possible. They all had close friends who were aware of their IBS and to whom they felt they could talk. Some parents had spoken to other parents to let them know of their child's IBS. They found that this made it easier for their children to visit friends or even spend the night at a friend's house, something many of them wouldn't have considered doing before.

Many of the children talked about how they sometimes felt down and sad because of their symptoms. Naturally they wondered why they had to have IBS, they worried about the pains coming on, and they were angry and frustrated by the restrictions put on their lives. However, the main feeling was one of optimism. One 15-year-old girl who had suffered with IBS for six years described the kind of determination we saw in all the children to live as normally as possible:

'. . . No way, no, it doesn't stop me doing anything like that [going out]. It used to when I was little, but now I've got to the stage where I just don't care any more because I've worked out that, even if I stayed at home, I'm going to have the pain. While I've got the pain, I seem to cope better when I'm with other people. When I'm with my family, I'm less strong, I think, because I know they'll be all soft on me . . . but when I'm with my friends, I'm harder and I have to get on with it. If I'm on the bus or I'm walking, I've got to keep walking whether the pain's there or not, but I generally forget about it, and if I'm having a good time, a really good time, I don't feel it, so it's better.'

Parents worry more than their children do!
All the children we spoke to seem to have been able to adapt well to life with IBS, having found ways, with the help of their friends and families, to cope with the problems that the illness brings. All the children were determined that IBS would not ruin their lives or stop them from doing the things they wanted to do, and none of them thought that their IBS would affect their future career plans. Many of the parents, on the other hand, found coping with a child with IBS difficult, frightening, frustrating and confusing, and they continued to feel helpless at being unable to ease the symptoms.

All of the parents and children we spoke to thought that it might be helpful to be able to talk to others with similar experiences, but very few of them had actually been able to do so. Joining a self-help or support group or contacting organizations such as the IBS Network (*see* page 358) is one way that people with similar experiences can contact each other and share valuable advice and information. It can help just to know that you are not alone in your fears and anxieties, and to know that there are many others out there with the same kinds of problems.

But perhaps most important of all is for parents to resist the temptation to pass on their fears and frustrations to their children. If parents have a problem with the IBS, the children must not be made to feel responsible.

What if your child seems to suffer from symptoms of IBS?

- Remember that only a small proportion of children suffer from IBS, although 16 per cent may suffer from one or two symptoms.
- It is better not to be unduly worried if your child occasionally suffers from some symptoms of irritable bowel. If you cannot help worrying, try not to transmit this to your child. Anxiety will make things worse.
- If, however, your child regularly complains of abdominal pain with bowel problems, it is important to take him or her to your GP to get a proper diagnosis. If symptoms change by becoming much worse or by the child having additional symptoms, go back to your GP.
- If your child *has* been diagnosed as having IBS, bear in mind that most children seem to cope extremely well. They will not worry as much as you will!
- It is important for your child not to feel different from his or her friends. Don't discourage him or her from going out with friends or becoming involved in school activities, just because you are worried.
- If the school is causing problems for your child – for instance, because of toilet inaccessibility or complaints about absence – visit the school to let them know of your child's IBS. In our experience, teachers and school nurses are very supportive once they know of a child's problems.

One IBS sufferer, who had had great difficulty with symptoms as a child, told us of the things that might have helped her at the time:

- Not being treated like a nuisance – 'Oh, you're not going to the toilet again, are you?'. . . 'Hurry up!'
- Not making the toilet a battleground.
- Being listened to and taken seriously, but not having the symptoms made too big an issue – it is important to take the lead from the child.
- Being able to talk about it. Not feeling that you had to hide your symptoms and the fear and anxiety that went with them.
- Being 'allowed' to go to the toilet whenever necessary.
- Some sort of relaxed, low-key counselling.

Chapter 13

Helping Yourself to Health: Self-help Groups and IBS

Christine P. Dancey

'*I believe the IBS Network is pioneering nothing short of a revolution in health care and that the medical profession should lend their support to this initiative.*' **Professor Nick Read, Northern General Hospital, Sheffield**

'Self-help' refers here to help which is initiated by patients or, in this case, by IBS sufferers themselves. In other words, you may get together with other sufferers from IBS and decide how best to help yourselves. You may want to do this by setting up small discussion groups, to inform and support each other. Together, you may decide to set up telephone helplines or befriender groups, or to communicate with each other by a newsletter or letter-writing. These are all forms of self-help: the common theme is that the activities are initiated and organized by the affected people themselves rather than by professionals such as doctors or health projects.

What are self-help groups?

Groups which are formed for the purpose of sharing personal experiences of a particular problem, and for giving mutual support

The author would like to thank the medical practitioners and coordinators of the IBS self-help groups who contributed to this chapter by giving their views on self-help.

and information, are called self-help groups or support groups. One 1989 study revealed that there were 6.25 million members of self-help groups in the United States, a figure predicted to rise to 10 million by 1999. Unfortunately, there has been no comparable research into overall numbers of self-help groups in Britain. However, a spokeswoman at the Self Help Centre in London (now, sadly, closed down) said that self-help groups are a growing phenomenon: for instance, in Nottingham in 1982 there were 82 groups, but by 1994 there were 165. Groups now exist for most chronic diseases: there are hundreds of distinct groups for conditions such as Alzheimer's disease, diabetes, cancer, tranquillizer addiction, alcoholism, impotence, hysterectomies and bereavement, to name but a few – and, since 1991, for IBS.

Self-help groups have been defined as 'usually formed by peers who have come together for mutual assistance in satisfying a common need, overcoming a common handicap or life-disrupting problem, and bringing about social and/or personal change'. This definition is particularly suitable to the groups which have been formed by IBS sufferers. They have generally come together in order to help each other deal with the physical symptoms and the psychological and social effects of irritable bowel syndrome, which, while not life-threatening, can be very disruptive of normal life. As a sufferer of IBS – and particularly if you are a long-time sufferer – you may realize that your symptoms could remain with you for some time, and you may need support in coping with them. Rather than allowing your symptoms to overwhelm you, you need to be able somehow to keep them in the background. This is the personal change which you, as an IBS sufferer, need, which can help you while you wait for social and medical change to come about – social change in the form of better knowledge about the problem and acceptance for IBS sufferers, and medical change in the form of better treatment and increased facilities for people with bowel problems.

Since groups are usually formed by the sufferers themselves, they are based on trust and reciprocity. IBS groups generally have no 'leader', being rather a group of people who act together as equals; if professionals are involved, they usually take on a minor role. Basically, such groups are run by the sufferers, for the sufferers. This is generally the case with groups of sufferers of any chronic disease or disorder.

Self-help groups may have been seen in the past as something peripheral, which *might* help, and could at least do no harm. However, such groups have gained acceptance over the years as a valid form of health care. Self-help groups are often set up in order to meet a need which is not being met by the NHS. According to Professor Nick Read:

'So many people suffer from IBS, far more than the Health Service can cope with. The situation is made worse by the fact that medical treatments for IBS seem not to be very effective for a large number of patients.'

Although self-help groups are run by the sufferers themselves, this does not mean that they cannot make use of medical expertise. Professionals often wish to work *with* self-help groups, rather than against them. In fact, professionals can assist self-help groups by referring people to them. Dr Chris Mallinson, consultant physician at the Lewisham Hospital NHS Trust in south London, says:

'I do find it helpful to have the IBS Network at hand. It has to be said that quite a lot of patients don't want to know about it to begin with, but increasingly we are able to put patients in touch.'

Other medical practitioners find that self-help groups can keep them in touch with what their patients think. This is what Professor David Wingate of the London Hospital Medical College has discovered:

'I have found the newsletter of the IBS Network to be useful in giving me some feedback on what patients think. One worry about talking to patients as a physician is that they are often guarded in expressing thoughts and opinions, and therefore, it is useful to have some inside information on what patients tell each other. Reassuringly, the concerns that are expressed are very similar to those that I hear.'

These sentiments are echoed by Professor Michael Farthing of St Bartholomew's Hospital, London:

'Publications like those of the IBS Network are useful for healthworkers as they often present the "patient's perspective" in a succinct and direct way.'

IBS groups often initiate contact with professionals, in order to use their expertise. Professionals can help with accommodation for groups' meetings; they can speak to the group regularly and keep them up to date with information, give them advice and perhaps write occasional articles for newsletters. However, group members generally prefer that professionals stay in the background, being non-directive and non-authoritarian.

What are self-help groups like?

Self-help groups in general differ in numbers, outlook and the way they run their meetings. IBS groups also differ, as each one is autonomous – that is, there is no one body which 'controls' local groups. Local IBS self-help groups are generally small, with between five and eight members at any one meeting, although often there may be 20 or 30 people 'on the books'; some even have as many as 45 people listed, although this is rare at present. Although some groups do not hold meetings (members talk to each other on the phone instead, or write letters), most meet once a month or every two months, usually at the home of one of the members. Some groups meet in a room made available to them by their local GP or hospital. Most groups started up by advertising for members in their local newspaper.

'We first met together in April 1992 and now meet about every two to three months at my home. We make it as positive, friendly, relaxed and informal as possible. The members of the group vary as symptoms and other commitments permit, but we usually average about six each time.' (*South-West Hertfordshire group coordinator*)

'The Exmouth and East Devon IBS Support Group was started in March 1992 at my home with just a few interested sufferers. We now have over 45 members and we meet monthly at Exmouth Hospital, where we have either a speaker or a general discussion. Members represent a good cross-section of the community and are of all ages, male and female, from all over Devon.' (*Exmouth and East Devon group coordinator*)

How can an IBS group help you?

'The major reason for a [support] group is to give hope, encouragement and support, especially as illness can seem very lonely – as if you are the only person in the world who suffers this way.'

Ian Forgacs, consultant at King's College Hospital, Dulwich

People with IBS often ask their doctors, or the IBS Network, how such groups can help them. Sometimes people phrase their questions in such a way that they seem prejudiced against such groups from the start. Some, for example, ask: 'How can a bunch of people moaning about their symptoms help get themselves better?' Others say: 'How can a group help me when the doctors themselves don't know how to help?' You may be reading this book now, wondering how meeting with a group of like-minded people could actually help you physically. Comments such as those quoted above show that the questioner feels that the only purpose of treatment is to relieve her or his symptoms directly, and also that the questioner has not considered that there might be a relationship between his or her symptoms and emotional and social support.

Large numbers of people are finding that, by organizing themselves into groups, they can help themselves in all sorts of ways. Self-help groups cannot alleviate symptoms in a direct manner, so anybody who comes to a group thinking that their symptoms will be relieved just by attending the group will be sadly disappointed. However, self-help groups *can* help indirectly. As you no doubt realize, symptoms may be made worse by stress, anxiety and lack of support from partners, friends, family and so on. Participants in studies researching IBS often say that stress makes their IBS worse. Indeed, anxiety and stress make *any* illness worse, not just IBS. So if you can manage to lessen your anxiety, and not feel so stressed about having IBS (and all sufferers understand how difficult this is), while your symptoms may not go away completely, they may be somewhat alleviated. Through reading this chapter, you will see that being part of a self-help group for IBS can help you with the stress and anxiety which you may find accompanies the condition.

This is how Professor Nick Read sees the benefits of self-help groups to IBS sufferers:

'There is a need to break the mould and explore new methods of managing IBS. It is here that the IBS Network and IBS self-help groups are such an important initiative. The treatment of IBS requires a holistic approach that involves psychology, nutrition, an examination of lifestyle, exercise, as well as medical factors. To go into all of this requires much more time than the average doctor has at his/her disposal. I believe that the most effective means by which the medical profession can tackle the epidemic of IBS is to encourage the establishment of a network of self-help groups throughout the country and to work closely with these groups to educate and facilitate the support of their members. It is not that the treatment of IBS is difficult, it's more than it requires insight into the way in which life events, stress, food and other factors all interact to produce disturbances in bowel function. These principles can be taught to sufferers of IBS who, through the self-help groups, can produce a network of support and confidence.'

What benefits will you gain by joining a group?

Researchers have tried to find out how members felt that their lives had improved as a result of joining self-help groups. Although this research was not conducted on IBS groups, the latter would be expected to produce similar benefits. One researcher asked 232 members from 65 different groups the benefits of belonging to such a group. Briefly, he found that:

- 80 per cent experienced an improvement in health.
- three-quarters reported positive changes in other aspects of their lives.
- members participated in social life more actively – half became more enterprising and more outgoing.
- a quarter reported positive changes in their relationships with partners.
- over half said they had greater knowledge of their illness.
- over half made use of that knowledge by being able to deal with medical professionals more effectively.
- three-quarters were able to reduce drug treatments as they learned of other ways of treating themselves.

This same researcher also listed benefits identified by other researchers. One found that 'helping others, help from others, coping strategies, sense of community, coping with public attitudes, factual information, spirit of hope, self-confidence and meeting others with similar problems' all gave benefit to members. In another study, the most frequently mentioned responses were that the group had provided social involvement and fellowship (43 per cent) and a supportive, accepting environment (83 per cent). According to another researcher, 76 per cent said that sharing thoughts and feelings was important, 68 per cent said that they felt supported, approved of and valued, and 63 per cent mentioned knowing that their problems, feelings and fears were not unique.

When we wrote *Overcoming IBS*, there were no published studies on the benefits of self-help groups for IBS sufferers, although there were plenty relating to other conditions. However, since then, researchers Annette Payne and Edward Blanchard at the State University of New York have been conducting studies to see if self-help groups for IBS can improve *symptoms* as well as psychological health. It's quite easy to see how self-help groups might help you feel better psychologically – after all, you are with people who understand you, you are making friends and so on. It's harder to see how your symptoms can improve. However, that's just what the researchers found. They ran a self-help group for sufferers of IBS, with members meeting weekly for just over an hour, for eight weeks. The researchers found that, at the end of the study, there was an average reduction in symptoms of 31 per cent! Just in case you might think these people would have got better anyway, the researchers compared the group with sufferers who wanted to join the group but had to wait a while (this is called a 'waiting list control'). Their average symptom reduction was only 10 per cent, so it seems that self-help groups *do* work.

The following sections describe some of the particular benefits gained by people who have joined IBS self-help groups.

'I know just how you feel'

The most immediate benefit is that, as a new member, you are able to talk about your symptoms without embarrassment, knowing that the other members will understand what you are going through. Those members who have been in self-help groups for some time are often amazed at the relief expressed by newcomers when they are able to talk about their symptoms, because they themselves have forgotten what it was like in the beginning, when they had no one to confide in. Most sufferers of IBS do not talk about their condition to their friends or family; if they do confide in someone, it is likely to be just one member of the family, and they try not to talk about it too much. Sufferers are often too embarrassed to talk about their problems.

However, as one of the purposes of a self-help group is for members to be able to talk about themselves and their problems, you should feel justified in talking about yourself to others in the group. Thus the immediate benefit for you is to be able to talk

– about your symptoms, your problems, and sometimes your anger at people who have not understood your predicament, often doctors and family. Often you may want to talk in depth about your feelings with regard to the medical profession. Talking in a non-judgemental atmosphere and having your views validated can provide an immediate relief.

'I thought I was the only one!'
Interacting in a self-help group relieves the isolation felt by people who previously knew no one with IBS – or rather, *thought* they knew no one: since IBS sufferers try to keep their condition secret, it is often the case that people do know others with the condition but do not realize it! Once people begin talking about their condition, they find that others will say: 'I suffered from that some years ago' or 'My sister has IBS really badly.' As IBS has had more publicity in the last few years, so there are many more people who know what it is. Once you have been in a group for some time, you will find that you gain confidence and are able to tell others of your problems. Trying to keep a condition like IBS secret is a source of stress in itself, and being open and honest about yourself relieves some of this. Often sufferers feel very alone and 'abnormal', and this sense of abnormality often leads in turn to a sense of isolation from others. Groups generally act to give members a sense of normality, which they often find they have lost as their symptoms have increased.

'We all talk freely about IBS and its many and varied symptoms without any embarrassment and are able to pass on tips to each other on ways of being able to talk about IBS openly and to be among others who know what it is like to suffer from this distressing condition.' (*Member of Farnham, Surrey self-help group*)

Access to more information about IBS
People generally join self-help groups because the medical profession has not met their needs in full, and groups can provide information and advice which has not been given by

such professionals. Since medical practitioners have a limited amount of time to spend with each patient with IBS, they cannot give each individual all the information he or she needs. When asked what the medical profession could have done to help them the most, IBS sufferers did not cite more or better drugs – they said that what they wanted most was information on IBS. Self-help groups are often able to give this.

'What I've found helps is . . .'
Members are often able to pass on tips on how to cope with particular problems or to answer questions which are troublesome. For example, you may be worrying about whether your symptoms are due to something more serious than IBS – cancer, for instance. Other sufferers will be able to reassure you on this point, with the knowledge they have gained over the past months or years. You may not have had hospital tests to exclude the more serious diseases yet, and you may be worried about going for tests; sometimes sufferers are terrified. Other members can often tell you all about these tests – they have been through them, and survived them. At other times, members will be able to give you support and advice in dealing with 'difficult' GPs. Often members feel intimidated by GPs and consultants and unable to put the questions they want to ask. Other members can help you through these problems.

Long-time members are able to share their experiences with you, showing you that they have managed to cope with their IBS, that they still find enjoyment in life, and that their IBS can be put in the background. This is very important, as members tend to join groups when they are feeling at their worst – indeed, this is often why they have joined – because joining a self-help group is sometimes seen as a last resort. This should not be the case; a self-help group really should be the *first* resort, because joining one gives you so many advantages, as members will tell you. Nevertheless, people do often come to groups at their lowest, worn down, depressed and anxious. Talking to long-time members, most of whom have improved over time, can be uplifting. Long-time members will often tell about the things which have helped them through their IBS, both psychological and medical. Often, when discussing which treatments helped them, long-time members are able to point newcomers in a promising direction. You may not have tried, or even thought of, a certain treatment before – members can give you the experience of their advice. Just being able to consider a range of treatments which *may* be beneficial, and which you could try, will give you hope.

'I've just read this great book'

One of the more popular discussions in IBS groups is about books and articles on IBS. Before 1989, there were hardly any books on IBS that were accessible to the layperson. The first general book on IBS was written by Rosemary Nicol in 1989 and is still extremely popular. Two more, published in 1990, were by Geoff Watts and Shirley Trickett; *Overcoming IBS*, written by the editors of this book, was published in 1993 and was followed by *Treating IBS* in 1995. During this time, a few specialist books on aspects of IBS have also appeared – for instance, *Herbal Remedies: Irritable Bowel* (1992) by D. Potterton and *Beat IBS through Diet* by the Stewarts, who have contributed a chapter to this book.

Between them, members of self-help groups generally have a good knowledge of these publications and can discuss them with new members, who are then in a better position to choose the book(s) which will suit them. Sometimes self-help groups are able to buy books which they can then lend to members.

'I thought it was my fault'

Another benefit of self-help groups is that members begin to believe that IBS is a disorder worth taking seriously. So many sufferers have felt that they are to blame for their IBS, and that others blamed them, too. Often they feel that IBS is not given as much consideration as other disorders. Many medics try to reassure IBS sufferers that IBS is a definite, positive, valid diagnosis; however, the people whom we have met through the IBS Network do not seem to have this view. Often they feel that their IBS is due to some personality deficit, some inability to cope properly. Members of self-help groups come to believe that IBS is a valid disorder, which should be dealt with properly, rather than a trivial complaint which they should be able to deal with. This helps them cope:

> 'Personally, I find that having a group gives IBS the recognition that it is not something trivial that some people have to deal with.' (*Member of Isle of Wight self-help group*)

'Now you're here, doctor, we'd like to ask . . .'
Most self-help groups invite professionals to speak at some of their meetings. Despite not being funded, they have been able to persuade professors of gastroenterology, dietitians specializing in IBS and complementary health practitioners to speak to them.

> 'To date we have had speakers on hypnotherapy, reflexology, aromatherapy, homoeopathy, acupuncture, physiotherapy – also a counsellor and a dietitian. But most of our members find the general discussion meetings of most benefit, and our discussions are both varied and informative – it does help to know that one does not suffer alone when GPs seem unable to help.' (*Member of East Devon self-help group*)
>
> 'At meetings we exchange ideas and experiences. Our invited guests have included an osteopath who followed naturopathic practice, an advocate of homoeopathy, a much improved sufferer who gave us hope and shared tips and coping strategies with us, and a minister and his wife (a leukaemia sufferer) who helped us to explore how faith can help with chronic health problems.' (*Member of South-West Hertfordshire self-help group*)

Since most IBS self-help groups are quite small, such meetings with professionals are fairly intimate and non-threatening. Members feel more able to ask questions about their IBS in this sort of setting than in a more formal one such as a hospital, where they would often feel intimidated. Also, sufferers have more confidence in a situation such as this because of the support of the others in the group. Gastroenterologists who have taken the opportunity to speak to these small groups have also found that they can talk in a friendly, relaxed way, more so than they would find appropriate in their consulting rooms. One of these is Dr Chris Mallinson of the Lewisham Hospital NHS Trust in south London:

'I think the visit to the local group emphasized what a tremendously broad network a group of this sort provides. It would have been almost impossible to categorize the patients that I met, given their variety of age and experience of IBS. Nevertheless, a thread runs through the group, as indeed it does through the comments in the articles in *Gut Reaction* [the IBS newsletter], which I read with interest – one of the threads being the complete lack of unanimity about any sort of treatment.'

'It helps to know someone's there'

All the above points relate to social and emotional support. Many sufferers do not feel that they have support from the medical profession, friends or families. Many keep their problems secret from others, especially their employers. Members of a group can help each other through mutual support – giving a shoulder to lean on, being at the end of a phone in times of crisis. Even when members are unable to attend a local self-help group, just knowing others are there, suffering from the same type of problems, gives them a sense of support.

'Perhaps our most important achievement has been the instigation of a local telephone contact list which enables us to help a much wider circle of sufferers who are either unable or unwilling to attend meetings.

'We have all found it very helpful to have the opportunity to share our concerns with others who really understand and are not shocked, embarrassed or judgemental about our condition. We don't have to keep "pretending".

'Instead of feeling isolated and ashamed, we feel reassured that there is always a friendly voice at the end of a telephone if needed and a ready supply of advice about treatments tried as well as ongoing updates of recent research from those currently undergoing specialist treatment.' (*Member of South-West Hertfordshire self-help group*)

Making friends

Some people in groups become close friends and see each other outside of group meetings. Some studies have shown that members who develop these out-of-group activities have a greater sense of well-being than people who do not do this. Of course, it could be that people who feel a greater sense of well-being are more likely to make friends and see each other outside of the group anyway.

'I have made many new friends. I know that the self-help group I created has helped me so much. I have people I can talk to when I have a bad attack of IBS.' (*Coordinator, High Wycombe self-help group*)

Benefits for the long-time member

The preceding sections have concentrated on the benefits of group membership from the point of view of the new member. But how do groups benefit the long-time member? After all, these people will have spoken about their symptoms and IBS-related problems, and generally feel no need to go over the same ground repeatedly. However, their need for emotional and social support, while it may have lessened during the time they have been in the group, will still be there. Also, such members feel a sense of satisfaction in knowing that they are of help to new, less secure members.

In theory, it is probably easier to see the benefits of relying on others for advice and support than to see how helping others can benefit you directly. Yet in 1988 a researcher who studied three different kinds of self-help groups (not IBS) found that people who *both* gave *and* received support were less depressed, and found greater benefits and group satisfaction, than people who *only* gave support or *only* received it!

'I take telephone calls from sufferers when they are feeling down. Just having someone to talk to helps a lot. I now have over 30 sufferers on my database who I write to every three months. I have great support from the Priory Centre, High Wycombe.' (*Coordinator, High Wycombe self-help group*)

Beginning to look outward

Long-time members, having made friends, often feel a sense of belonging, and often feel the need to keep the group going most strongly. The needs and interests of such members are different from those of new entrants: perhaps not needing any more to talk about themselves, or requiring crisis intervention, they often begin to look outward from the group, and to focus on bettering the lot of IBS sufferers in general. In other words, once you feel more confident of yourself and are able to feel secure in your own coping mechanisms for IBS, then you are able to move forward to helping in a more general sense. For instance, some members want to help raise the profile of the condition by talking to other groups about IBS, or by writing to their local MPs about toilet facilities in public places, or by offering to talk to the media about IBS – in other words, raising the political profile of IBS. Over recent years, for instance, two members of IBS Network groups have been on television to talk about their IBS, and four have given telephone interviews for women's magazines. Such activities benefit all IBS sufferers and, as such, are likely to be a source of satisfaction to members, which in turn increases their own confidence and self-esteem.

Clare, the previous coordinator of the Wandsworth group, decided to speak out about her IBS on a London television programme, *Capital Woman*, for several reasons. Here she explains exactly what these were:

'I was hoping that the four-minute slot on *Capital Woman* might lead to a whole programme devoted to IBS. There was so much more I wanted to say – I needed four hours, not four minutes!

'I agreed to do the programme because I was tired of reading about how IBS is a stress-related illness. Personally, the only stress I have is the illness itself. I wanted the world to know just how awful IBS is, and I wanted people to actually *see* that I really look quite ordinary – I don't have green skin with purple spots, I'm not neurotic and externally I look well. The more people who know about IBS, the better chance we have about finding the answer. Maybe more doctors will become interested and take up the challenge of finding out what it is and how to put it right. I'm not prepared to take this lying down. I'm going to go on talking about it, writing about it, whatever it takes, until the answer is found.'

What self-help groups can't do

Self-help groups cannot cure IBS. One of the reasons for some people feeling that groups cannot help them is that they start with unrealistic expectations of the group – they are hoping it will mean their symptoms will disappear.

Some members often feel too ill to travel to a meeting, especially as some groups are thinly scattered. For instance, the coordinator of the North-West London group says:

'I read at the weekend in an article on ME [now known as chronic fatigue syndrome] self-help groups – "We are the only self-help group that nobody attends as we are all too sick to get there." I know what the writer means and I sympathize with her, but I think if people make the effort to get to a meeting, it may be of reward to them and to us.'

It is true that some people may not gain much from a self-help group. These are usually people who are different in certain respects from the rest of the members: for example, occasionally a sufferer is referred to a group with a diagnosis of IBS but has symptoms very different from the rest of the group. Betty was referred to a London self-help group as an IBS sufferer by a local GP. When talking to her, the group found that she suffered from nausea but had no abdominal pain and no bowel problems – yet her GP had told her that she suffered from IBS. Although the group were very sympathetic to Betty, and tried to help her, it was clear that she was very different from the rest and so felt out of place. The more similar you are to the rest of the group, the more likely you are to feel part of it, and therefore benefit from it.

Professor Wingate feels that self-help groups are not beneficial to everyone:

'"A problem shared . . ." may be true and there is no doubt that some patients benefit. I do not think that this is true of all patients, and there are some theoretical or even actual negative aspects . . . Affiliation to a patient network could mean, for some people, affiliation to a state of chronic invalidism. This is, of course, true of other conditions; a crutch can either be used as a badge of disability or an accessory to enable its owner to lead a normal life.'

However, Professor Wingate feels that the advantages outweigh the disadvantages:

'On balance, I believe that self-help groups are a good thing because they underline the autonomy of patients. They also lift some of the burdens of looking after this disorder from physicians.'

Funding

Since self-help groups are meeting a definite need in the community, and are supporting care by the NHS, I believe that such groups should be supported by grants from local councils or health authorities. Self-help groups are perceived as having a wide range of benefits by the people who attend them, and no doubt help some people who would otherwise use the NHS to a greater extent. Given adequate finance, self-help groups could perhaps become involved in preventative work rather than dealing primarily with sufferers when they are at their lowest.

At present, however, most groups are largely self-supporting.

All such groups need funds in order to exist – for basic needs such as tea, coffee and biscuits, and also for more costly items such as stationery and postage, telephone calls, and paying travelling expenses to speakers. Often group members contribute subscriptions to help with running costs, but still most groups are low on funds:

> 'We have no funds as such but to raise money for postage, refreshments, etc. at the last few meetings, each member has brought a small item to raffle and this helps with costs. Our members are very keen to keep the group going, but like all groups, we need new members with new ideas.' (*Member of Essex self-help group*)

With adequate finances groups can be proactive – they can recruit more effectively, they can publicize their existence much more widely (through the Family Practitioners Committee, for instance; charges vary, but it can cost £25 for them to send out your literature to the doctors in their area) and they can disseminate information to the general public by leaflets and posters through stalls at charity fairs. Groups can use such funds for speakers who make a charge for their time, and for buying copies of IBS-related books to lend to members. All such activities cost money, and groups could do so much more if they had funding.

If you start a group, or already belong to one, it is worth writing to your local council to ask whether any grants exist to help your group get off the ground. One IBS group did this (Sydenham, in south London) and in 1991 was awarded £1,000 from Lewisham Council, enabling it to buy books for members to borrow, to have their literature sent out to all GPs in the borough, to buy stamps, stationery, etc. and to pay speakers' expenses – and generally not to worry about finance for some time to come.

Belonging to a national organization

> 'I'm a new member, and when I started reading all the newsletters, I cried. I cried, "What a relief, I'm not going mad after all!"' (*Letter to IBS Network, 1994*)

Often local organizations are 'held together' by a parent organization – that is, a national body which produces a newsletter and gives advice and support to individuals and local groups. This is the case with, for instance, the NACC (National Association for Crohn's Disease and Colitis), the ME Association (for myalgic encephalitis/chronic fatigue syndrome) and the Endometriosis Society, as well as the IBS Network. Groups such as these produce regular newsletters, with contributions from professionals and members. Members may or may not wish to join a local self-help group, and many do not, but they still wish to receive information and advice from the parent organization. This is the case with the IBS Network. Despite the absence of personal contact which the self-help group can give you, you will still feel that you 'belong' to an organization which supports and cares for you:

> '. . . as all sufferers will heartily agree, IBS is depressing, painful, embarrassing and little researched, or so it would appear. That is why most of us welcome all the help we can give to and receive from others. This society seems to be well organized and to fulfil a long-felt need. Shared experiences can provide not only ourselves, but also the medical profession with valuable information.' (*Letter in* Gut Reaction, *no. 11*)

Also, a quarterly newsletter can give you information, advice and the knowledge that there are hundreds of people with exactly the same problems as you have. Just knowing that there are other people who are coping with IBS should make you feel less isolated.

> 'What a wonderful power for good you have created. *Gut Reaction* is such a help. You have turned the ignorance, pain, trauma and despair of IBS into something we can now come to grips with – because we are sharing it! To read of others' mind-blowing problems helps us deal with our own, and we no longer feel freaks. Thank you.' (*Letter in* Gut Reaction, *no. 12*)

Members know there are the opportunities for them to join in self-help groups or befriending schemes (discussed later in this chapter) if they so wish, and this in itself makes them feel more secure.

Starting a group

You may want to join a group, but find there isn't one in your area. If you are thinking of starting a group, the first thing to do is to think about premises. Do you want to have the group meet at your home? There are definite advantages in this. The home is generally a more comfortable environment for people to meet in than a doctor's surgery, hospital or community flat. Also, you do not need to go out at night to your meeting! However, some people prefer somewhere more neutral to meet. You could ask your GP whether she or he has a spare room that you could use for your meetings, or make contact with the gastroenterology department of your local hospital, which may be able to offer you a room in which to meet. Otherwise, try to find an advice centre or voluntary organization in your area, and ask their advice. The advantages to having somewhere like this to meet are, of course, that your group will be able to take it in turns to open up, make the coffee, etc., and you may be able to share the responsibility for the group. Also, groups which meet in hospitals seem to be more successful in terms of numbers – maybe this is because people perceive groups like this as having more 'validity' because they are seen to be backed up by the medical profession!

Once you have somewhere to meet, then you need to find a few people to come to your first meeting. Set a date and time for this. Ring or write to your local newspaper telling them what you are doing. Put up posters in your GP's surgery, health stores, and libraries. (The IBS Network can help you with posters.) Make sure everyone is clear about the place, date and time. Decide how long you are going to meet for – most groups meet for one-and-a-half to two hours. Organize refreshments, and have a rough idea about what you want to do.

The first meeting is the easiest; people want to introduce

themselves, and talk through their symptoms and problems. You will want to discuss what everyone wants out of the group, possible speakers, and other issues relating to the actual running of the group. Be sure to set a definite date and time for the next meeting.

If you are thinking of joining a new group or setting up one yourself, it is important not to imagine that everyone setting up groups has experience in these matters, is efficient and knows what they are doing! Most people who set up groups have had absolutely no experience of setting up or running one. They took the plunge and managed. So can you!

Successful groups

In research on self-help groups, three things were identified by one researcher, K. I. Maton, as especially important in successful groups. These are:

- the role each member plays
- rules and regulations
- core members

The role each member plays
If each member has a clearly defined role – for instance, one person makes the tea, another organizes the speakers, another greets new members and so on – each member will feel a greater commitment to the group. Maton found, too, that in groups which were run like this, members had a greater sense of well-being. Also, coordinators of IBS groups are less likely to leave if they feel supported in what they are doing.

Rules and regulations
According to Maton, a certain amount of organization at meetings is necessary if members are actually to benefit from them. For some groups, this may mean following a set agenda rather than having members just chat about anything which comes to mind.

Rules and regulations can be minimal, but they should exist. For instance, one self-help group for sufferers of multiple sclerosis has 11 guidelines which they believe help the group to survive. These are:

1 This self-help group belongs to you, and its success rests largely with you.
2 Enter into the discussions enthusiastically.
3 Give freely of your experiences.
4 Confine your discussion to the problem being dealt with.
5 Say what you think.
6 Only one person should talk at a time.
7 Avoid private conversation while someone else is speaking.
8 Be patient with other members.
9 Appreciate the other person's point of view.
10 Do not break confidentiality. If you do, you will be asked to leave the group.
11 A member must attend at least one regular self-help group meeting between socials to qualify to attend the socials.

Some people may feel they prefer the group to just meet and chat, but with no clear sense of direction many groups lose members, fail to recruit and eventually close down.

Core members

Although members of a self-help group have equal responsibility, it does seem that only a few individuals in each group 'lead' (or perhaps I should say 'do the work'!). Such people are important in the group because they often have a considerable influence on organization, so it is important that such 'core' members are capable.

Coordinators often complain that it is easy to set up a group, but harder to keep it going. Groups must continually recruit new members if they are to survive as other members eventually leave. Also, if group coordinators take too much responsibility for the group, others can become dependent on them: the coordinator may then feel that he or she is doing too much, may become ill or just plain fed up, and may no longer want to be involved. Also, others in the group feel a lessening of responsibility for the group, as they have no hand in running it.

To ensure that the group remains of interest to everyone, the members need to discuss every so often what they want out of the group. Most individuals in groups want expert speakers. This involves work – finding out which professionals have an interest in IBS, writing to them, maintaining contact with them and asking them to speak at the group. Once the speaker has agreed to come at a set time, members need to organize publicity – perhaps posters in local surgeries and libraries – arrange for refreshments and make sure everything is running smoothly on the night. Nothing is more embarrassing than turning up with an invited speaker and finding only two people have arrived, due to a series of mishaps.

Everyone needs to be encouraged to do something, so that there is a feeling of togetherness.

Befriending schemes and penpals

Sometimes it has not been possible to set up a group in a particular area of the country, despite a willing coordinator and good publicity. This is not the fault of the people who try to set up groups. Setting up a group, and keeping it running, on limited resources can be quite difficult. Some people have found that they have had a great response to local advertising – quite often coordinators find they have 20 or 30 replies to a small piece in the local newspaper, and other members wanting to join through seeing publicity in doctors' surgeries, libraries and so on. Other coordinators, despite doing everything possible, are not so lucky:

'I tried, I really did. I had publicity in the free local paper covering thousands of homes, I put adverts in shops in my village and the surrounding villages, and of the dozen names supplied by the IBS Network, only one was willing or able to come. Many reasons were given, but basically the North-east is just too vast an area to host a self-help group. You need lots of more localized groups. Trying to find a venue for a meeting when members live 60 miles apart is virtually impossible, but that is the state at the moment. If anyone wants to ring me, or write to me, that is fine. In actual fact, I have started writing to a lady who sounded very desperate in her first letter to me, and much appreciated the letter I wrote back to her. It seemed to end her sense of isolation in trying to cope with a condition that is so embarrassing to talk about. I was also contacted by another lady who asked if I could give her any advice, or indeed minded if she started a group of her own. In actual fact, she helped me more than I helped her. I hope to meet this lady soon to see if we can organize a Newcastle-based group. Anyway, if we manage to do that, I will be delighted.'

This coordinator was obviously very disappointed that her efforts were seemingly unrewarded. However, although she has not managed to start a group yet, with continued publicity she may eventually be able to do so.

Sometimes, as in the case of the coordinator quoted above, although it is not possible to start or continue a self-help group, contacts are made by telephone or letter which offer support to those involved. In the example above, the coordinator has found a source of support in two of the people she contacted, and they will also benefit from her experience. Other coordinators have also found themselves (accidentally!) acting as befrienders while attempting to set up a group.

Sometimes befriending schemes are the support network of choice for many people. There are several reasons why some sufferers prefer these to group meetings, including:

- they are not able or willing to travel large distances, often at night, in order to attend a group.
- they prefer one-to-one contact.
- they prefer to be more anonymous.

The befriending schemes run by the IBS Network are essentially different from penpal schemes in that befrienders offer the benefit of their experience and advice to someone who tends to be newly diagnosed as having IBS, and who feels they need contact with someone who is coping well with IBS, in order to see them through the bad times. The schemes that are run for IBS sufferers tend to work by post or phone, since there are not enough befrienders or befriendees to match people up according to area. Neither are befrienders or befriendees matched on other qualities, again unlike penpal schemes. Such schemes have benefits in their own right; they are not second-best substitutes for self-help groups. Befriendees feel that they have someone on whom they can rely, and who will be there for them. The befriender often feels more useful giving help to one particular person than acting in a group. Often the befriendee is more open at first in letter-writing and phone calls than they would be in a face-to-face meeting.

Such relationships can lead to many of the benefits described above for self-help groups. Whether such schemes are generally successful is not known, as until now they have not been monitored.

Penpal schemes are similar, except that, of course, the relationship is more equal from the beginning. Participants advertise for sufferers with specific qualities, and therefore can communicate with the sort of person they require. Again, how successful these schemes are is not known, as they, too, have not been monitored.

Summary

Treating yourself by self-help, and being part of an organization of IBS sufferers, may make you feel a lot better, both psychologically and even physically. You may gain more confidence in yourself and your ability to cope, both with social situations and in relationships. You will have a lot more information, and so be in a better position to deal with medical practitioners. You will be able both to give and to receive emotional and social support, and other sufferers can help you through the bad times.

Group activities are likely to decrease depression, anxiety and stress and therefore have an indirect effect on symptoms, breaking the vicious cycle of symptoms leading to stress, leading to an aggravation of symptoms. Although a self-help group cannot cure your IBS, it can have a positive impact on your life overall, and should be considered as part of the total treatment of irritable bowel syndrome.

Chapter 14

Conclusion and Recommendations

Susan Backhouse and Christine P. Dancey

'I am writing to tell you that I feel so much better after coming to the self-help group that I do not need to come any more.'

Having had a glimpse into the lives of other IBS sufferers and looked at the debates around the causes of IBS, you will be wanting to know if there is anything you can do to help alleviate your suffering. The more information you have about IBS, the more you will feel able to take control. The following is a brief round-up of everything we have recommended in the previous chapters, along with stories from people who have recovered or almost recovered from IBS, which will show you that eliminating IBS is indeed possible.

Medication

While some people respond quite well to drugs, in our experience the relief from symptoms does not last. Drugs may help in the short term, but in the long term, we must try to encourage the medical profession into finding the causes of IBS, and therefore finding a proper cure. However, until this happens, you must decide whether you are going to take medications on a regular basis or for emergencies only, and if so, which. The accent here is on informed choice – why take a drug you know nothing about just because your GP suggests it? Make sure you ask your doctor how the drug works and what side-effects are likely. Make sure he or she explains it in simple language; otherwise you may forget what was said as soon as you walk out of the surgery. Appendix IV lists the common drugs used in IBS and explains what they do and the most common side-effects. This should help you in your decision-making.

Melanie found that drugs helped her over some of the bad times:

'My doctor gave me Prothiaden, which calmed me and cured my IBS for three months. Although I hate the idea of tranquillizers, I think I've come to the conclusion that I prefer them to the discomfort and real suffering of IBS.'

Belle found some of the drugs useful for a time, but does not take them now:

'I had chronic pain and diarrhoea. None of the diarrhoea tablets worked, and eventually, after I collapsed on the stairs with exhaustion, the doctor was called. His words as he left my house echoed in my head for ages – "I don't know what to do with you." After a while, we tracked down a private specialist who told me to listen to my body and do what it asks. She placed me on Colofac and Colpermin three times a day, and told me to avoid dairy products as much as possible. I also have a bottle of codeine phosphate which, although it is my lifesaver, doesn't work for everyone. Since I started all this, I am pleased to say that I have made a full recovery now. I am off all tablets.'

Complementary medicine

We cannot recommend any particular complementary therapy which will help IBS sufferers. While some have been said to alleviate the symptoms of IBS, many people still continue to suffer. By all means experiment with different therapies – they are all worth a try – but be careful how you spend your money!

Complementary therapies do not generally have the same risk of side-effects as does conventional drug treatment, and even if the therapy does not eliminate your symptoms, at the very least you will probably experience an increased feeling of well-being which will help you cope better with your IBS. Ironically, some traditional medical doctors doing research into IBS now feel that a combination of different treatments and a more holistic approach is the way forward for IBS patients.

Although complementary medicine can be very expensive, some practitioners do charge on a sliding scale for people on a low income.

Lifestyle

We know that, for some people, stress is a trigger factor in IBS, and for all of us, stress makes any illness worse. It therefore pays to try to alter your lifestyle so as to minimize stress. This may be hard to do, especially if you are trying to hold down a job, look after a family and perhaps have financial or other worries as well. There are various books you can read that give advice on relieving stress. A course in stress management may help you, and you may be able to find one at your local adult education institute. Try to include activities in your life which will help you relax – yoga or other relaxing exercise, painting, meditating, etc. Find interests which will suit you and which you enjoy.

June told us how her IBS has completely disappeared now:

'I am fast approaching my sixtieth year and would not wish to continue to 70 with that complaint, thank you! Now I am definitely not a person who suffers from stress, or so I thought. Nevertheless, as luck would have it, my doctor's practice was providing a six-week "Coping with Stress" course at that time, which I promptly joined. I don't know whether it was the effect of being among people who really suffered from stress or the yoga-type relaxation exercises we were advised to do, but the IBS disappeared! Now and again, when I am overworked and rushing around more than usual, I do feel a very slight twinge –

but that's my warning to slow down, even stop altogether. The memory of that pain is still with me and nothing is worth having that back again.'

Diet

We are asked about diet more than any other topic in our work with IBS sufferers. The short answer is that there is no one diet which will suit all IBS sufferers – you must find out which one suits you best. You should make sure you have a nourishing, well-balanced diet, which is particularly important for people who are often unwell. Variety is the key: do not restrict yourself so much that you allow yourself to be short of nutrients.

Support from others

It is most important to surround yourself with people who are sympathetic and will offer you practical and emotional support when you need it. We advise you to make sure people know of your problems. If they do not take you seriously, laugh at your symptoms or undermine your confidence, perhaps you should think twice about having them as friends. Make sure you assert yourself and ask for support, both emotional and practical, at times when you need it. Many times, people are not sympathetic because they just do not understand your problems and what you are going through. Perhaps they could read this book, or at least look at the following tips on how to deal with the IBS sufferer.

Tips for friends and family

- It may at times be hard to live with a sufferer of IBS. Try to be patient and reassuring. Your partner, relative or friend may suffer with low self-esteem because of her or his IBS. Offer encouragement by telling her or him that you think she or he copes with her or his symptoms well.
- If your partner, friend or relative begins to panic or get a bad

pain, speak calmly and reassuringly to her or him. Remind her or him to breathe deeply and, if possible, sit her or him down somewhere quiet where she or he can relax.

✒ If she or he cannot get to the toilet in time and has an accident, reassure her or him that it doesn't matter and that it happens to many people. Keep the event low-key without denying the distress that she or he may feel. Of course, some people are able to treat an occasional accident as mere inconvenience.

• It helps if you can listen to the sufferer when she or he needs to talk, but there may be times, too, when you can help by distracting her or him.

• It is important for her or him to be reassured that she or he is still attractive to you or that you don't find her or him a nuisance or a bore (depending on your relationship!).

• If you live with someone with IBS, be careful not to make the toilet a battleground. Avoid making insensitive comments about smells, noises, the time she or he takes on the toilet, the number of times she or he has to go back, and the inappropriate occasions when emergencies can occur – such as just as you are about to leave to catch a train, or in the middle of a rush-hour jam on the M25. Believe it or not, this will only make it worse!

Paige is 39 years old, married, with a son and daughter. She describes how her husband speeded her recovery:

'My IBS started about ten years ago, abroad. I still don't know why, but I had an "accident" when I was out. It was awful; I was so embarrassed. I had abdominal pains and the other symptoms, but there was really nowhere safe to go. After that, I started looking for toilets everywhere – I started having panic attacks on the tube and trains, I didn't know what was happening to me. My doctor thought it was all nerves and sent me to a psychiatrist, but he did no good, he didn't understand. Eventually I found it difficult to go out at all, even in the car. Peter was really understanding, though. If we had to come home straight away, he never complained. He never made me feel a nuisance or a bother. He was always sympathetic, and he went to great pains to reassure me that it wasn't all in my head, I wasn't going mad. He really helped me through. I can't explain it properly; I don't really know how I got better. All I know is that I wouldn't be OK today if it wasn't for him.'

Self-help groups

If there is a self-help group in your area, join it. Even if you only go occasionally you will meet people in the same situation as yourself, people who understand, and you may pick up some tips for helping your symptoms that you haven't come across before. See Chapter 13 for details of the advantages of self-help groups for people with IBS.

Your GP

Many of our respondents felt their GPs were not sympathetic to their needs. If you feel the same way, then *change your doctor*. People often write to us about their problems with their GPs, but very few people change to another one. Why is this? If your doctor is not meeting your needs, if you do not feel comfortable with him or her, why stay? Ask your friends and neighbours what they think of their doctors, and ask for a pre-registration interview so that you can find out if the new one is suitable.

Recovery

Through reading this book, you have learned how sufferers live and cope with their condition. However, the problem with writing a book such as this one is that the people who recover do not generally join IBS groups, or write in with their stories! It is important to realize that many people do recover; one study carried out in 1985 found that, after a year, 12 per cent of IBS patients were symptom-free, and a further third of them were improved. Only 2 per cent became worse. A follow-up study two to three years later found that half showed substantial improvement; and after six years, another third of them had no problems. So you can see that people can, and do, get better.

A dual approach

The medical profession as a whole needs to change the way it looks at treating IBS sufferers. As mentioned already, a psychological approach as well as conventional drug treatment has been found to be very valuable for some people. Here is what Dr K. W. Heaton thinks of the dual approach:

'I think the medical profession is slowly progressing in the direction of the dual approach to IBS. However, the great majority of gastroenterologists are completely untrained in psychological treatments. There is also still much uncertainty as to when such treatment should be initiated, how it should be tailored to the individual person and how long it should be continued. A major problem is the severe deficiency of clinical psychologists or even counsellors in the NHS, especially the hospital service.'

Come out!

The best way we can help ourselves in the long term is to increase awareness of IBS among the public, the medical profession, employers, friends and family. We shouldn't have to feel embarrassed about having IBS. The more we talk about it, the more people will understand. When you first have IBS, you may think you do not know anyone else who has it, but once you begin to confide in people, you will often find they say, 'I think I've got that,' or 'I had that for two years some time ago,' or 'My cousin/sister/mother has that.' It's amazing how many people you will hear about who have IBS. However, some people will have never heard of it, and this is your chance to let them know what IBS is. Increased awareness of IBS can only give good results: it will lead to employers being more sympathetic, and friends and family being more supportive. GPs who at present have little understanding of IBS may begin to see what a devastating effect it can have on people's lives, and how belittled we sufferers can be made to feel. The people who run our councils and are closing down public toilets need educating about IBS, and it is only by all of us raising public awareness that things will improve.

And finally . . .

Here are some points to remember for all-round physical and mental health.

- It is important to remember that, in order for the healing process to take place, you need to maintain a positive attitude. Easier said than done, you cry! And don't we know it. However, the more you can do yourself to improve your health, the better. Taking responsibility is part of taking control, and those of us with IBS soon realize that we can't rely on the medical profession. It's up to us. Make sure that you are open to experiencing an improvement in your symptoms. In other words, don't assume, at any time, that you will feel bad before you actually do.
- If you've found it difficult to talk about your IBS, consider making contact with other sufferers through the IBS Network, as penpals, phone pals, or meeting them personally. It is important to have someone to turn to.
- All treatment for IBS should take into account the whole person – mind and body.
- Remember that stress can make all illnesses worse, not just IBS.
- Avoid resorting to laxatives. If they are used regularly, the bowel becomes lazy and will eventually be unable to function without them.
- Avoid antibiotics that aren't necessary. In fact, only take medical drugs if you really have to. This includes both prescription and over-the-counter drugs. Some can make the symptoms of IBS worse in the long term.
- Smoking can cause a number of problems for anyone with

abdominal trouble. It intensifies gas and stimulates intestinal activity. In addition, the nicotine reduces the blood flow to the digestive system, which can aggravate abdominal pain and spasms.

- Recreational or street drugs have a negative effect on health.
- Take regular physical exercise. Try to do something that you enjoy! You will no doubt experience an increased sense of well-being that will help you cope with your life in general, as well as IBS. Aim for three to four episodes of moderately strenuous exercise for 40 to 60 minutes each week. If this is new to you, work up to it gradually. If you can't manage that, any amount of regular exercise is worthwhile. And here's something to think about – Dr Vernon Coleman, in his book *Bodypower*, says, 'One of the ironies of modern living is that many people who don't take enough exercise, and who use gadgets daily to help avoid exercise, spend a lot of money on rowing machines, exercise bicycles and other devices designed to help them get some exercise!'
- Mental exercise is also important. There is no doubt that mental and physical health are bound up together. Stimulate your mind with creativity, hobbies, reading. Again, do things you enjoy.
- Both mental and physical exercise can help to take your mind off your symptoms. This is particularly important to those of us who know there is a direct connection between thinking about our IBS and suddenly wanting to dash to the toilet!
- Concentrate on the areas of your life where you feel in control. You may not be able to go to football matches with your friends, but you can build the model train set you always wanted. You may not be able to be relied upon to go on your child's school coach trip, but you can be counted on for a cuddle and a bedtime story. Carry this through to all areas of your life – at work, at home, in your relationships.
- Remember that life can be enjoyed and that it is possible to experience pleasure even if you are unwell. When you feel really low, concentrate on the areas of your life which make you feel good and know that you are helping your body to heal.

Even if you cannot cure yourself of all of your symptoms, we hope that the information in this book will help you overcome the anxiety, distress and isolation you may have felt because of your condition. You *can* overcome the disabling physical and psychological effects of IBS, even while your symptoms remain. Be optimistic – research is being carried out today which may one day make life easier for everyone with IBS. Meanwhile, we must help ourselves.

Appendix I

Further reading

Irritable bowel syndrome

K. W. Heaton, F. Creed and N. L. M. Goeting (eds), *Current Approaches towards Confident Management of Irritable Bowel Syndrome*, Duphar Medical Relations, Southampton, 1991.

R. McCloy and E. McCloy, *The IBS: Clinical Perspectives*, Meditext Ltd, London, 1988.

R. Nicol, *Coping Successfully with Your Irritable Bowel Syndrome*, Sheldon Press, London, 1989.

R. Nicol, *The Irritable Bowel Diet Book*, Sheldon Press, 1990.

R. Nicol, *The Irritable Bowel Stress Book*, Sheldon Press, 1991.

Barbara Rowlands, *The Troubled Gut*, Headline Publishing, London, 1996.

Maryon Stewart and Alan Stewart, *Beat IBS through Diet*, Vermillion, London, 1994.

W. Grant Thompson, *Gut Reactions: Understanding symptoms of the digestive tract*, Plenum Press, London, 1989.

Shirley Trickett, *Irritable Bowel and Diverticulosis: A self-help plan*, Thorsons, London, 1990.

Geoff Watts, *The Irritable Bowel Syndrome: A practical guide*, Cedar Press, London, 1990.

Nutrition and diet

J. Brostoff and L. Gamlin, *The Complete Guide to Food Allergy and Intolerance*, Bloomsbury, London, 1989.

Stephen Davies and Alan Stewart, *Nutritional Medicine*, Pan, London, 1987.

L. Galland, *Allergy Prevention for Kids*, Bloomsbury, London, 1989.

D. Grant and J. Joice, *Food Combining for Health*, Thorsons, London, 1984.

Rachel Haigh, *The Neal's Yard Bakery Wholefood Cookbook*, Neal's Yard Bakery Co-operative.

Miscellaneous

A. Broome and H. Jellicoe, *Living with Your Pain: A self-help guide to managing pain*, Methuen, London, 1987.

Vernon Coleman, *Stress and Relaxation*, Hamlyn, London, 1993.

P. J. Donoghue and M. Siegel, *Sick and Tired of Feeling Sick and Tired: Living with invisible chronic illness*, Norton, London, 1994.

G. Jacobs, *Candida Albicans: Yeast and your health,* Optima, London, 1990.

D. Potterton, *Herbal Remedies: IBS*, Foulsham, Slough, 1992.

Newsletter

What Doctors Don't Tell You: a monthly newsletter covering thoroughly researched health topics. Available from: 4 Wallace Road, London N1 2PG.

Appendix II

Useful addresses

Bowel disorders

Australian Crohn's & Colitis Association (ACCA), PO Box 201, Mooroolbark, 3138 Victoria, Australia. Tel: (+61) 3 726 9008. Newsletters, workshops and support groups.

British Digestive Foundation, 3 St Andrews Place, Regent's Park, London, NW1 4LB.

British Society of Gastroenterology, 3 St Andrews Place, Regent's Park, London, NW1 4LB.

Continence Foundation, 2 Doughty Street, London, WC1N 2PH. SAE and donation towards costs appreciated.

Crohn's & Colitis Foundation of America, 386 Park Avenue South, 17th Floor, New York, NY 10016–8804, USA. Tel: (+1) 212 685 3440 or 1+ 800 932 2423. Books, information, newsletters and support groups.

Crohn's & Colitis Foundation of Canada (CCFC), 21 St Clair Avenue East, Suite 301, Toronto, Ontario M4T 1L9, Canada Tel: (+1) 416 920 5305 or 1 800 387 1479.

Crohn's & Colitis Support Group, 32 Bloomfield Terrace, Lower Hutt, New Zealand.

Crohn's & Colitis Support Group, PO Box 52043, Kingsland, Auckland, New Zealand.

Crohn's Disease & Colitis Association of South Australia, 32 Reid Avenue, Tranmere, 5073, South Australia. Contact secretary Maggie Noble for information about IBS.

The IBS Network, Northern General Hospital, Sheffield, S5 7AU. Tel: 0114 2611531 (answerphone). Send large SAE for information pack.

IBS Self-Help Group, 3332 Yonge Street, PO Box 94074, Toronto, Ontario M4N 3RI, Canada. Contact Jeffrey Roberts on (+1) 416 932 3311 or via email at jdr@io.org.

International Foundation for Bowel Dysfunction, PO Box 17864, Milwaukee, Wisconsin 53217, USA. Produces a newsletter, Participate, for people affected by bowel dysfunction or incontinence.

Intestinal Disease Foundation, 1323 Forbes Avenue, Suite 200, Pittsburgh, PA 15219, USA. Tel: (+1) 412 261 5888. Support and education for those with any intestinal disease.

Irish Society for Colitis & Crohn's Disease (ISCC), Carmichael Centre, North Brunswick Street, Dublin 7, Republic of Ireland. Tel: (+353) 1 872 1416.

National Digestive Diseases Information Clearinghouse, 2 Information Way, Bethesda, MD 20892, USA. Tel: (+1) 301 654 3810. Government-funded information agency.

National Incontinence Helpline, 0191 213 0050 (Mon–Fri 14.00– 19.00hrs). A confidential service for people whose lives are affected by incontinence. The telephone line is staffed by health professionals.

Northwestern Society of Intestinal Research, c/o Vancouver Hospital & Health Sciences Centre, 855 West 12th Avenue, Vancouver, BC V5Z 1MP, Canada. Tel: (+1) 604 875 4875. A charity: informational brochures and a support group for those with IBS.

South African Crohn's & Colitis Association, PO Box 2638, Cape Town 800, Republic of South Africa. Tel: (+27) 21 25 2350.

Pain

Campain, 26 Weston Rise, Caister, Norfolk, NR30 5AT. (Charity created by doctors and health professionals aiming to change attitudes towards pain and improve its relief.)

Self-Help In Pain (SHIP), 33 Kingsdown Park, Whitstable, Kent, CT5 2DT. Helpline: 01227 264677.

Unwind, Pain and Stress Management, 'Melrose', 3 Alderlea Close, Gilesgate, Durham, DH1 1DS. Non-profit making. Tel/fax: 0191 3842056. Self Help programmes (tapes, books, charts etc.) for pain and stress management available by mail. Send for factsheets enclosing large (A5) SAE.

Nutrition, allergy and food intolerance

Action Against Allergy, Greyhound House, 23–24 George St, Richmond, Surrey, TW9 1JY.

Institute for Optimum Nutrition, 5 Jerdan Place, London, SW6 1BE.

National Society for Research into Allergy, 26 Welwyn Road, Hinckley, Leics, LE10 1JY.

Register of Nutritional Therapists, Hatton Green, Warwick, CV35 7LA.

Society for the Promotion of Nutritional Therapy, PO Box 47, Heathfield, E. Sussex, TN21 8ZX. Tel: 01435 867007. Fax: 01435 868033. email: 100045.255@compuserve.com. Send £1.00 plus SAE for information about nutritional therapy and a list of nutritional therapists in your area who may be able to help you overcome IBS.

Foresight (The Association for Promotion of Preconceptual Care), Mrs Barnes, 28 The Paddock, Godalming, Surrey, GU7 1XD. Primarily an organization to promote good health of parents prior to conception, but publishes a booklet, *Findout*, listing all additives and E numbers and their known dangers.

National Centre for Organic Gardening, Ryton-on-Dunsmore, Coventry, CV8 3LG. (Information on local wholefood and organic suppliers.)

Producers and suppliers of dairy-free, gluten-free and other products

Allergycare, Pollard's Yard, Wood St, Taunton, Somerset, TA1 1UP. Tel: 01823 325023. Fax: 01823 325024. Mail order foods for people with allergies and/or on special diets. Free catalogue on request.

Berrydales, Berrydale House, 5 Lawn Road, London, NW3 2XS. Tel: 0171 722 2866. Fax: 0171 722 7685. email: 106023.215@compuserve.com. Supplies dairy-, gluten- egg and sugar-free chocolate and chocolate novelties (both through health stores and by mail order). Publishes quarterly magazine, *The Inside Story,* which concentrates on dietary problems in relation to health. Also produces various associated booklets.

Biocare Ltd, 17 Pershore Road South, Birmingham, B30 3EE. Mail order suppliers of nutritional supplements.

Cirrus Associates, Little Hintock, Kington Magna, Gillingham, Dorset, SP8 5EW. Tel/fax: 01747 838165. email: cirrussw@aol.com. Runs a small mail order service for people suffering with diet or environment-related illness. Issues updated newsletter six-monthly to self-help organizations, private clinics and individuals containing detailed information about all the products and services they offer. Write or phone for advice or further information.

The Candida Shop, Natural Ways, Arfryn Caergeiliog, Anglesey, Gwynedd, LL65 3NL. Sells various products and advises on candida problems.

Higher Nature Ltd., Burwash Common, East Sussex, TN19 7LX. Orders: 01435 882880. Enquiries: 01435 883484. Fax: 01435 883720. Sells nutritional products, vitamins, aloe vera, etc.

Nutricia Dietary Products Ltd., 494–496 Honeypot Lane, Stanmore, Middx, HA7 1JH. Suppliers of gluten-free products.

Sunnyvale Organic Bread and Cakes, Everfresh Natural Foods, Gatehouse Close, Aylesbury, HP19 3DE. Foods suitable for gluten-free, vegan and yeast-free diets.

Trufree Foods, Larkhall Natural Health, 225 Putney Bridge Road, London, SW15 2PY. Gluten free products, including bread and cake mixes, and a free handbook for coeliacs and gluten-free/wheat-free dieters, *Getting Safely Started.*

Ultrapharm Ltd., Centenary Business Park, Henley-on-Thames, Oxfordshire, RG9 1DS. Tel: 01491 578016. Fax: 01491 571704. Bakers and suppliers of fresh gluten-free products. The range includes bread, biscuits, cakes and sweet and savoury pastry products.

Complementary/Holistic Medicine

Alternative Health Information Bureau, 12 Upper Station Road, Radlett, Herts, WD7 8BX. Tel/fax: 01923 857670.

The Dr. Edward Bach Healing Centre, Mount Vernon, Bakers Lane, Brightwell cum Sotwell, Wallingford, Oxon, OX10 0PZ. General retail mail order: 0171 495 2404. Trade and professional enquiries: 0181 780 4200. General information, publications, etc: 01491 834678.

British Acupuncture Association and Register, 34 Alderney Street, London, SW1. Tel: 0171 834 1012/6229. They will send you a list of their members. Their members are not allowed to advertise but you can find practitioners in the Yellow Pages. They advise looking for the designation MCBAcA or FBAcA (Membership or Fellowship of the BAAR). All their members are qualified in another form of medicine apart from acupuncture. Members can issue sickness certificates.

The British College of Acupuncture, 8 Hunter Street, London, WC1N 1BN. Tel: 0171 833 8164 or 0171 837 6429. They run a teaching clinic where treatment is available at reduced fees under the supervision of qualified practitioners.

British College of Naturopathy and Osteopathy, Frazer House, 6 Netherhall Gardens, London, NW3 5RR. Tel: 0171 435 7830.

British Complementary Medicine Association, Mental Health Unit, St Charles Hospital, Exmoor Street, London, W10 6DZ. Tel: 0116 242 5406 (answer machine).

British Holistic Medical Association, 179 Gloucester Place, London, NW1 6DX.

The British Homoeopathic Association, 27A Devonshire Street, W1N 1RJ. Please send SAE with all enquiries. Tel: 0171 935 2163.

British Hypnotherapy Association, 1 Wythburn Place, London, W1. Send SAE with enquiries.

The British School of Reflexology, The Holistic Healing Centre, 92 Sheering Road, Old Harlow, Essex, CM17 0JW.

British Society of Medical and Dental Hypnosis, 42 Links Road, Ashstead, Surrey, KT21 2HJ.

Colonic Irrigation Association, 16 England Lane, London, NW3 4TG. Tel: 0171 438 1595.

Institute for Complementary Medicine, PO Box 194, London, SE16 1QZ. Tel: 0171 237 5165: advice on finding reputable practitioners.

The International Federation of Aromatherapists, Stamford House, 2–4 Chiswick High Road, London, W4 1TH. Tel: 0181 742 2605. They can provide a directory of courses and members. There is a charge (as of 1997) of £2.50 per booklet.

International Federation of Reflexology, The Holistic Healing Centre, 92 Sheering Road, Old Harlow, Essex, CM17 0JW.

International Register of Oriental Medicine (UK), 4 The Manor House, Colley Lane, Reigate, Surrey, RH2 9JW. Members are designated by the initials MIROM or IROM after their names.

The International Society of Professional Aromatherapists, The House, 82 Ashby Road, Kingsly, Leicestershire, LE10 ISN. Tel: 01455 637987.

General Council and Register of Naturopaths, Goswell House, Goswell Street, Street, Somerset, BA16 0JG. Tel: 01458 840072.

National Institute of Medical Herbalists, 56 Longbrook Street, Exeter, Devon, EX4 6AH. Tel: 01392 426022. Fax: 01392 498963.

The Royal London Homoeopathic Hospital, Great Ormond

Street, London, WC1N 3HR. Tel: 0171 831 9199. (Homoeopathic prescriptions are available on the NHS.)

Hypnotherapy

Physicians practising Gut-Directed Hypnotherapy within the
NHS:

Dr P.J. Whorwell, BSc MD FRCP, Consultant Physician and
Senior Lecturer in Medicine, Withington Hospital, Nell
Lane, West Didsbury, Manchester, M20 8LR.

Dr P. Cann, FRCP, Consultant Physician and Gastroenterologist, Dept of Medicine, Middlesbrough General Hospital,
Ayresome Green Lane, Middlesbrough, Cleveland, TS5
5AZ.

Dr Alastair Forbes, BSc MD MRCP, Consultant Physician and
Gastroenterologist, St Mark's Hospital, City Road, London,
EC1V 2PS.

Dr I Cobden, MD FRCP, Consultant Physician and Gastroenterologist, North Tyneside District Hospital, North Shields,
Tyne and Wear, NE29 0LR.

The Register of Approved Gastrointestinal Psychotherapists
and Hypnotherapists: for explanatory pamphlet and list of
registered therapists in your area please send a large SAE to:
Elizabeth Taylor, coordinator, 5 Stonefold, Rising Bridge,
Accrington, Lancs, BB5 2DP.

Research:

If you have IBS and would like to participate in research studies
concerned with IBS, then please write to The IBS Research Team,
Psychology Dept., University of East London, London, E15 4LZ.
Most studies simply require the completion of questionnaires.

*Whilst every care has been taken in compiling this list, the
authors cannot accept responsibility for any error or mis-statement
contained therein.*

Appendix III

The IBS Network

The IBS Network was founded in 1991 by Susan Backhouse and Christine Dancey in order to help alleviate the distress, suffering and isolation associated with irritable bowel syndrome. Until then, there had been no self-help organization for sufferers of the condition.

Members receive the quarterly journal *Gut Reaction*, which includes information about the growing network of local IBS self-help groups. There are also 'befriending' and penpal schemes for members.

For more information, please send a large SAE to: IBS Network, St John's House, Hither Green Hospital, Hither Green Lane, London SE13 6RU.

You can also get a lot of information from the following websites on the Internet, though bear in mind that Internet sites frequently move or change.

- The IBS Network:
  http://www.uel.ac.uk/pers/C.P.Dancey/ibs.html
- Irritable Bowel Syndrome:
  http://www.geocities.com/Athens/Acropolis/3590/
- Irritable Bowel Syndrome (IBS) Self-Help Group (Canada):
  http://www.ibsgroup.org

Appendix IV

Glossary of drug treatments

Alimix
Cisapride. Facilitates or restores gastric motility. Do not take if pregnant, or with anti-cholinergic drugs. Side-effects can include abdominal cramps, rumbling noises in digestive system and diarrhoea.

alverine citrate
See Spasmonal.

amitryptyline hydrochloride
Tricyclic anti-depressant. Has a sedative effect. Side-effects: as for dothiepin.

Bisacodyl
See Dulco-Lax.

Bolvidion
Mianserin. Anti-depressant. Not for nursing mothers. May cause drowsiness.

Buscopan
Hyoscine. An anti-cholinergic anti-spasmodic. Can cause blurred vision, dry mouth.

Carbellon
Anti-cholinergic/antacid/anti-flatulent. Contains magnesium hydroxide, charcoal, peppermint oil.

chlordiazepoxide
See Librium.

codeine phosphate
Used as an analgesic to relieve pain. Codeine is a weak narcotic – low potential for addiction.

Colofac	Mebeverine hydrochloride. Anti-spasmodic.
Colpermin	Anti-spasmodic. Helps to relieve discomfort due to excessive wind by encouraging eructation (belching). Contains peppermint oil. Can be bought over the counter.
Colven	Anti-spasmodic and bulking agent, for IBS. Contains mebeverine hydrochloride.
diazepam	*See* Valium.
Diconal	Dipipanone. Opiate. Used for moderate to severe pain. Should not be used when pregnant. Do not use with alcohol. Side-effects: drowsiness, dry mouth. Addictive.
dicyclomine	*See* Merbentyl.
dolmatil	Sulpiride. Sedative used primarily to treat schizophrenia. Side-effects: muscle spasms, dry mouth, urine retention, weight gain, drowsiness, menstrual changes, jaundice. Not to be used with a variety of other drugs including alcohol, painkillers, tranquillizers and anti-depressants.
dothiepin	Prothiaden. Tricyclic anti-depressant. Side-effects: dry mouth, constipation, blurred vision, drowsiness, sleeplessness, dizziness, weight change, loss of libido (sex drive).
Dulco-Lax	Bisacodyl. Tablets or suppositories for treatment of constipation or to empty the bowel prior to medical examination.
Duphalac	Lactulose. Osmotic laxative to treat constipation. Take with plenty of water.

Fybogel	Ispaghula. Bulking agent to counteract constipation.
hyoscine	*See* Buscopan.
imipramine	Tofranil. Tricyclic anti-depressant. Side-effects: as for dothiepin.
Imodium	Loperamide. Opium-based anti-diarrhoeal agent. Slows down the passage of intestinal contents so that more water is reabsorbed into the body.
Isogel	Ispaghula. Bulking agent for constipation or diarrhoea.
ispaghula	*See* Fybogel, Isogel, Regulan.
Kolanticon	Aluminium hydroxide, magnesium oxide, dicyclomine, dimethicone. For gastrointestinal spasms, flatulence, hyperacidity. Can cause constipation, dry mouth.
lactulose	*See* Duphalac.
Lentizol	*See* Amitriptyline hydrochloride.
Librium	Chlordiazepoxide. Tranquillizer – treats anxiety. Causes drowsiness. Side-effects: confusion, unsteadiness, changes in vision and sex drive, retention of urine. Addictive. Not to be used long term, and withdrawal should be gradual.
Loperamide	*See* Imodium.
mebeverine hydrochloride	*See* Colofac.
Merbentyl	Dicyclomine. Anti-cholinergic anti-spasmodic for bowel and stomach spasm. Can cause blurred vision, dry mouth.
Mogadon	Nitrazepam. Sleeping tablet. Sedation may carry through to next day. Side-effects: confusion, unsteadiness, rash, changes in vision and sex

	drive, retention of urine. Not to be used long term, withdraw gradually. Not to be used with alcohol, other tranquillizers or anti-convulsants.
Mianserin	*See* Bolvidion.
Motival	Fluphenazine and nortriptyline. Anti-psychotic and tricyclic anti-depressant for anxiety/depression. Side effects: as for dothiepin.
nitrazepam	*See* Mogadon.
Normacol Plus	Frangula and sterculia. Bulking agent.
Prothiaden	*See* Dothiepin.
Regulan	Ispaghula. Bulking agent to relieve constipation due to lack of dietary fibre.
Senokot	Senna. Stimulant to treat constipation. Increases colonic mobility. May cause colicky pain in the long term. Should only be used sparingly.
Spasmonal	Alverine citrate. Anti-spasmodic. Can cause dry mouth, blurred vision, confusion.
Sulpiride	*See* Dolmatil.
Tofranil	*See* Imipramine.
Tryptizol	Amitriptyline hydrochloride. Side effects: as for dothiepin.
Valium	Diazepam. Tranquillizer – treats anxiety. Causes drowsiness. Side-effects: reduced reactions. Not to be used long term, and withdrawal should be gradual.

Index